Clinical Laboratory Mathematics

Mark D. Ball, Ph.D., SC(ASCP)[CM]

Specialty Chemistry Development Coordinator
Pathology Laboratories
Northwestern Memorial Hospital
Chicago, Illinois

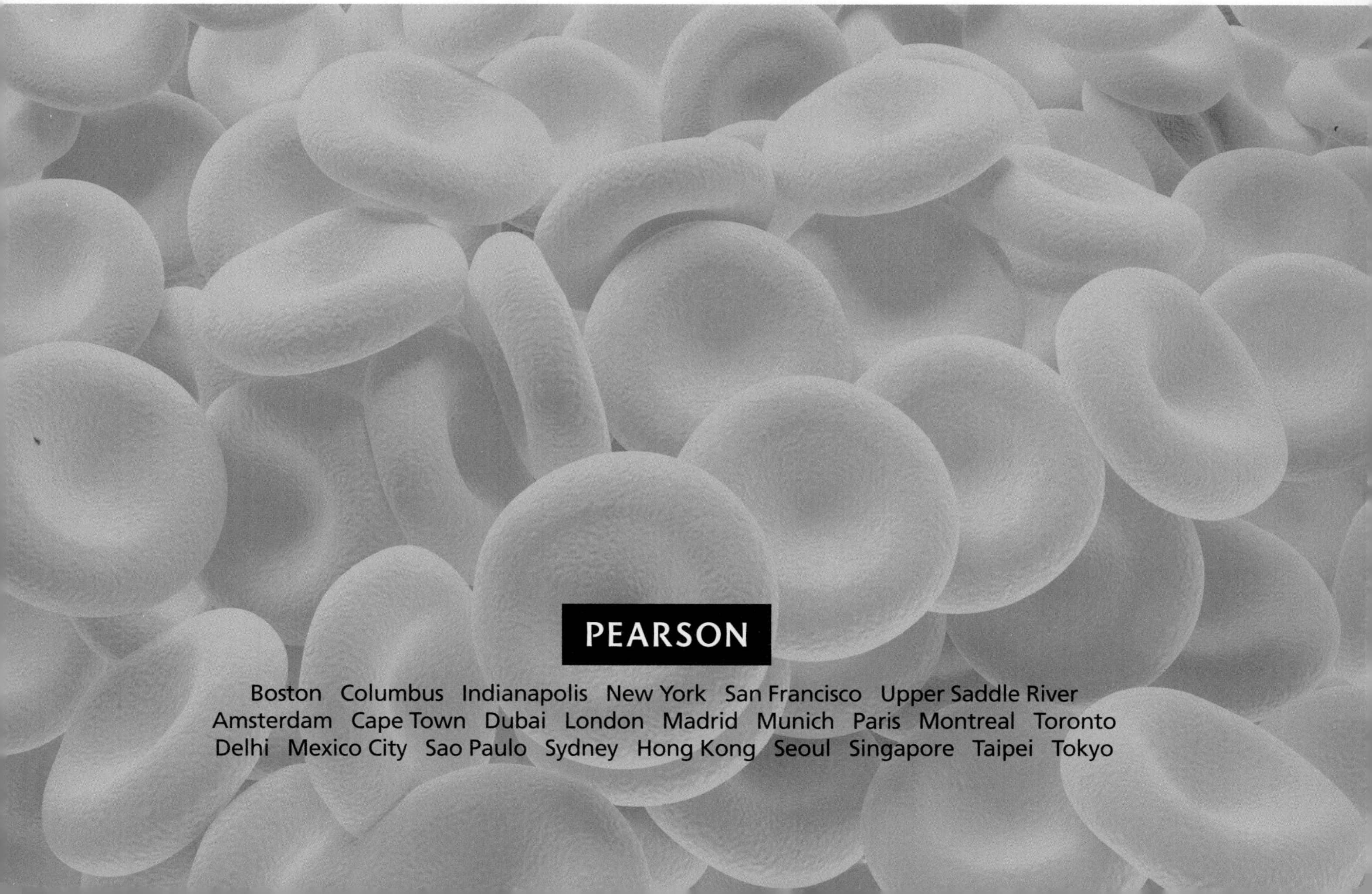

PEARSON

Boston Columbus Indianapolis New York San Francisco Upper Saddle River
Amsterdam Cape Town Dubai London Madrid Munich Paris Montreal Toronto
Delhi Mexico City Sao Paulo Sydney Hong Kong Seoul Singapore Taipei Tokyo

Publisher: Julie Levin Alexander
Publisher's Assistant: Regina Bruno
Editor-in-Chief: Marlene McHugh Pratt
Executive Editor: John Goucher
Editorial Project Manager: Melissa Kerian
Editorial Assistant: Erica Viviani
Development Editor: Joanna Cain, Auctorial Pursuits
Director of Marketing: David Gesell
Executive Marketing Manager: Katrin Beacom
Marketing Coordinator: Alicia Wozniak
Senior Managing Editor: Patrick Walsh
Project Manager: Patricia Gutierrez
Senior Operations Supervisor: Lisa McDowell
Senior Art Director: Mary Siener
Text design: Candace Rowley
Cover design: Carly Schnur
Cover Art: Cover Art and Chapter Opener image bioraven / Shutterstock.com
Media Producer: Amy Peltier
Lead Media Project Manager: Lorena Cerisano
Full-Service Project Management: Patty Donovan, Laserwords, Inc.
Composition: Laserwords, Inc.
Printer/Binder: Courier Kendallville
Cover Printer: Lehigh-Phoenix Color/Hagerstown
Text Font: Minion Pro Display 10/12

Credits and acknowledgments borrowed from other sources and reproduced, with permission, in this textbook appear on the appropriate page within text.

Library of Congress Cataloging-in-Publication Data
Ball, Mark D.
Clinical laboratory mathematics / Mark D. Ball.—1st ed.
p. ; cm. — (Pearson clinical laboratory science series)
Includes index.
ISBN-13: 978-0-13-234437-1
ISBN-10: 0-13-234437-8
I. Title. II. Series: Pearson clinical laboratory science series.
[DNLM: 1. Clinical Laboratory Techniques--methods--Problems and Exercises. 2. Mathematics--methods--Problems and Exercises. 3. Problem Solving--Problems and Exercises. QY 18.2]
610.72'4--dc23

2012036467

10 9 8 7 6 5 4 3 2 1

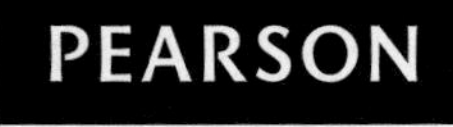

ISBN 10: 0-13-234437-8
ISBN 13: 978-0-13-234437-1

Contents

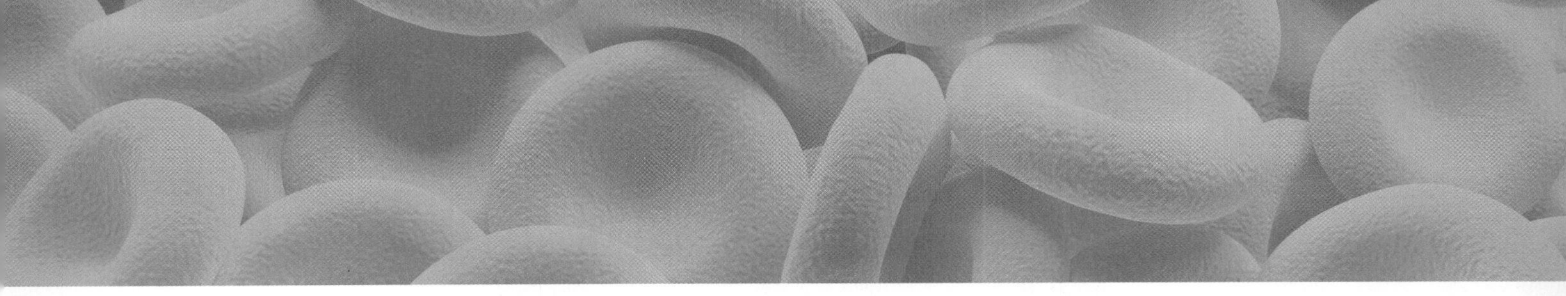

Foreword

Clinical Laboratory Mathematics is part of Pearson's Clinical Laboratory Science series of textbooks, which is designed to balance theory and practical applications in a way that is engaging and useful to students. The author of *Clinical Laboratory Mathematics* presents highly detailed technical information and effective tools that will help beginning learners envision themselves as members of a healthcare team, while helping advanced learners and practitioners continue their education. The synergy of theoretical and practical information in this text enables learners to analyze data and synthesize conclusions. Additional applications and instructional resources are available at *www.myhealthprofessionskit.com*.

We hope that this book, as well as the entire series, proves to be a valuable educational resource.

Elizabeth A. Gockel-Blessing (formerly Zeibig), PhD, MLS(ASCP)^{CM}
Clinical Laboratory Science Series Editor, Pearson Health Science
Interim Associate Dean for Student and Academic Affairs, Department of Clinical Laboratory Science, Doisy College of Health Sciences, Saint Louis University

Preface

Clinical Laboratory Mathematics is a comprehensive textbook on the mathematical techniques and theories of clinical laboratory science. It is written for students at any point on the trajectory toward an undergraduate or graduate degree in the discipline, from an associate's degree to a doctorate. Students and practitioners of related disciplines will also find the book useful: pathologists, medical students, nurses, pharmacists, biochemists, biomedical engineers, and physician assistants.

Going well beyond the notion of "relevance," this book tries to convey the conviction that learning mathematics is not only helpful, but often critical, in the high-technology milieu of a clinical laboratory. It repeatedly highlights the reasons for developing a battery of mathematical tools: (1) to handle unfamiliar mathematical problems that arise in the course of laboratory work; (2) to follow the reasoning in seminars, papers, and discussions; (3) to detect mathematical errors made by individuals; (4) to recognize instrument malfunctions or method anomalies through mathematical irregularities; (5) to adapt new methods, ideas, and technologies that require some mathematical competence; and (6) to shift smoothly into research-oriented work, whether in the form of short-term projects in a routine laboratory, long-term projects in a research laboratory, or method development at a diagnostics company.

Therefore, the book integrates real-world examples of mathematical tools at work in the clinical laboratory. To achieve this goal, practice problems are strategically designed to have the student confront scenarios involving mathematical questions that have both context and consequence. Such problems offer the student a chance to think under the circumstances that a laboratory professional might encounter on the job, requiring him or her to solve a mathematical problem while coming to appreciate the importance of correct calculation and the repercussions of error.

The book supports both self-guided study and the more traditional lecture-discussion format. Meeting the needs of either approach, or of any approach in-between, is a matter not only of organizing the topics logically, but also of liberally cross-referencing so that students see connections and common motifs. This technique promotes comprehension while lessening the burden of brute memorization.

The book includes online resources (*www.myhealthprofessionskit.com*) intended to meet the needs of advanced users: (1) chapter appendices, which elaborate topics introduced in the main text, and (2) advanced topics, which emerge from frequently asked questions and from the main text.

Because some instructors start their courses with a review of arithmetic, and because some students seek such a review, the first chapter deals with addition, subtraction, multiplication, division, fractions, decimals, percentages, algebra, and ratios. Furthermore, it includes strategies for speeding up calculations without relying on electronics. Subsequent chapters cover increasingly complex and specialized topics, with the online appendices carrying those topics to the greatest depth.

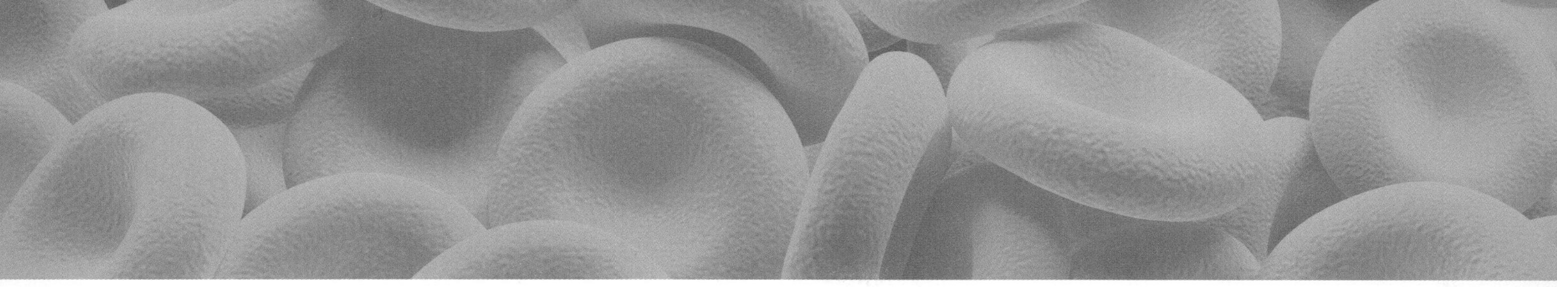

Reviewers

James E. Daly, MEd, MT(ASCP)
Lorain County Community College
Elyria, Ohio

Amy Gatautis, MBA, MT(ASCP)SC
Cuyahoga Community College
Cleveland, Ohio

Amy Kapanka, MS, MT(ASCP)SC
Hawkeye Community College
Cedar Falls, Iowa

Pamela Lonergan MS, MT(ASCP)SC
Norfolk State University
Norfolk, Virginia

Leslie Lovett, MS, MT(ASCP)
Pierpont Community and Technical College
Fairmont, West Virginia

Stephen Olufemi Sodeke, PhD, MA
Tuskegee University
Tuskegee, Alabama

Kathleen Paff, MA, MT(ASCP)
Kellogg Community College
Battle Creek, Michigan

Travis M. Price, MS, MT(ASCP)
Weber State University
Ogden, Utah

Susan Schoffman, MPH, MT(ASCP), CLS(NCA)
Tulsa Community College
Tulsa, Oklahoma

Dick Y. Teshima, MPH, MT(ASCP)
University of Hawaii at Manoa
Honolulu, Hawaii

Darius Y. Wilson, EdD
Southwest Tennessee Community College
Memphis, Tennessee

Patricia Wright, MT(ASCP)
Southeastern Community College
Whiteville, North Carolina

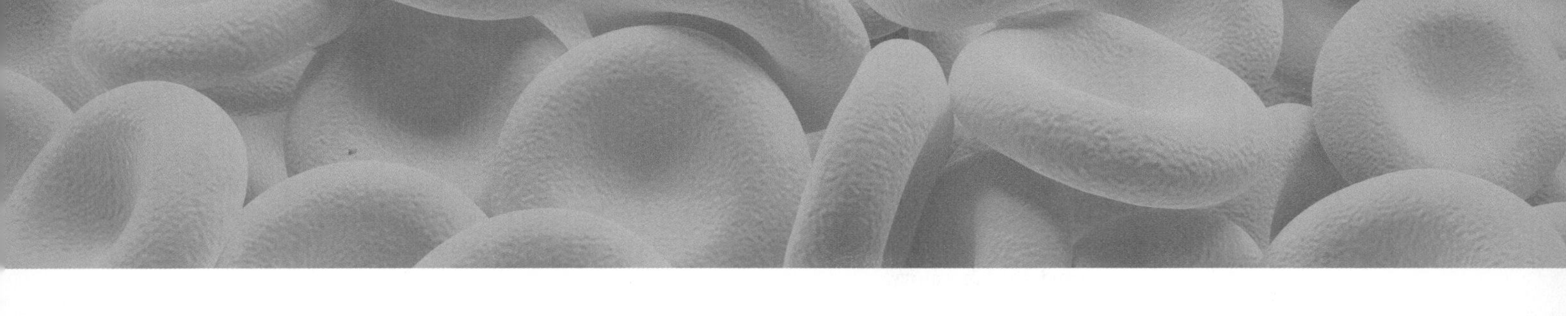

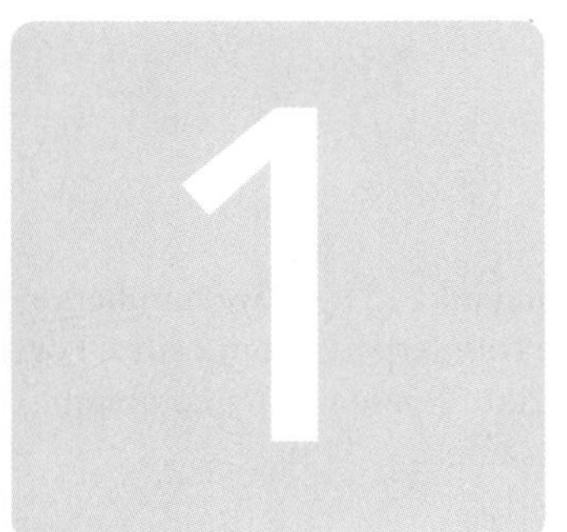

1 Arithmetic and Algebra

Learning Objectives

At the end of this chapter, the student should be able to do the following:

1. To add, subtract, multiply, and divide positive and negative numbers
2. To multiply, divide, and reduce fractions
3. To add and subtract fractions
4. To express fractions as decimal numbers and to express improper fractions as mixed numbers
5. To simplify complex fractions
6. To interconvert percentages, decimal numbers, and fractions
7. To calculate a specified percentage of a number
8. To express change properly as a percentage
9. To solve an equation algebraically for an unknown variable
10. To calculate and interpret ratios
11. To solve equations of two ratios for an unknown variable by cross-multiplication

Key Terms

associative property
canceling
commutative property
complex fraction
denominator
difference
distributive property
factor
improper fraction
least common denominator
mixed number
numerator
opposite
percentage
product
proper fraction
quotient
ratio
reciprocal
reducing
sum

Chapter Outline

Arithmetic is the manipulation of numbers through addition, subtraction, multiplication, and division. Algebra is the strategic manipulation of relationships in order to find the unknown value of a certain quantity. In medical decisions, the importance of having reliable information is self-evident. Therefore, mastering the basic skills of arithmetic and algebra is critical to ensuring the accuracy of every result that leaves the laboratory.

ADDITION

In the problem

$$a + b = c$$

variable *c* is referred to as the **sum** of *a* and *b*.

In the operation of addition, positive numbers represent a "putting in" and negative numbers a "taking out." Therefore, we regard a positive number and its negative counterpart as **opposites**. For example, the opposite of "7" is "−7," and the opposite of "−200" is "200." Consequently, combining a positive number with a negative number amounts to a decrease. For example,

$$5 + (-3) = 2$$

A simple way to approach a problem like this is to refer to a number line. Adding a negative number is the same as moving leftward. In this case, we start at the "5" and then move to the left by "3," which brings us to "2."

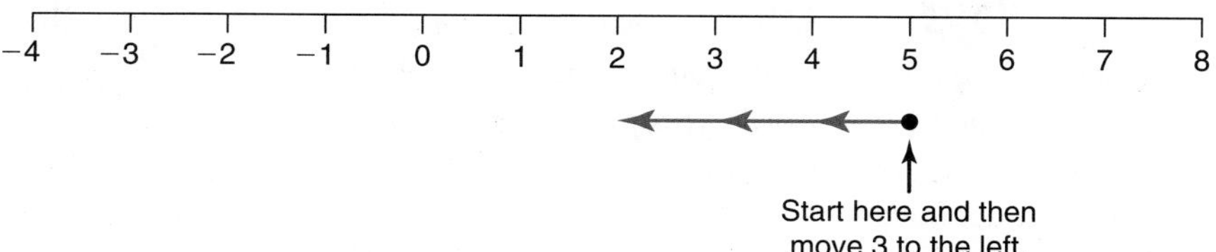

Adding a negative number to a negative number follows the same rule, that is, a leftward movement:

$$-2 + (-3) = -5$$

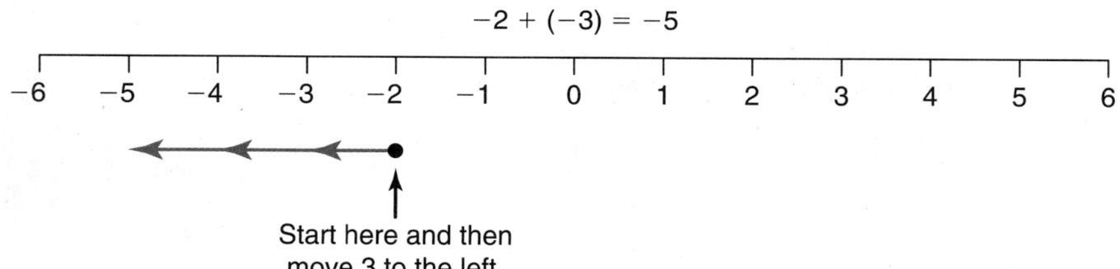

To clarify this procedure with an analogy, envision a beaker of water on a tabletop. Let the number "1" be a unit of heat and the number "−1" be a unit of cold. Adding a positive number to another positive number puts units of heat into the water, causing the temperature to rise. Adding a negative number to a positive number, however, introduces units of cold to the water, bringing the temperature down.

Addition is commutative. In other words, the order in which we add two numbers together does not affect the sum. Thus, this equation shows the **commutative property** of addition, that is, adding *a* and *b* gives the same result as adding *b* and *a:*

$$a + b = b + a$$

For example,

$$3 + 6 = 6 + 3 = 9$$

and

$$-0.721 + 0.0044 = 0.0044 + (-0.721)$$

The grouping of numbers in addition also does not affect the sum. This fact reflects the **associative property** of addition, meaning the sum of *a* and *b* plus *c* is equal to *a* plus the sum of *b* and *c*, as represented in this equation:

$$(a + b) + c = a + (b + c)$$

For example,

$$(2 + 8) + 5 = 2 + (8 + 5) = 15$$

and

$$(-1 + 9) + 3 = -1 + (9 + 3) = 11$$

☑ CHECKPOINT 1-1

1. Evaluate the following expressions.
   (a) $16 + (-9)$ (b) $(-4) + 10$ (c) $1.7 + (-3.4)$ (d) $(-58) + (-4)$
2. Evaluate the following expressions.
   (a) $(-9) + 5 + (-2)$ (b) $13.5 + 0.2 + (-0.8)$
   (c) $0.0556 + (-0.0102) + 0.0433$ (d) $(-128) + (-128) + 256$

1. (a) 7 (b) 6 (c) −1.7 (d) −62
2. (a) −6 (b) 12.9 (c) 0.0887 (d) 0

SUBTRACTION

In the problem

$$a - b = c$$

variable *c* is referred to as the **difference** between *a* and *b*.

Subtracting a positive number from a positive number is intuitive:

$$13 - 8 = 5$$

In fact, we define subtraction as the addition of an opposite:

$$a - b = a + (-b)$$

Subtracting a negative number from a positive number, however, may seem counterintuitive:

$$13 - (-8) = 21$$

Here, we are subtracting the opposite of 8 from 13. If we were subtracting 8 itself, then we would bring the total down to 5, that is, $13 - 8 = 5$. Instead, we are subtracting a "taking out," a process that amounts to a "putting in." Therefore, subtracting a negative number has the same effect as adding its opposite:

$$13 - (-8) = 13 + 8 = 21$$

Our beaker-of-water analogy might prove helpful here. We can say that subtracting a negative is the same as withdrawing units of cold from the water, the result of which is an *increase* in the temperature.

☑ CHECKPOINT 1-2

Evaluate the following expressions.
(a) $10 - (-2)$ (b) $(-3) - 5$ (c) $40 - 46$ (d) $(-18) - (-30)$

(a) 12 (b) −8 (c) −6 (d) 12

MULTIPLICATION

In the problem

$$a \times b = c$$

variables *a* and *b* are called the **factors**, and variable *c* is referred to as the **product** of *a* and *b*.

Multiplication is a shortcut for addition:

$$6 \times 4 = 24$$

What this operation does is to add together six fours or four sixes:

$$6 \times 4 = 4 + 4 + 4 + 4 + 4 + 4 = 6 + 6 + 6 + 6 = 24$$

There are three common ways to symbolize multiplication:

$$a \times b = a \cdot b = ab$$

Like addition, multiplication is commutative. The order in which we multiply two numbers together does not affect the product:

$$a \times b = b \times a$$

For example,

$$6 \times 5 = 5 \times 6 = 30$$

The grouping of numbers in multiplication also does not affect the product. Thus, the associative property of multiplication is

$$(a \times b) \times c = a \times (b \times c)$$

For example,

$$(3 \times 7) \times 2 = 3 \times (7 \times 2) = 42$$

As in addition and subtraction, multiplying two positive numbers together makes sense. Equally logical, though, is multiplying a positive number by a negative number:

$$6 \times (-4) = -24$$

What this operation does is to add together six negative fours or negative-six fours:

$$6 \times (-4) = (-4) + (-4) + (-4) + (-4) + (-4) + (-4) = -24$$

$$(-6) \times 4 = -24$$

What does it mean to add together negative-six fours? Fortunately, our beaker-of-water analogy is useful here, too. Regard the operation not as an *addition* of negative-six fours but as a *subtraction* of six fours, giving −24. In other words, we are subtracting four units of heat six times, for a total of 24 units of heat out of the water. The result is a *lower* temperature. Therefore, a negative times a positive is a negative.

Another way to approach this problem is to apply the commutative property of multiplication:

$$(-6) \times 4 = 4 \times (-6) = -24$$

Written as such, the problem tells us simply to add together four negative sixes:

$$4 \times (-6) = (-6) + (-6) + (-6) + (-6) = -24$$

Finally, consider the multiplication of two negative numbers:

$$(-6) \times (-4) = 24$$

To understand this, we can extend our analogy from above and treat the operation as a subtraction of six negative fours, giving 24. In other words, we are subtracting, or withdrawing, four units of cold six times, pushing the temperature *up*. Therefore, a negative times a negative is a positive.

Table 1-1 ★ summarizes the four possible sign combinations in multiplication.

★ **TABLE 1-1** The Four Sign Combinations in Multiplication

Rule	Analogy
positive × positive = positive	Adding units of heat raises the temperature
positive × negative = negative	Adding units of cold lowers the temperature
negative × positive = negative	Subtracting units of heat lowers the temperature
negative × negative = positive	Subtracting units of cold raises the temperature

☑ CHECKPOINT 1-3

Evaluate the following expressions.

(a) 4×9 (b) $2 \times (-6)$ (c) $(-10) \times 3$ (d) $(-5) \times (-4)$
(e) $1.5(2)$ (f) $33 \cdot (-3)$ (g) $(-8)(-8)$ (h) $(-4.04) \cdot 2$

(a) 36 (b) −12 (c) −30 (d) 20
(e) 3 (f) −99 (g) 64 (h) −8.08

DIVISION

In the problem

$$a \div b = c \quad \text{or} \quad \frac{a}{b} = c$$

variable c is referred to as the **quotient** of a and b, that is, c is the result of dividing a by b.

We define division in terms of multiplication:

$$a \div b = a \cdot \frac{1}{b} \quad \text{or} \quad \frac{a}{b} = a \cdot \frac{1}{b}$$

The two quantities b and $1/b$ are **reciprocals** of each other. Reciprocals are two numbers whose product is 1:

$$b \times \frac{1}{b} = 1$$

If $a \div b = c$, then $b \times c = a$. One important consequence of this relationship is a prohibition against dividing by zero. *Division by zero is undefined* because there are no values for a and c that satisfy this equation:

$$\frac{a}{0} = c$$

If a, for example, is 25, then c does not exist, because there is no value for c that, when multiplied by zero, gives 25:

$$c \times 0 \neq 25$$

Of course, *zero divided by any number is zero* because any nonzero value for b satisfies these equations:

$$\frac{0}{b} = 0 \quad \text{or} \quad b \times 0 = 0$$

Because we define division in terms of multiplication, the sign rules are the same. Table 1-2 ★ summarizes those rules.

★ **TABLE 1-2** The Four Sign Combinations in Division

Rule
positive ÷ positive = positive
positive ÷ negative = negative
negative ÷ positive = negative
negative ÷ negative = positive

☑ **CHECKPOINT 1-4**

Evaluate the following expressions.

(a) $\frac{18}{-3}$ (b) $2.4 \div 0.3$ (c) $\frac{-160}{-4}$ (d) $(-49) \div 7$

(e) $5\left(\frac{1}{10}\right)$ (f) $\frac{0.54}{-9}$ (g) $-35\left(\frac{1}{7}\right)$ (h) $25 \div (-75)$

(a) −6 (b) 8 (c) 40 (d) −7

(e) 0.5 (f) −0.06 (g) −5 (h) −0.33

FRACTIONS

A fraction is nothing more than a representation of a division. The top number is the **numerator** and the bottom number is the **denominator**. The denominator specifies the number of equal parts into which we divide something, and the numerator specifies the number of those equal parts.

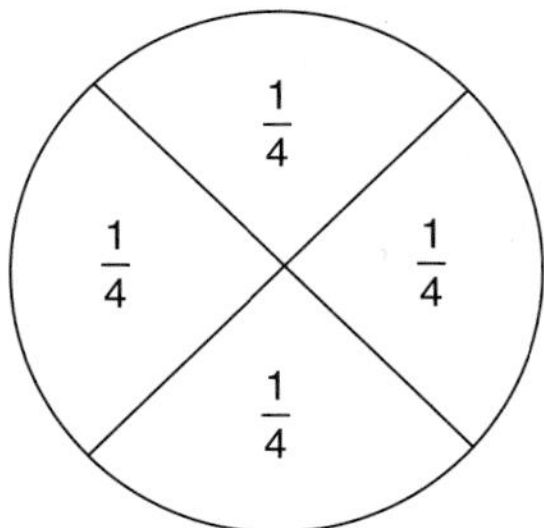

In the above diagram, for example, we divide the circle into four equal parts, and each part is one of the four. For each part, therefore, the denominator is 4 and the numerator is 1.

As a division, the fraction "$\frac{1}{4}$" tells us that (1) we divided one whole thing (a circle in this case) into four equal parts, and (2) we are considering one of those parts.

Multiplying Fractions

To multiply fractions, multiply the numerators and multiply the denominators. For example,

$$\frac{2}{3} \times \frac{3}{4} = \frac{6}{12}$$

What this equation tells us is that 2/3 of 3/4 is the same as 6/12. Figure 1-1 ■ depicts this relationship.

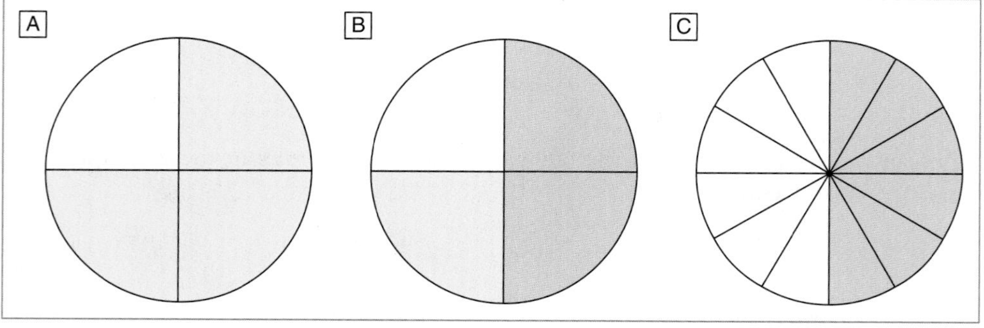

■ **FIGURE 1-1** A depiction of the equation $\frac{2}{3} \times \frac{3}{4} = \frac{6}{12}$. Two-thirds of 3/4 is the same as 6/12. Panel *A:* Three-fourths of the circle is yellow. Panel *B:* This represents 2/3 of 3/4: 2/3 (in green) of the original 3/4 (in green and in yellow). Panel *C:* Six-twelfths (in green) of the whole circle, which is the same as the green area in panel *B.*

Multiplying a fraction by a whole number is straightforward; just treat the whole number as a fraction with "1" in the denominator. For example,

$$\frac{4}{5} \times 10 = \frac{4}{5} \times \frac{10}{1} = \frac{40}{5} = 8$$

Dividing Fractions

To divide a fraction, multiply it by the reciprocal of the other number:

$$\frac{2}{3} \div 3 = \frac{2}{3} \times \frac{1}{3} = \frac{2}{9}$$

What these equations tell us is that dividing 2/3 of an object into three equal parts gives 2/9 of that object. For example, consider a circle (Figure 1-2 ■).

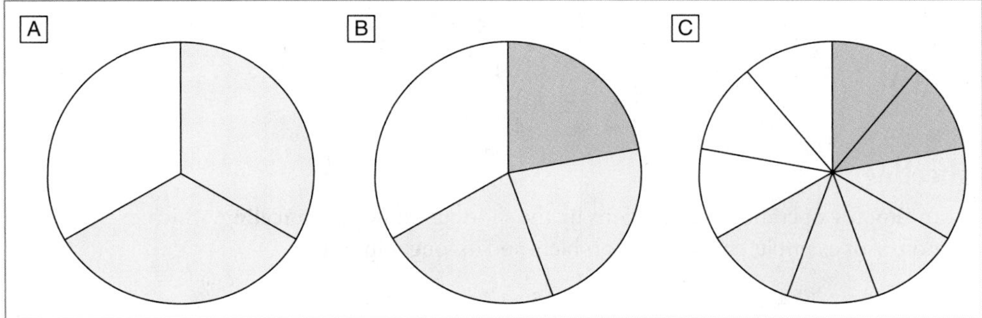

■ FIGURE 1-2 A depiction of the equations $\frac{2}{3} \div 3 = \frac{2}{3} \times \frac{1}{3} = \frac{2}{9}$. Two-thirds divided by 3 is the same as 1/3 of 2/3, which equals 2/9. Panel *A:* Two-thirds of the circle is blue. Panel *B:* One-third (in purple) of the original 2/3 (in purple and in blue). Panel *C:* Two-ninths (in purple) of the whole circle, which is the same as the purple area in panel *B.*

☑ CHECKPOINT 1-5

1. Evaluate the following expressions.

   (a) $\frac{3}{5} \times \frac{4}{9}$ (b) $\frac{2}{7} \times \frac{1}{2}$ (c) $\frac{1}{4} \times \frac{2}{3}$ (d) $25 \times \frac{4}{5}$

2. Evaluate the following expressions.

   (a) $\frac{8}{9} \div 2$ (b) $\frac{1}{2} \div \frac{3}{5}$ (c) $6 \div \frac{2}{3}$ (d) $\frac{3}{7} \div \frac{4}{7}$

1. (a) $\frac{12}{45}$ (b) $\frac{2}{14}$ (c) $\frac{2}{12}$ (d) $25 \times \frac{4}{5} = \frac{100}{5} = 20$

2. (a) $\frac{8}{9} \div 2 = \frac{8}{9} \times \frac{1}{2} = \frac{8}{18}$ (b) $\frac{5}{6}$ (c) 9 (d) $\frac{21}{28}$

Reducing Fractions

Generally, fractions should be **reduced** (or "simplified") so that the numerator and denominator are as small as possible, that is, until the only number evenly divisible into both of them is "1."

Sometimes the reduction is comparatively easy to see, as in the following example.

$$\frac{2}{4} \text{ reduces to } \frac{1}{2}$$

In the fraction $\frac{2}{4}$, the "2" divides evenly into the "4"; therefore, the "2" reduces to a "1" and the "4" reduces to a "2."

Here is another simple example:

$$\frac{5}{20} \text{ reduces to } \frac{1}{4}$$

The "5" divides evenly into the "20"; therefore, the "5" reduces to a "1" and the "20" reduces to a "4."

In more complex reductions, it helps to write out the factors. Three examples follow.

$$\frac{18}{32} = \frac{2}{2} \times \frac{9}{16} = 1 \times \frac{9}{16} = \frac{9}{16}$$

$$\frac{9}{15} = \frac{3}{3} \times \frac{3}{5} = 1 \times \frac{3}{5} = \frac{3}{5}$$

$$\frac{16}{64} = \frac{16}{16} \times \frac{1}{4} = 1 \times \frac{1}{4} = \frac{1}{4}$$

Canceling

We can simplify operations on fractions by the shortcut known as **canceling**, which exploits simple reductions. For example, consider this problem and its long solution:

$$\frac{4}{5} \times \frac{15}{16} = \frac{4 \times 15}{5 \times 16} = \frac{15 \times 4}{5 \times 16} = \frac{15}{5} \times \frac{4}{16} = 3 \times \frac{1}{4} = \frac{3}{4}$$

Now consider the same problem simplified by canceling:

$$\frac{\cancel{4}^{1}}{{}_{1}\cancel{5}} \times \frac{\cancel{15}^{3}}{{}_{4}\cancel{16}} = \frac{1 \times 3}{1 \times 4} = \frac{3}{4}$$

The "4" in the numerator divides evenly into the "16" in the denominator; as a result, the "4" becomes a "1" and the "16" a "4." We say that the "4" cancels out. Likewise, the "5" in the denominator divides evenly into the "15" in the numerator; accordingly, the "5" becomes a "1" and the "15" a "3." We say that the "5" cancels out.

Here is another example:

$$\frac{\cancel{7}^{1}}{{}_{2}\cancel{16}} \times \frac{\cancel{8}^{1}}{{}_{3}\cancel{21}} = \frac{1 \times 1}{2 \times 3} = \frac{1}{6}$$

☑ CHECKPOINT 1-6

Reduce the following fractions.

(a) $\frac{4}{6}$ (b) $\frac{16}{36}$ (c) $\frac{28}{56}$ (d) $\frac{9}{12}$ (e) $\frac{5}{20}$

(a) $\frac{2}{3}$ (b) $\frac{4}{9}$ (c) $\frac{1}{2}$ (d) $\frac{3}{4}$ (e) $\frac{1}{4}$

Adding and Subtracting Fractions

To add (or subtract) fractions, add (or subtract) the numerators but not the denominators. Furthermore, *the denominators must all be the same.*

Consider the simple addition of 1/4 and 1/4, which is highlighted in pink in the diagram below.

$$\frac{1}{4} + \frac{1}{4} = \frac{2}{4}$$

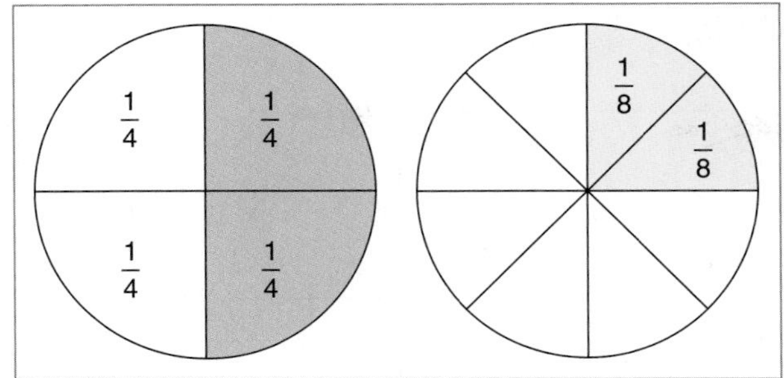

■ FIGURE 1-3 Adding fractions entails adding the numerators but not the denominators. Clearly, the proportion of 2/4 (pink) is greater than the proportion of 2/8 (orange). Therefore, $\frac{1}{4} + \frac{1}{4} = \frac{2}{4} \neq \frac{2}{8}$.

It is logical to add only the numerators together because we clearly have two-fourths of the circle. As Figure 1-3 ■ shows, adding the denominators would be meaningless: it is impossible to arrive at two-eighths by adding together 1/4 and 1/4. Therefore, *adding or subtracting fractions requires a common denominator.*

If two denominators are different, we must equalize them before addition or subtraction. To accomplish this, we find the **least common denominator**, which is the single lowest number into which each denominator divides evenly. For example, in the problem

$$\frac{2}{3} + \frac{1}{4}$$

the least common denominator is "12." To prove this, we construct a chart of multiples:

Multiples of 3:	3	6	9	12	15	18	21
Multiples of 4:	4	8	12	16	20	24	28

Therefore, the addition problem above becomes

$$\frac{g}{12} + \frac{h}{12}$$

The next step is to find the numerators g and h that correspond to the new denominator:

$$\frac{2}{3} = \frac{g}{12} \quad \text{and} \quad \frac{1}{4} = \frac{h}{12}$$

In the first equation (for numerator g), the original denominator of 3 was multiplied by 4 to give the least common denominator of 12. Therefore, we also multiply the numerator by 4:

$$\frac{2}{3} \times \frac{4}{4} = \frac{8}{12}$$

In the second equation (for numerator h), the original denominator of 4 was multiplied by 3. Therefore, we also multiply the numerator by 3:

$$\frac{1}{4} \times \frac{3}{3} = \frac{3}{12}$$

Now we may perform the addition:

$$\frac{2}{3} + \frac{1}{4} = \frac{8}{12} + \frac{3}{12} = \frac{11}{12}$$

Figure 1-4 ■ illustrates this addition of fractions, showing that combining 2/3 with 1/4 gives the same fraction as 11/12.

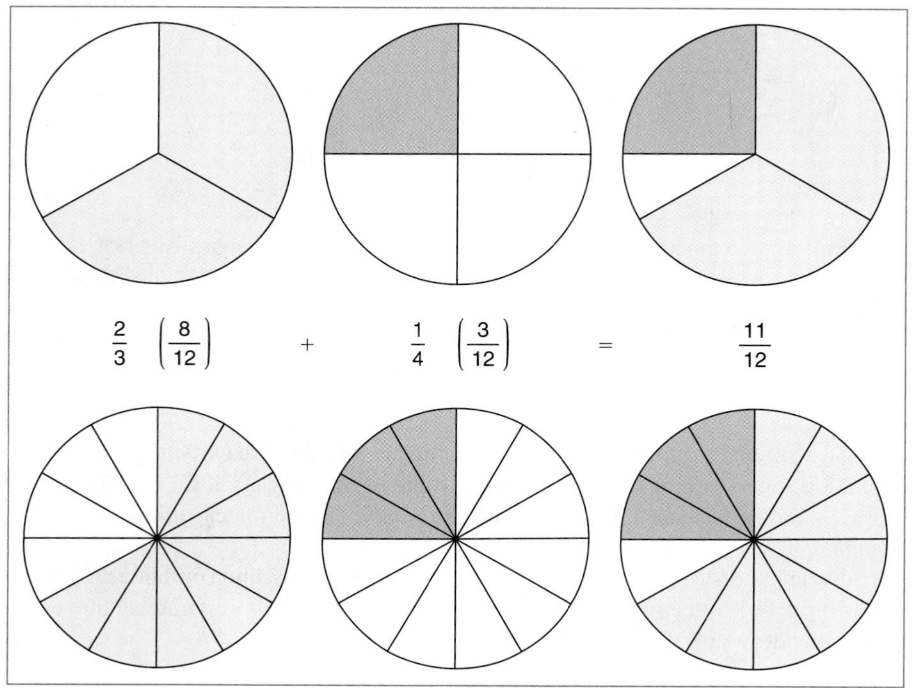

■ **FIGURE 1-4** An illustration of the equation $\frac{2}{3} + \frac{1}{4} = \frac{11}{12}$, showing the need for a common denominator. The area of the circle covered by the addition of 2/3 (blue) and 1/4 (purple) is the same as the area covered by 11/12 (blue and purple).

☑ CHECKPOINT 1-7

1. Evaluate the following expressions.

   (a) $\frac{1}{5} + \frac{4}{9}$ (b) $\frac{2}{3} + \frac{2}{9}$ (c) $\frac{3}{8} + \frac{1}{2}$ (d) $\frac{1}{3} + \frac{2}{5}$

2. Evaluate the following expressions.

   (a) $\frac{3}{4} - \frac{1}{2}$ (b) $\frac{6}{7} - \frac{8}{9}$ (c) $\frac{4}{5} - \frac{2}{3}$ (d) $\frac{1}{2} - \frac{1}{4}$

1. (a) $\frac{9}{45} + \frac{20}{45} = \frac{29}{45}$ (b) $\frac{8}{9}$ (c) $\frac{7}{8}$ (d) $\frac{11}{15}$

2. (a) $\frac{3}{4} - \frac{2}{4} = \frac{1}{4}$ (b) $\frac{-2}{63}$ (c) $\frac{2}{15}$ (d) $\frac{1}{4}$

Expressing Fractions as Decimal Numbers

Because fractions are divisions, we may express them as decimals. For example, the fraction $\frac{1}{2}$ is the same as 0.5:

$$\frac{1}{2} = 2\overline{)1.0}^{\,0.5}$$

This is consistent because 0.5 is the same as 5/10, which reduces to 1/2:

$$0.5 = \frac{5}{10} = \frac{5}{5} \times \frac{1}{2} = \frac{1}{2}$$

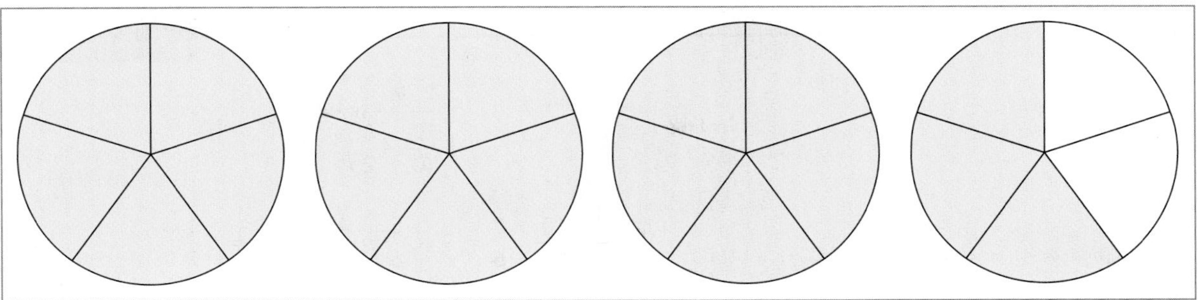

■ FIGURE 1-5 A depiction of the improper fraction $\frac{18}{5}$ and its equivalent mixed number $3\frac{3}{5}$. Each wedge represents 1/5 of a circle. Clearly, 18/5 constitutes three whole circles and an additional 3/5 of another circle.

Another example is $\frac{3}{5}$, which is equal to 0.6:

$$\frac{3}{5} = 5\overline{)3.0}\quad(0.6)$$

Like the preceding decimal, this one is consistent because 6/10 reduces to $\frac{3}{5}$:

$$0.6 = \frac{6}{10} = \frac{2}{2} \times \frac{3}{5} = \frac{3}{5}$$

Improper Fractions

An **improper fraction** is one in which the numerator is greater than the denominator. This is the opposite of a **proper fraction**, whose denominator is larger than its numerator. Any improper fraction has a value greater than 1, a fact that allows us to express it as a whole number with a proper fraction. This is called a **mixed number**.

An example of improper fractions is

$$\frac{18}{5}$$

Carrying out the division, we see that 5 goes into 18 three times, with a remainder of 3 (Figure 1-5 ■). Accordingly, the equivalent mixed number is

$$\frac{18}{5} = 3 + \frac{3}{5} = 3\frac{3}{5}$$

Another example is $\frac{58}{7}$:

$$\frac{58}{7} = 8 + \frac{2}{7} = 8\frac{2}{7}$$

Complex Fractions

A **complex fraction** is one in which the numerator and/or the denominator is itself a fraction. Simplifying complex fractions is a matter of applying rules already articulated. Consider the following three examples.

EXAMPLE 1

$$\frac{2}{3}\Big/\frac{5}{8}$$

$$\frac{2}{3} \times \frac{8}{5} = \frac{16}{15} = 1\frac{1}{15}$$

EXAMPLE 2

$$\frac{9}{\left(\frac{12-6}{10\div 2}\right)}$$

$$9\times\frac{10\div 2}{12-6}=9\times\frac{5}{6}=\frac{45}{6}=7\frac{3}{6}=7\frac{1}{2}$$

EXAMPLE 3

$$\frac{0.8}{\frac{1}{2}} \qquad 0.8\times\frac{2}{1}=1.6$$

☑ CHECKPOINT 1-8

1. Express the following fractions as decimal numbers (to two places).
   (a) $\frac{3}{7}$ (b) $\frac{2}{3}$ (c) $\frac{4}{5}$ (d) $\frac{1}{6}$
2. Express the following improper fractions as mixed numbers.
   (a) $\frac{3}{2}$ (b) $\frac{8}{3}$ (c) $\frac{25}{7}$ (d) $\frac{19}{4}$
3. Simplify the following complex fractions.
   (a) $\frac{2}{3}\Big/\frac{6}{7}$ (b) $18\div 2\Big/\frac{(14\times 2)}{7}$ (c) $\frac{48}{\left(\frac{6}{7}\right)}$

1. (a) 0.43 (b) 0.67 (c) 0.80 (d) 0.17
2. (a) $1\frac{1}{2}$ (b) $2\frac{2}{3}$ (c) $3\frac{4}{7}$ (d) $4\frac{3}{4}$
3. (a) $\frac{7}{9}$ (b) $2\frac{1}{4}$ (c) 56

PERCENTAGES

The usefulness and importance of percentages as a mathematical tool cannot be overstated. The term "per cent" comes from the Latin *per centum*, meaning "through a hundred." A **percentage** represents a number of parts out of every 100 parts; it is symbolized by "%".

Consider two simple examples. If four out of 100 patients test positive for human immunodeficiency virus (HIV), then we say that 4% of the patients tested positive. If 52 out of every 100 persons are female, then we say that 52% are women.

The decimal equivalent of a percentage is the quotient itself. The following example shows that 25% is the same as 25 out of 100, which, in turn, is the same as 0.25, or twenty-five-hundredths:

$$25\%=\frac{25}{100}=0.25$$

Therefore, *to convert from a percentage to a decimal, divide the number by 100 and drop the "%" sign. To convert from a decimal to a percentage, multiply the number by 100 and add the "%" sign.*

Percentages also give us a means of standardizing proportions when the total number of parts is not 100. For example, suppose that last year 240 of 2000 patient specimens tested positive for antibodies against *Helicobacter pylori*, the bacterium that causes gastric ulcers. Suppose that, in the preceding year, 72 of 900 tested positive. In which year were there more positives out of every 100 specimens?

To answer this question, we recognize that for last year the result of 240 out of 2000 is a fraction:

$$\frac{240}{2000}$$

The same is true for the preceding year, with 72 out of 900:

$$\frac{72}{900}$$

To compare the two directly, therefore, we must set each denominator to 100 and then find the corresponding numerator:

$$\frac{240}{2000} = \frac{?}{100} \text{ and } \frac{72}{900} = \frac{?}{100}$$

The straightforward way to solve this problem is to perform the division and express the result as a percentage. For last year:

$$\frac{240}{2000} = 2000\overline{)240.00}\;\;0.12$$

$$0.12 = 12\%$$

The decimal number "0.12" tells us that 12/100, or 12 out of 100, patient specimens last year tested positive for antibodies against *H. pylori*. The fraction $\frac{12}{100}$ is the same as 12%. For the preceding year:

$$\frac{72}{900} = 900\overline{)72.00}\;\;0.08$$

$$0.08 = 8\%$$

The decimal number "0.08" tells us that 8/100, or 8 out of 100, patient specimens the preceding year tested positive for antibodies against *H. pylori*. The fraction $\frac{8}{100}$ is the same as 8%.

Solving Percentage Problems

In essence, percentage problems are multiplications. For example, when we ask what 20% of 300 is, we are asking what 20/100 of 300 is. That, in turn, is the same as asking how much we have after dividing 300 into 100 equal parts and then taking 20 of those parts:

$$20\% \text{ of } 300 = 0.20 \times 300 = \frac{20}{100} \times 300 = \frac{300}{100} \times 20 = 60$$

Consider the following examples.

EXAMPLE 1

What is 25% of 400?

$$25\% \text{ of } 400 = 0.25 \times 400 = \frac{25}{100} \times 400 = \frac{400}{100} \times 25 = 100$$

EXAMPLE 2

What is 72% of 0.663?

$$72\% \text{ of } 0.663 = 0.72 \times 0.663 = \frac{72}{100} \times 0.663 = \frac{0.663}{100} \times 72 = 0.477$$

EXAMPLE 3

The number "144" is 48% of what other number? Let us call the unknown number "*a*." Solving this problem requires understanding from the outset that

$$48\% \text{ of } a = 0.48 \times a = 144$$

Therefore, dividing 144 by 0.48 reveals the value of *a:*

$$a = \frac{144}{0.48}$$

$$a = 300$$

We check our result in the original equation:

$$0.48 \times 300 = 144$$

$$144 = 144$$

Two Caveats

The first caveat is about the decimal point. It is easy to misplace it in a percentage calculation, especially when the percentage itself is less than 1. Remember that converting a percentage to a decimal number entails moving the decimal point two places to the left, that is, dividing the percentage by 100. For example, 0.1% of 5000 is

$$0.1\% \text{ of } 5000 = 0.001 \times 5000 = \frac{1}{1000} \times 5000 = 5$$

Notice that the decimal number of 0.001, which is the same as 0.1%, involves the thousandths place. Notice the pattern in the factors of 10, which the section on shortcuts discusses later:

Percentage of 5000	Decimal Equivalent	Fraction Equivalent	Numerical Value
100	1	1/1 (= 100/100)	5000
10	0.1	1/10 (= 10/100)	500
1	0.01	1/100	50
0.1	0.001	1/1000 (= 0.1/100)	5
0.01	0.0001	1/10,000 (= 0.01/100)	0.5

The second caveat concerns a common error among expressions of change reported as percentages. Consider this statement:

> "Two years ago, our laboratory ran the test for varicella-zoster virus on 500 patient specimens. Last year, that number fell to 400. Thus, there was a 20% decrease."

That conclusion is correct. The number of tests started at 500 but went down by 100. Therefore, the decrease itself is 20% of the starting number:

$$\frac{100}{500} = 0.20 = 20\%$$

Now consider this statement:

"Two years ago, 30% of the specimens we tested for varicella-zoster virus were positive. Last year, 50% were positive. Thus, there was a 20% increase in the number of positive results."

This conclusion is wrong. There was not a 20% increase in the number of positive test results or in the percentages themselves.

Consider first the number of positive test results. Two years ago, that number was

$$30\% \text{ of } 500 = 0.30 \times 500 = 150$$

Last year, however, the number of positive test results was

$$50\% \text{ of } 400 = 0.50 \times 400 = 200$$

Clearly, the number of positive test results went up from 150 to 200, an increase of 50. Thus, relative to the starting number, the increase itself is actually

$$\frac{50}{150} = 0.33 = 33\%$$

We can say, then, that the number of positive test results increased by 33%, *not* by 20%.

Now consider the percentage values themselves. Of the specimens tested, 30% were positive 2 years ago, and 50% were positive last year. The percentage went up from 30 to 50, an increase of 20. *However*, relative to the starting percentage, the increase itself is actually

$$\frac{20}{30} = 0.67 = 67\%$$

We can say, then, that the percentage of test results that were positive increased by 67%, *not* by 20%. *What we say instead is that there was an increase of 20 percentage points.*

In summary, the accurate and meaningful way to articulate the change we observed above is that there was (a) a 33% increase in the number of positive results, and (b) an increase of 20 percentage points.

☑ CHECKPOINT 1-9

1. Express the following as percentages.

   (a) 0.88 (b) $\frac{1}{4}$ (c) 0.61 (d) $\frac{3}{10}$

2. Express the following as decimal numbers.

   (a) 19.5% (b) 0.44% (c) 54.03% (d) 0.012%

3. Evaluate the following expressions.

   (a) 20% of 400 (b) 63% of 0.932 (c) 0.5% of 1000 (d) 1% of 10

1. (a) 88% (b) 25% (c) 61% (d) 30%
2. (a) 0.195 (b) 0.0044 (c) 0.5403 (d) 0.00012
3. (a) 80 (b) 0.587 (c) 5 (d) 0.1

ALGEBRA

The practical purpose of algebra is to find the unknown value of some variable. The strategy behind this goal is two-fold: (1) to write a suitable mathematical equation that includes the target variable, and (2) to isolate the target variable on one side of the equation and the numbers on the other side.

In so doing, we apply two rules: (1) carry out the opposite of whatever operations appear on the same side as the target variable, and (2) maintain the equality by performing the same operation on each side of the equals sign.

For our first example, consider this simple equation with a variable, x, whose value is unknown:

$$x + 4 = 7$$

To isolate x on one side of the equation and the numbers on the other, we carry out the opposite of the operation that appears on the same side as x. Because 4 is added to x on the left side, we subtract it. But in order to maintain the equality, we subtract it also from the other side:

$$x + 4 - 4 = 7 - 4$$

$$x = 3$$

The next example involves multiplication:

$$3x = 18$$

Because x is multiplied by 3, we divide each side by 3:

$$\frac{3x}{3} = \frac{18}{3}$$

$$x = 6$$

We next try an equation involving division:

$$\frac{x}{9} = 5$$

Because x is divided by 9, we multiply each side by 9:

$$\frac{x}{9} \cdot 9 = 5 \cdot 9$$

$$x = 45$$

Now let us consider an equation involving more than one operation on x:

$$3x + 6 = 18$$

There are two operations on the left side of the equation: multiplication and addition. We perform their opposites, division and subtraction, but only one at a time. First, we subtract 6 from each side of the equation, giving

$$3x + 6 - 6 = 18 - 6$$

$$3x = 12$$

Next, we divide each side by 3:

$$\frac{3x}{3} = \frac{12}{3}$$

$$x = 4$$

It is always wise to check the final result by substituting it into the original equation. In this case, we put "4" back into "$3x + 6 = 18$"; our result is correct because it satisfies the equation:

$$3(4) + 6 = 18$$

$$12 + 6 = 18$$

$$18 = 18$$

In our final example, we consider a more-complex equation:

$$\frac{\frac{1}{2}x - 10}{5} = 30$$

On the left side of the equation, there is division by 5, subtraction of 10, and multiplication by $^1/_2$. To isolate x, we perform their opposites. First, we multiply each side by 5:

$$\frac{\frac{1}{2}x - 10}{5} \cdot 5 = 30 \cdot 5$$

$$\frac{1}{2}x - 10 = 150$$

Second, we add 10:

$$\frac{1}{2}x - 10 + 10 = 150 + 10$$

$$\frac{1}{2}x = 160$$

Third, we multiply by 2:

$$\frac{1}{2}x \cdot 2 = 160 \cdot 2$$

$$x = 320$$

Finally, we check our result in the original equation:

$$\frac{\frac{1}{2}(320) - 10}{5} = 30$$

$$\frac{160 - 10}{5} = 30$$

$$\frac{150}{5} = 30$$

$$30 = 30$$

Operational Properties

We have already seen the commutative and associative properties of addition and multiplication:

Commutative property: $a + b = b + a$

$a \times b = b \times a$

Associative property: $(a + b) + c = a + (b + c)$

$(a \times b) \times c = a \times (b \times c)$

Now we introduce the **distributive property:**

$$a(b + c) = ab + ac$$

We have distributed the variable a to the variables inside the parentheses, b and c. We can verify this property by assigning arbitrary values to the variables, and in doing so we see that the left and right sides of the equation are indeed equal:

$$3(5 + 8) = 3(5) + 3(8)$$

$$3(13) = 15 + 24$$

$$39 = 39$$

Using the distributive property, let us now solve some equations algebraically.

EXAMPLE 1

$$4(x + 8) = 48$$

There are two equally effective approaches to this problem.

Approach 1

Divide each side by 4, giving

$$\frac{4(x + 8)}{4} = \frac{48}{4}$$

$$x + 8 = 12$$

(continued)

Next, subtract 8 from each side:

$$x + 8 - 8 = 12 - 8$$
$$x = 4$$

Approach 2

Apply the distributive property:

$$4x + 4(8) = 48$$
$$4x + 32 = 48$$

Then subtract 32 from each side:

$$4x + 32 - 32 = 48 - 32$$
$$4x = 16$$

In the final step, divide each side by 4:

$$\frac{4x}{4} = \frac{16}{4}$$
$$x = 4$$

Check the result by substituting it back into the original equation:

$$4(4 + 8) = 48$$
$$4(12) = 48$$
$$48 = 48$$

EXAMPLE 2

$$\frac{2(x - 7)}{4} = 2.5$$

There are three effective approaches to solving this problem, one of which involves the distributive property.

Approach 1

Multiply each side by 4:

$$\frac{2(x - 7)}{4} \times 4 = 2.5 \times 4$$
$$2(x - 7) = 10$$

Divide each side by 2:

$$\frac{2(x - 7)}{2} = \frac{10}{2}$$
$$x - 7 = 5$$

Add 7 to each side:

$$x - 7 + 7 = 5 + 7$$
$$x = 12$$

Approach 2

Reduce the fraction on the left side by canceling the "2" in the numerator:

$$\frac{2(x - 7)}{4} = 2.5$$

$$\frac{1(x - 7)}{2} = 2.5$$

$$\frac{x - 7}{2} = 2.5$$

Then multiply each side by 2:

$$\frac{x - 7}{2} \times 2 = 2.5 \times 2$$

$$x - 7 = 5$$

Finally, add 7 to each side:

$$x - 7 + 7 = 5 + 7$$

$$x = 12$$

Approach 3

Multiply each side by 4 (the same step as in approach #1):

$$\frac{2(x - 7)}{4} \times 4 = 2.5 \times 4$$

$$2(x - 7) = 10$$

Next, apply the distributive property:

$$2x - 2(7) = 10$$

$$2x - 14 = 10$$

Then add 14 to each side:

$$2x - 14 + 14 = 10 + 14$$

$$2x = 24$$

Finally, divide each side by 2:

$$\frac{2x}{2} = \frac{24}{2}$$

$$x = 12$$

Check the result by substituting it back into the original equation:

$$\frac{2(12 - 7)}{4} = 2.5$$

$$\frac{2(5)}{4} = 2.5$$

$$\frac{10}{4} = 2.5$$

$$2.5 = 2.5$$

EXAMPLE 3

$$2(x + 9) + 3x = 14$$

Notice that the variable x appears in two terms on the left side of the equation. Therefore, we must combine them in order to isolate x. Our first step, then, is to distribute the "2":

$$2x + 2(9) + 3x = 14$$
$$2x + 18 + 3x = 14$$

Realize that $2x = x + x$ and that $3x = x + x + x$. Therefore, our equation above becomes

$$x + x + 18 + x + x + x = 14$$
$$5x + 18 = 14$$

The next step is to subtract 18 from each side:

$$5x + 18 - 18 = 14 - 18$$
$$5x = -4$$

The final step is to divide each side by 5:

$$\frac{5x}{5} = \frac{-4}{5}$$
$$x = -0.8$$

Checking the result in the original equation shows it to be correct:

$$2(-0.8 + 9) + 3(-0.8) = 14$$
$$2(8.2) + (-2.4) = 14$$
$$16.4 - 2.4 = 14$$
$$14 = 14$$

☑ CHECKPOINT 1-10

Solve each of the following equations for x.

(a) $3x + 5 = 17$ (b) $\frac{x - 5}{8} = 2$ (c) $0.25x - 1 = 4$

(d) $\frac{2}{3}x + 4 = 8$ (e) $4(x + 1) = 56$ (f) $\frac{3(x - 5)}{9} = -1$

(a) $x = 4$ (b) $x = 21$ (c) $x = 20$

(d) $x = 6$ (e) $x = 13$ (f) $x = 2$

RATIOS

A **ratio** is a quotient of two numbers. It provides a convenient summary of how those two numbers compare with each other. The numerator and denominator may have the same units (e.g., minutes, grams, milliliters, dollars, milligrams per deciliter), or they may have different units, in which case the quotient is technically a *rate*. When saying "the ratio of *a* to *b*," we mean this quotient:

$$\frac{a}{b}$$

Ratios figure prominently in laboratory calculations, especially those involving concentrations and dilutions, which later chapters in this book cover. Let us consider several examples now.

EXAMPLE 1

Automated instrument *A* takes 90 minutes to run the test for parathyroid hormone. Automated instrument *B* takes 40 minutes. What is the ratio of the time required to run the test on *A* to that on *B*? What does it mean mathematically?

$$\frac{90 \text{ min}}{40 \text{ min}} = 2.25$$

The ratio of 2.25 tells us that instrument *A* takes 2.25 times as long as instrument *B* to run the test for parathyroid hormone. The division cancels out the units because they are the same in the numerator and denominator. Notice that this ratio is also an improper fraction (a subject discussed earlier in the chapter), which we can convert to a mixed number:

$$\frac{90 \text{ min}}{40 \text{ min}} = \frac{9}{4} = 2 + \frac{1}{4} = 2\frac{1}{4}$$

Because $2.25 = 2\frac{1}{4}$, the two results and their interpretation are the same whether we ultimately call the quotient a "ratio" or an "improper fraction."

EXAMPLE 2

On a given date, the number of platelets in a fixed volume of patient *X*'s blood was 120. Three months later, after a course of drug therapy, the count was 480. What is the ratio of the count after therapy to the count before therapy? What does it mean mathematically?

$$\frac{480 \text{ platelets}}{120 \text{ platelets}} = 4$$

After therapy, there were four times as many platelets in a fixed volume of patient *X*'s blood as there were before therapy. In other words, the ratio tells us that the count quadrupled.

EXAMPLE 3

A reagent for a particular assay in your laboratory comes from the manufacturer in powder form. You must reconstitute it in water before use. The instructions specify adding 3 milliliters of water to 0.60 grams of powder. What is the ratio of the volume of water to the weight of powder? What does it mean mathematically?

$$\frac{3.0 \text{ milliliters}}{0.60 \text{ grams}} = 5.0 \text{ milliliters/gram}$$

What this ratio means is that every gram of powder requires 5 milliliters of water. This information would help us calculate the volume of water needed to reconstitute any amount of powder we might have at a given time. Notice that, because the units in the numerator differ from those in the denominator, the division does not cancel them out; they appear in the quotient.

EXAMPLE 4

The assay for a particular protein in plasma requires mixing 11 parts of reagent *A* with 0.20 parts of reagent *B*. What is the ratio of the volume of reagent *A* to reagent *B*? What does it mean mathematically?

$$\frac{11 \text{ parts reagent } A}{0.20 \text{ parts reagent } B} = 55 \text{ parts reagent } A/\text{part reagent } B$$

This ratio tells us that each part of reagent *B* requires 55 parts of reagent *A*. As in example 3 above, this information would help us calculate the volume of either reagent needed when we know the volume of the other.

Cross-Multiplication

Cross-multiplication is a technique for solving problems that equate two ratios. Although it is just a specific instance of the broader rules of algebra presented earlier, it is so useful that it deserves special attention.

Consider first a simple example in which we solve for an unknown, *x*:

$$\frac{2}{3} = \frac{x}{18}$$

In reading this equation, we say that 2 is to 3 as *x* is to 18. In other words, 2 has the same relationship to 3 as *x* has to 18.

Applying the rules of algebra discussed earlier, we perform the opposite of the operation on *x*, and we do so on each side of the equation. In this case, therefore, we multiply by 18:

$$\frac{2}{3} \cdot 18 = \frac{x}{18} \cdot 18$$

$$\frac{36}{3} = x$$

$$12 = x$$

Checking the final result by substituting it in the original equation verifies our algebra:

$$\frac{2}{3} = \frac{12}{18}$$

$$\frac{2}{3} = \frac{6}{6} \times \frac{2}{3}$$

$$\frac{2}{3} = 1 \times \frac{2}{3}$$

$$\frac{2}{3} = \frac{2}{3}$$

In cross-multiplication, we multiply the denominator on one side of the equation by the numerator on the other side and the numerator on one side by the denominator on the other:

$$\frac{2}{3} \times \frac{12}{18}$$

This gives us

$$2 \times 18 = 3 \times 12$$

$$36 = 36$$

Now let us use cross-multiplication to solve the same problem:

$$\frac{2}{3} = \frac{x}{18}$$
$$2 \times 18 = 3x$$
$$36 = 3x$$
$$\frac{36}{3} = \frac{3x}{3}$$
$$12 = x$$

Here is an example from the laboratory. Suppose an assay requires mixing 0.30 parts of reagent *A* with 7.0 parts of reagent *B*. If the number of patient specimens we have requires 0.52 parts of reagent *A*, how much reagent *B* must we use?

We know the ratio of the volumes of reagents *A* and *B*, and we know how much *A* we need in this run of the assay. So, the volume of *B* is our target:

$$\frac{0.30 \text{ parts reagent } A}{7.0 \text{ parts reagent } B} = \frac{0.52 \text{ parts reagent } A}{x}$$

Cross-multiplying gives

$$(0.30 \text{ parts } A) \cdot x = (7.0 \text{ parts } B)(0.52 \text{ parts } A)$$
$$\frac{(0.30 \text{ parts } A) \cdot x}{0.30 \text{ parts } A} = \frac{(7.0 \text{ parts } B)(0.52 \text{ parts } A)}{0.30 \text{ parts } A}$$
$$x = (7.0 \text{ parts } B)(1.73)$$
$$x = 12.1 \text{ parts } B$$

We can also use cross-multiplication to solve percentage problems. In fact, example 3 under "Solving Percentage Problems" employed this technique without identifying it as cross-multiplication. The question was this: 144 is 48% of what number? To set up the proper equation, we say that 48 is to 100 as 144 is to *a:*

$$\frac{48}{100} = \frac{144}{a}$$

Cross-multiplying gives

$$48a = 144 \times 100$$
$$48a = 14{,}400$$
$$a = 300$$

☑ CHECKPOINT 1-11

1. Calculate each of the following ratios, including the units.

   (a) $\frac{622 \text{ miles}}{38 \text{ gallons}}$ (b) $\frac{49 \text{ bananas}}{21 \text{ bananas}}$ (c) $\frac{2{,}400{,}000 \text{ red blood cells}}{4000 \text{ white blood cells}}$ (d) $\frac{0.33 \text{ grams}}{2.64 \text{ grams}}$

2. Solve each of the following equations for *x*.

   (a) $\frac{6}{60} = \frac{x}{28}$ (b) $\frac{102}{773} = \frac{x}{90}$ (c) $\frac{2}{30} = \frac{9}{x}$ (d) $\frac{0.5}{10} = \frac{x}{25}$

3. Solve the following problems.
   (a) What is 24% of 330?
   (b) What is 66% of 0.827?
   (c) The number "5" is 40% of what other number?
   (d) The number "0.22" is 75% of what other number?

1. (a) 16.4 miles/gallon (b) 2.3 (c) 600 red blood cells/white blood cell (d) 0.125
2. (a) 2.8 (b) 11.9 (c) 135 (d) 1.25
3. (a) 79.2 (b) 0.546 (c) 12.5 (d) 0.293

Summary

1. Arithmetic is the manipulation of numbers through addition, subtraction, multiplication, and division. Algebra is the strategic manipulation of relationships in order to find the unknown value of a certain quantity.
2. A positive number and its negative counterpart are *opposites*. Adding a negative number is the same as subtracting its opposite, that is, moving leftward on the number line.
3. The *commutative property* of addition is the fact that the order in which we add two numbers together does not affect the sum, as shown in this equation:

$$a + b = b + a$$

4. The grouping of numbers in addition does not affect the sum. This fact reflects the *associative property* of addition, represented by the equation

$$(a + b) + c = a + (b + c)$$

5. Subtracting a negative number has the same effect as adding its opposite.
6. There are three ways to symbolize multiplication:

$$a \times b = a \cdot b = ab$$

7. Multiplication is commutative. The order in which we multiply two numbers together does not affect the product:

$$a \times b = b \times a$$

8. The grouping of numbers in multiplication does not affect the product. Thus, the *associative property* of multiplication is

$$(a \times b) \times c = a \times (b \times c)$$

9. Multiplication and division follow the same rules governing sign:

Rule
positive × or ÷ positive = positive
positive × or ÷ negative = negative
negative × or ÷ positive = negative
negative × or ÷ negative = positive

10. We define division in terms of multiplication:

$$a \div b = a \cdot \frac{1}{b} \quad \text{or} \quad \frac{a}{b} = a \cdot \frac{1}{b}$$

11. The two quantities b and $1/b$ are *reciprocals* of each other. The product of two reciprocals is 1:

$$b \times \frac{1}{b} = 1$$

12. Division by zero is undefined.
13. Zero divided by any number is zero.
14. A fraction is nothing more than the representation of a division. The top number is the *numerator* and the bottom number is the *denominator*.
15. To multiply fractions, multiply the numerators and multiply the denominators.
16. To divide a fraction, multiply it by the reciprocal of the other number.
17. You have *reduced* fractions fully when the numerator and denominator are as small as possible, that is, when the only number evenly divisible into both of them is "1."
18. To add (or subtract) fractions, add (or subtract) the numerators but not the denominators. Moreover, adding or subtracting fractions requires a common denominator.
19. An *improper fraction* is one in which the numerator is greater than the denominator. This is the opposite of a *proper fraction*, whose denominator is larger than its numerator.
20. A *percentage* represents a number of parts out of every 100 parts; its symbol is "%".
21. To convert from a percentage to a decimal, divide the number by 100 and drop the "%" sign. To convert from a decimal to a percentage, multiply the number by 100 and add the "%" sign.
22. The practical purpose of algebra is to find the unknown value of some variable. The strategy is two-fold: (1) to write a suitable mathematical equation that includes the target variable, and (2) to isolate the target variable on one side of the equation and the numbers on the other side.
23. Algebra has two practical rules: (1) carry out the opposite of whatever operations appear on the same side as the target variable, and (2) maintain the equality by performing the same operation on each side of the equals sign.
24. The *distributive property* is shown in the equation

$$a(b + c) = ab + ac$$

25. A *ratio* is a quotient of two numbers. It provides a convenient summary of how those two numbers compare with each other.
26. In cross-multiplication, we multiply the denominator on one side of the equation by the numerator on the other side and the numerator on one side by the denominator on the other.

Practice Problems

1. (LO 1) Solve the following problems.

(a) $6 + (-9)$ (b) $-7 + 10$
(c) $6.5 - 8.5$ (d) $33.9 + (-52.6)$
(e) $0.224 + 0.035$ (f) $13.006 - 0.909$
(g) $-125 - (-250)$ (h) $-1.79 - 0.53$
(i) $-219 + 221$ (j) $0.00501 + (-0.00623)$
(k) $9701 + 330$ (l) $72.2 - (-17.8)$

2. (LO 1) Evaluate the following expressions.

(a) $2 \times (-3.5)$ (b) $-5 \cdot 18$
(c) $(-20)(-4)$ (d) $0.50 \cdot 66$
(e) -7.1×3 (f) $183 \times (-2)$
(g) $-10 \cdot (-33)$ (h) $(0.0049)(-2)$
(i) $6600 \cdot 0.25$ (j) 1.5×0.3
(k) $-500 \times (500)$ (l) $(-10{,}000)(0.01)$

3. (LO 2, 4, 5) Evaluate the following expressions.

(a) $18 \div 9.1$ (b) $10 \times \frac{3}{4}$
(c) $\frac{0.492}{-3}$ (d) $\frac{-50}{-25}$
(e) $3.6 \div (-9)$ (f) $\frac{7500}{3}$
(g) $\frac{41}{-0.7}$ (h) $\frac{1}{4}(-0.022)$
(i) $200 \div \frac{1}{2}$ (j) $2.096 \div (-4.192)$
(k) $\frac{346}{2/3}$ (l) $\frac{9/16}{0.2}$

4. (LO 2, 4, 5) Evaluate the following expressions. Express each answer as a reduced fraction or a mixed number.

(a) $\frac{1}{4} \times \frac{3}{5}$ (b) $\frac{6}{7} \times 10$
(c) $\frac{3}{4} \div \frac{1}{2}$ (d) $\frac{2}{5} \div 7$
(e) $-2 \div \frac{8}{9}$ (f) $\frac{4}{16} \Big/ \frac{3}{4}$
(g) $\frac{5}{6} \div \frac{1}{4}$ (h) $7\left(\frac{1}{3}\right)$
(i) $\frac{9}{10} \div 2$ (j) $\frac{3/4}{8}$
(k) $\frac{18/27}{2/3}$ (l) $\frac{4000}{\frac{4}{5}}$

5. (LO 2, 3, 4) Evaluate the following expressions. Express each answer as a reduced fraction or a mixed number.

(a) $\frac{1}{2} + \frac{4}{5}$ (b) $\frac{2}{3} - \frac{1}{4}$ (c) $2\frac{2}{3} + \frac{7}{8}$
(d) $\frac{9}{10} - \frac{4}{5}$ (e) $1\frac{1}{2} + \frac{3}{4}$ (f) $\frac{10}{13} - \frac{2}{3}$
(g) $10\frac{2}{3} + 1\frac{5}{6}$ (h) $\frac{6}{7} - \frac{1}{8}$ (i) $\frac{4}{5} + \frac{1}{10}$

6. (LO 4) Express the following fractions as decimal numbers.

(a) $\frac{2}{3}$ (b) $\frac{4}{5}$ (c) $\frac{7}{8}$
(d) $\frac{2}{5}$ (e) $\frac{1}{4}$ (f) $\frac{7}{28}$

7. (LO 6) Complete the following table.

Percentage	Decimal Number	Fraction
12		
	0.04	
		$\frac{3}{4}$
	0.91	
0. 55		
		$\frac{1}{3}$

8. (LO 7) Evaluate the following expressions.

(a) 19% of 200 (b) 63% of 0.112
(c) 0.7% of 88 (d) 110% of 60
(e) 0.01% of 30,000 (f) 33% of 0.0174

9. (LO 9) Solve each equation for x.

(a) $2x - 13 = 6$ (b) $\frac{x}{6} + (-0.37) = 5$
(c) $120 + 6x = 138$ (d) $5(x + 2) - 1 = 59$
(e) $\frac{2}{8(x + 4)} = 0.03125$ (f) $\frac{1}{4}x - 6.00 = -5.93$

10. (LO 11) Solve each equation for x.

(a) $\frac{46}{12} = \frac{x}{36}$ (b) $\frac{0.33}{7} = \frac{3.3}{x}$
(c) $\frac{450}{81.2} = \frac{x}{29.2}$ (d) $\frac{1000}{50} = \frac{600}{x}$
(e) $\frac{0.098}{0.345} = \frac{x}{1.035}$ (f) $\frac{24}{6} = \frac{192}{x}$

Contextual Problems

1. (LO 1, 9) The Friedewald formula provides a calculated estimate of the concentration of LDL cholesterol in serum, given three other measured concentrations:

$$\text{conc. of LDL cholesterol} = (\text{total conc. of cholesterol}) - (\text{conc. of HDL cholesterol}) - \left(\frac{\text{conc. of triglycerides}}{5}\right)$$

where LDL is low-density lipoprotein and HDL is high-density lipoprotein. Each concentration has units of "milligrams per deciliter," symbolized by "mg/dL."

   (a) Compute the concentration of LDL cholesterol when the total concentration of cholesterol is 190 mg/dL, the concentration of HDL cholesterol is 36 mg/dL, and the concentration of triglycerides is 288 mg/dL.

   (b) Compute the concentration of LDL cholesterol when the total concentration of cholesterol is 260 mg/dL, the concentration of HDL cholesterol is 22 mg/dL, and the concentration of triglycerides is 317 mg/dL.

   (c) Compute the total concentration of cholesterol when the concentration of LDL cholesterol is 101 mg/dL, the concentration of HDL cholesterol is 46 mg/dL, and the concentration of triglycerides is 150 mg/dL.

   (d) Compute the concentration of triglycerides when the total concentration of cholesterol is 208 mg/dL, the concentration of LDL cholesterol is 129 mg/dL, and the concentration of HDL cholesterol is 59 mg/dL.

2. (LO 10, 11) You are running an assay that requires preparation of the working reagent by mixing stock reagent *A* with stock reagent *B* in a ratio of 0.5 to 3. Each patient specimen requires 0.10 volumes of stock reagent *A*. If you have 23 patient specimens, calculate the volume of stock reagent *B* you need.

3. (LO 2, 7) Your laboratory is conducting an experiment, for which you have been saving patient specimens. There are 624 specimens in all. You randomly select 1/3 of the specimens to run on your automated instrument (group 1). Another 1/3 you ship to a laboratory out of state to be run on their instrument (group 2). The final third, however, you must divide in half; 1/2 remains in storage (group 3) and the other half undergoes a different test in your laboratory (group 4).

   (a) If 1/4 of the specimens in group 4 are not useable because of clotting, how many good specimens remain in that group?

   (b) Three-eighths of the group 2 specimens give uninterpretable results in their test. How many specimens does this represent?

   (c) To confirm the results, you decide to rerun a randomly selected 25% of the specimens in group 1. How many specimens does this represent?

4. (LO 1) The hematocrit is the volume of whole blood occupied by packed red blood cells (RBCs). To ascertain this value, blood is loaded into a capillary tube and centrifuged; the resulting volume taken by the RBCs is expressed sometimes as a percentage of the total volume. The hemoglobin concentration should be three times the RBC count, and the hematocrit should be three times the hemoglobin concentration plus or minus 3:

$$\text{hemoglobin} = \text{RBC count} \times 3$$

$$\text{hematocrit} = (\text{hemoglobin} \times 3) \pm 3$$

These relationships are collectively called the "rule of 3," a quick way for the hematology technologist or the physician to check results for the presence of errors and of a disease state. In performing these calculations, we use the numbers only and we ignore the units. For example, the following data satisfy the rule of 3:

RBC count = 4.1   hemoglobin = 12.3   hematocrit = 37

   (a) Do the following data satisfy the rule of 3?

   RBC count = 4.8   hemoglobin = 13.6   hematocrit = 45

   (b) Do the following data satisfy the rule of 3?

   RBC count = 5.1   hemoglobin = 15.3   hematocrit = 46

   (c) In order to satisfy the rule of 3, what should the value of the RBC count be?

   hemoglobin = 14.0   hematocrit = 41

5. (LO 7) Albumin is one of many plasma proteins. It has various physiological roles, including the maintenance of osmotic pressure and the transport of fatty acids, hormones, vitamins, and other substances. The concentration of albumin is normally between 3.4 and 5.0 grams per deciliter (g/dL). When outside that range, a disease may be present.

   Consider a patient specimen. If albumin is 56.0% of the total plasma protein, and if the concentration of total plasma protein is 7.0 g/dL, then does the albumin concentration in this specimen fall within the expected range?

6. (LO 7) The concentration of glucose in cerebrospinal fluid (CSF) is usually 60–75% of the concentration in plasma. A concentration below this range is consistent with meningitis and other diseases of the central nervous system.

   Consider a patient whose plasma glucose concentration is 81 milligrams per deciliter (mg/dL). If the CSF glucose concentration is 54 mg/dL, does it fall within the expected range?

7. (LO 1, 7, 8, 9) If a whole blood specimen is allowed to stand, the cells metabolize glucose at such a rate that its concentration decreases 7% in 1 hour. Consider a whole blood specimen that has been standing on a bench for an hour since it was drawn. If the plasma glucose concentration of that sample is 61 milligrams per deciliter (mg/dL), approximately what was its value at the time of collection?

8. (LO 2, 3, 4, 6, 8) Your laboratory uses the solvent acetonitrile in its assays involving the technique of high-pressure liquid chromatography (HPLC). For today's run, you can see that you will need $\frac{3}{4}$ of the acetonitrile currently in the bottle. However, a colleague from another laboratory borrows half of your acetonitrile for his own HPLC, leaving the other half with you.
   (a) He uses $\frac{1}{3}$ of what he borrowed and returns the remainder to you. Between your half and what he returns to you, do you have enough acetonitrile for today's run?
   (b) What your colleague returns to you is 1/5 of the amount that was in the bottle before he borrowed it. Between your half and the 1/5 he is returning, do you have enough acetonitrile for today's run?
   (c) Your laboratory's consumption of acetonitrile in the last 6 months (period 2) was 4.6 liters (L), an increase of 30% over the preceding 6 months (period 1). How much acetonitrile did your laboratory consume in period 1?
9. (LO 10, 11) Your laboratory's chromatographic assay for a certain drug uses a solvent that is prepared by mixing 400 milliliters (mL) of methanol with 90 mL of water.
   (a) You discover that you have only 320 mL of methanol in stock. What volume of water should you mix with it to prepare the solvent?
   (b) Your colleague prepared the solvent by mixing 600 mL of methanol with 135 mL of water. Is that ratio correct?
   (c) In an experiment she wants to carry out, your laboratory director has asked you to double the ratio of methanol to water. For this experiment, how much water should you mix with 500 mL of methanol?

Appendix

Mind Over Calculator: A Few Tips for Calculating Without Electronics

In the clinical laboratory, as in all of science and technology, it is not only possible, but also easy, to depend too much on calculators. The laboratorian must be poised to (1) catch his or her own errors, as well as those of colleagues, supervisors, trainees, nurses, physicians, and anyone else who does something that results in a calculation; (2) estimate numbers in order to follow technical papers or presentations and to save time and money in the laboratory; and (3) notice anomalies in test results in order to detect instrument malfunctions or procedural mistakes.

This appendix offers some strategies for carrying out mental calculations—without a calculator—whether the goal is an accurate value or just a rough estimate. *In every case, the key is to look for relationships among the numbers that might simplify the arithmetic.*

ADDITION AND SUBTRACTION PROBLEMS

EXAMPLE 1

$$21 + 58 - 6 + 33 = ?$$

For a rough estimate, rounding off is an effective start. Recognize 21 as being close to 20, 58 close to 60, and 33 close to 30.

$$20 + 60 + 30 = 110$$

Then subtract the 6:

$$110 - 6 = 104$$

This is close to the exact answer of 106.

To get the exact answer instead, break the problem into two simpler problems: the first one combining the tens and the second one combining the ones. Then bring the two results together.

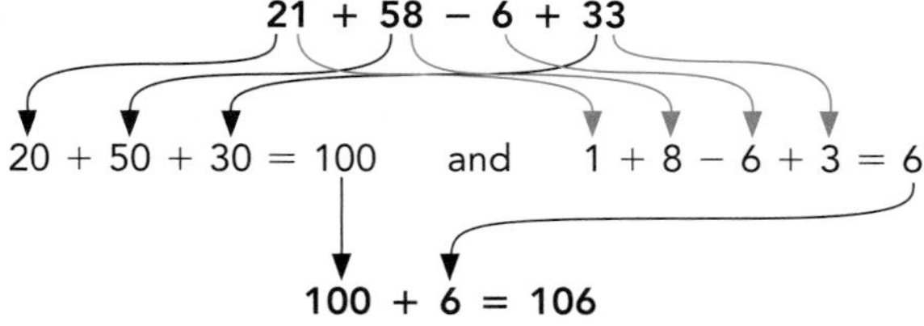

EXAMPLE 2

$$\begin{array}{r} 2253 \\ 3677 \\ +\ 6014 \\ \hline ? \end{array}$$

Rough estimate

The thousands place makes the sum at least 11,000 (2000 + 3000 + 6000). This may be close enough for some purposes. If not, continue to the next step.

More-refined estimate

The hundreds place adds 800 more (200 + 600), bringing the sum to at least 11,800. If this estimate is still not satisfactory, continue.

Even-more-refined estimate

The tens place adds 130 more (50 + 70 + 10), bringing the sum to at least 11,930. This is close to the correct sum of 11,944.

Exact sum

To the sum in the step above, just add the ones:

$$11{,}930 + (3 + 7 + 4)$$
$$11{,}930 + 14$$
$$11{,}944$$

EXAMPLE 3

$$\begin{array}{r} 31.8 \\ 14.2 \\ +\ 70.6 \\ \hline ? \end{array}$$

For the exact sum, use the same strategy as in example 1 above: break the problem into three simpler problems, one for each place (tens, ones, tenths). Then combine the three results.

Tens		*Ones*		*Tenths*
30 + 10 + 70	and	1 + 4 + 0	and	0.8 + 0.2 + 0.6

$$110 + 5 + 1.6 = 116.6$$

For a close estimate of the sum, round the numbers off:

$$\begin{array}{r} 32 \\ 14 \\ +\ 71 \\ \hline ? \end{array}$$

Next, as above, break the problem into two simpler problems: the first one combining the tens and the second one combining the ones. Then bring the two results together.

$$30 + 10 + 70 = 110 \quad \text{and} \quad 2 + 4 + 1 = 7$$
$$110 + 7 = 117$$

MULTIPLICATION PROBLEMS

EXAMPLE 1

$46 \times 9 = ?$

To arrive at the product, just remember the essence of multiplication. This particular problem consists of nine forties with an additional six nines:

$$\underbrace{40 + 40 + 40 + 40 + 40 + 40 + 40 + 40 + 40}_{9 \times 40} + \underbrace{9 + 9 + 9 + 9 + 9 + 9}_{6 \times 9}$$

In other words, 46×9 is

$$(9 \times 40) + (6 \times 9)$$
$$360 + 54$$
$$414$$

EXAMPLE 2

$81 \times 6 = ?$

Use the same strategy as in example 1 above. This problem is

$$(6 \times 80) + (1 \times 6)$$
$$480 + 6$$
$$486$$

EXAMPLE 3

$103 \times 13 = ?$

Break this problem down into

$$(100 \times 13) + (3 \times 13)$$
$$1300 + 39$$
$$1339$$

EXAMPLE 4

$42 \times 15 = ?$

This multiplication is the same as the following.

$$\underbrace{42 \times 5}_{} \times 3$$
$$(40 \times 5) + (2 \times 5)$$
$$200 + 10$$
$$= 210$$

$$210 \times 3$$
$$(200 \times 3) + (10 \times 3)$$
$$600 + 30$$
$$= 630$$

EXAMPLE 5

$0.30 \times 250 = ?$

This problem breaks down to

$$0.1 \times 3 \times 250 = \frac{1}{10} \times 3 \times 250$$

Therefore, it is possible to take either of two approaches.

Approach 1

Take 1/10 of 250, which is 25, and then multiply by 3:

$$\frac{1}{10} \times 250 = 25$$

$$25 \times 3 = 75$$

Approach 2

Multiply 250 by 3, which is 750, and then divide by 10:

$$250 \times 3 = 750$$

$$\frac{750}{10} = 75$$

EXAMPLE 6

$482 \times 56 = ?$

Rough estimate

Start by rounding off the numbers to 500 and 60:

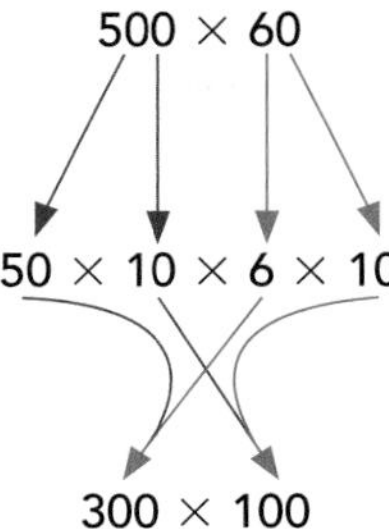

30,000

More-refined estimate

To get a bit closer, recognize 56 as being about halfway between 50 and 60. So, multiply 500 by 50 and then split the difference with the rough estimate from above:

$$500 \times 50 = 25{,}000$$

The product is about halfway between 25,000 and 30,000, which is 27,500, closer to the exact answer (26,992).

EXAMPLE 7

$290 \times 0.65 = ?$

To solve this problem exactly (188.5), use the strategy in example 5 above. For a rough estimate, however, begin by rounding off 290 to 300 and then breaking the problem down:

$$300 \times 0.65$$

$$300 \times (0.60 + 0.05)$$

Now apply the distributive property of multiplication:

$$(300 \times 0.60) + (300 \times 0.05)$$

Realize that 0.60 is the same as 60%, which is six times 10%:

$$10\% \text{ of } 300 = 0.10 \times 300 = 30$$

$$6 \times 30 = 180$$

Realize that 0.05 is the same as 5%, which is half of 10%:

$$10\% \text{ of } 300 = 0.10 \times 300 = 30$$

$$5\% \text{ of } 300 = \frac{30}{2} = 15$$

$$\mathbf{180 + 15 = 195}$$

EXAMPLE 8

$0.033 \times 0.12 = ?$

You may rewrite this problem:

$$33 \times \frac{1}{1000} \times 12 \times \frac{1}{100}$$

$$33 \times 12 \times \frac{1}{100{,}000}$$

Consequently, using the strategy in example 3 or 4 above, multiply 33 by 12 and then move the decimal point five places to the left; the result is 0.00396.

For a rough estimate, however, round 33 down to 30 and multiply by 12:

$$30 \times 12 = 360$$

Now, to divide by 100,000, move the decimal point five places to the left:

$$0.00360$$

DIVISION PROBLEMS

EXAMPLE 1

$480 \div 30 = ?$

This problem breaks down to

$$\frac{480}{10 \times 3} = \frac{480}{10} \times \frac{1}{3}$$

First, $\frac{480}{10} = 48$. Then, $\frac{48}{3} = 16$.

EXAMPLE 2

$$\frac{\mathbf{240}}{\mathbf{0.6}} = \mathbf{?}$$

Apply the rule of multiplying by the reciprocal:

$$240 \times \frac{10}{6}$$

First, multiply 240 by 10 and then divide by 6:

$$240 \times 10 = 2400$$

$$\frac{2400}{6} = 400$$

EXAMPLE 3

$$\frac{\mathbf{834}}{\mathbf{3.2}} = \mathbf{?}$$

Round 834 to 830 and 3.2 to 3. Then, break the problem down:

$$\frac{830}{3} = \frac{800 + 30}{3} = \frac{800}{3} + \frac{30}{3}$$

This quotient is between 250 ($3 \times 250 = 750$) and 300 ($3 \times 300 = 900$), though closer to 250. Thus, round it off to 250.

This quotient is 10.

$$\mathbf{250 + 10 = 260}$$

This is very close to the exact quotient of 260.625.

PERCENTAGE PROBLEMS

EXAMPLE 1

20% of 380 = ?

Recognize 20% as $2 \times 10\%$. Because 10% of 380 is 38, 20% is twice that number, or **76**.

EXAMPLE 2

15% of 440 = ?

Recognize 15% as being 10% plus another 5%:

$$15\% \text{ of } 440 = 0.15 \times 440 = (0.10 \times 440) + (0.05 \times 440)$$

So, 10% of 440 is 44. The additional 5% is half of whatever 10% happens to be. Half of 44 is 22. Therefore, add 44 and 22 together, and the result is 15% of 440, or **66**.

EXAMPLE 3

63% of 2000 = ?

Recognize 2000 as being twice 1000, which is an easy number to manage. Next, 63% of 1000 is 630. Therefore, 63% of 2000 is simply twice that number, or **1260**.

$$63\% \times 1000 \times 2 = 0.63 \times 1000 \times 2 = 630 \times 2 = 1260$$

EXAMPLE 4

9.4% of 660 = ?

Round 9.4% off to 10%—an easier number to manage. Thus, 10% of 660 is **66**, which may suffice as a rough estimate of the exact answer, which is **62.04**. To get closer, though, there are several alternatives.

Alternative 1

Take 9% of 660, but that does not lend itself to fast computation. So, recognize 9% as being 1 percentage point less than 10%:

$$10\% \text{ of } 660 - 1\% \text{ of } 660 = 9\% \text{ of } 660$$

But how much is 1% of 660? We recognize 1 as being 1/10 of 10:

$$1 = 0.1 \times 10$$

Thus, 1% of 660 is 1/10 of whatever 10% of 660 happens to be.

$$1\% \text{ of } 660 = 0.1 \times (10\% \text{ of } 660)$$

Because 10% is 66, 1% is 6.6:

$$\begin{aligned} 1\% \text{ of } 660 &= 0.1 \times 66 \\ &= 6.6 \end{aligned}$$

For convenience, round 6.6 up to 7. Then subtract 7 from 10%, which is 66, and the result is **59**:

66 ← This is 10% of 660.
−7 ← This is about 1% of 660.
59 ← This is about 9% of 660.

Not surprisingly, 59 is a bit closer to the exact answer than is 66.

Alternative 2

Subtracting 1 percentage point from the 10% value is too much because 9.4% is closer to 9.5% than it is to 9.0%. So, let us go from 10% down to 9.5%. In other words, instead of subtracting 1 percentage point from 10%, let us subtract only half a percentage point. Because, as we calculated above, 1 percentage point is 6.6, then half a percentage point is 3.3, which is close to 3. So, we subtract 3 from 66:

66 ← This is 10% of 660.
−3 ← This is about 0.5% of 660.
63 ← This is about 9.5% of 660.

The result, **63**, is even closer to the exact answer.

Alternative 3

Take 1% of 660 and then multiply it by 9. Thus, 1% of 660 is 6.6, which is close to 7. Then, 9×7 is **63**, the same result as that from alternative 2.

PEARSON
myhealthprofessionskit™

Go to www.myhealthprofessionskit.com <http://www.myhealthprofessionskit.com/> to access the Companion Website created for this textbook. Simply select "Clinical Laboratory Science" from the choice of disciplines. Find this book and log in using your username and password to access additional practice problems, answers to the practice and contextual problems, additional information, and more.

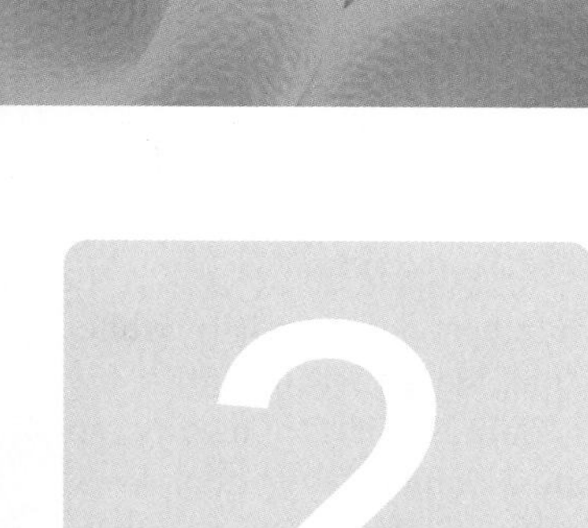

Exponential Notation and Logarithms

Learning Objectives

At the end of this chapter, the student should be able to do the following:

1. Explain the usefulness of exponential notation and logarithms
2. Write, evaluate, and interconvert exponential and logarithmic expressions; transform integers and decimal numbers into logarithms and back; and execute calculations involving exponents and logarithms
3. Use positive and negative exponents and exponential notation
4. Select and apply algebraic rules for exponents and logarithms
5. Compare and contrast logarithmic and arithmetic scales
6. Exploit the advantages of logarithmic scales
7. Plot and interpret logarithmic scales
8. Explain the benefits of transforming data into logarithms
9. Use natural logarithms and explain their relationship to base-10 logarithms

Key Terms

antilogarithm
argument
arithmetic scale
base
common logarithm
e
exponent
exponential notation
exponential term
logarithm
logarithmic scale
natural logarithm
scientific notation
semilogarithmic plot
significand

Chapter Outline

As we noted in the previous chapter, multiplication is a shortcut for addition. For example, the operation "3×4" represents the addition of three fours or of four threes:

$$3 \times 4 = 4 + 4 + 4 = 3 + 3 + 3 + 3 = 12$$

Now we introduce exponentiation as a shortcut for multiplication. For example, the operation "3^4" represents the multiplication of four threes:

$$3^4 = 3 \times 3 \times 3 \times 3 = 81$$

In a similar sense, **logarithms** offer a shortcut for expressing numbers exponentially, while reducing multiplication and division down to addition and subtraction. Since their invention by John Napier in 1614, logarithms have firmly established themselves not only as objects of theoretical interest but also as powerful tools for practical mathematicians, a group that includes laboratorians (technologists, scientists, technicians, etc.). Thus, there are sound reasons for understanding **exponents** and logarithms. The following are five situations in which they are used; the reasons for their usefulness are covered later.

1. Analytical spectroscopy—a paramount technique in the clinical laboratory—is based on the absorbance of light by the substance being quantified. The equations of this technique involve exponents and logarithms.
2. Exponents and logarithms appear in the equations describing *first-order processes*. These include (a) radioactive decay, which pertains to radioimmunoassay, (b) some chemical reactions exploited in manual or automated assays, and (c) the elimination of some drugs from the blood, important in therapeutic drug monitoring.
3. The growth of bacterial cultures is exponential, and some of the equations involve logarithms.
4. We express the acidity of blood, urine, and other aqueous solutions as *p*H, which is a logarithmic quantity. Moreover, we capture the strength of an acid or base in the value of its *pK*, which is also logarithmic.
5. Some diagnostic tests, such as viral loads and hormone levels, either express the results as logarithms or use logarithms to compute the results.

EXPONENTS AND LOGARITHMS

Consider this equation:

EQUATION 1

$$10^4 = 10,000$$

What this means is that the number "10" multiplied by itself four times is the same as the number "10,000":

$$10 \times 10 \times 10 \times 10 = 10,000$$

The term "10^4" in Equation 1 is read as "ten to the fourth," "ten to the fourth power," or "ten to the power of four."

In Equation 1, the number "10" is the **base** and "4" is the exponent:

$$10^4 = 10,000$$

Base (10) — Exponent (4)

Therefore, we call "4" the "logarithm of 10,000 to the base 10." In other words, "4" is the exponent to which 10 must be raised to give 10,000. We write this relationship as

EQUATION 2

$$\log_{10} 10,000 = 4$$

Inversely, we call "10,000" the "**antilogarithm** of 4 to the base 10." In other words, "10,000" is the result of raising 10 to an exponent of 4. We write this relationship as

$$\text{antilog}_{10}\ 4 = 10,000$$

The general equation, then, is

EQUATION 3

$$b^n = x$$

where b is the base and n is the exponent. Like Equation 1, we call this the exponential form of the relationship. Like Equation 2, however, the logarithmic form of the relationship has this equation:

$$\log_b x = n$$

EQUATION 4

in which x is called the **argument** of the logarithm. Thus, Equations 3 and 4 give the same information but in different forms.

When the base is 10, we often omit the subscript from the notation. Thus, $\log_{10} x = n$ is the same as $\log x = n$. Base-10 logarithms are also called **common logarithms** to distinguish them from **natural logarithms** (see below).

Be aware, though, that the base is not restricted to a value of 10. For example, $2^5 = 32$, which in logarithmic form is $\log_2 32 = 5$. The logarithm of 32 to the base 2 is 5, meaning that "5" is the exponent to which 2 must be raised to give 32:

$$2^5 = 2 \times 2 \times 2 \times 2 \times 2 = 32$$

Likewise, $6^3 = 216$. In logarithmic form, this is

$$\log_6 216 = 3$$

☑ CHECKPOINT 2-1

1. In exponential form, write this relationship: $\log_{10} 100{,}000 = 5$.
2. In logarithmic form, write this relationship: $2^8 = 256$.
3. Evaluate the following logarithms.
   (a) $\log_{10} 100$ (b) $\log_3 27$ (c) $\log_5 625$ (d) $\log_2 8$
4. Evaluate the following antilogarithms.
   (a) $\text{antilog}_{10}\, 3$ (b) $\text{antilog}_{10}\, 6$ (c) $\text{antilog}_2\, 5$ (d) $\text{antilog}_4\, 3$

1. $10^5 = 100{,}000$
2. $\log_2 256 = 8$
3. (a) 2 (b) 3 (c) 4 (d) 3
4. (a) 1000 (b) 1,000,000 (c) 32 (d) 64

NEGATIVE EXPONENTS

All the exponents in the previous section are positive, and their interpretation is clear: the exponent is the number of times we multiply the base by itself. But there are also negative exponents, and their interpretation at first may not make sense: how do we multiply the base by itself a negative number of times?

The answer is that a negative exponent symbolizes the reciprocal of the base that has been raised to the *positive* exponent:

$$b^{-n} = \frac{1}{b^n}$$

Consider the number 10^{-3}, for example:

$$10^{-3} = \frac{1}{10^3} = \frac{1}{1000} = 0.001$$

Likewise, the number 10^{-8} is

$$10^{-8} = \frac{1}{10^8} = \frac{1}{100{,}000{,}000} = 0.00000001$$

EXPONENTIAL NOTATION (SCIENTIFIC NOTATION)

Whether the exponent is positive or negative, working with a base of 10 is bothersome when a large number of zeros is involved. After all, who wants to write "1,000,000,000,000" when "10^{12}" is so much faster? Moreover, miscounting zeros is a pitfall when writing out numbers that contain many of them. When dealing with simple powers of 10, therefore, use the following two rules for converting between integers or decimal numbers and their shorter exponential equivalents.

1. **A positive exponent is the number of zeros following the "1."** A positive exponent is the number of places we move the decimal point to the *right* of the "1." For example, 10^6, which is $10 \times 10 \times 10 \times 10 \times 10 \times 10$, equals 1,000,000. The exponent is "6," and there are six zeros after the "1," which means we moved the decimal point six places to the right of the "1." Similarly, the number 10^2 is 100, with two zeros after the "1"; the decimal point was moved two places to the right of the "1." The number 10^9 is 1,000,000,000. Reasoning from the integer to the exponential form, we see that 1,000,000 is the same as 10^6, and 1000 is 10^3.
2. **A negative exponent is the number of decimal places in the number.** A negative exponent is the number of places we move the decimal point to the *left* of the "1." For example, 10^{-3}, which is the same as $1/10^3$, equals 0.001. The exponent is "-3," and there are two decimal places preceding the "1," which means that we moved the decimal point three places to the left of the "1." Similarly, 10^{-1} is 0.1, with only one decimal place; the decimal point was moved one place to the left of the "1." The number 10^{-8} is 0.00000001. Converting from the decimal number to the exponential form, we see that 0.000001 is 10^{-6}, and 0.01 is 10^{-2}.

☑ CHECKPOINT 2-2

1. Write the exponential equivalent of 10,000,000,000.
2. Write the exponential equivalent of 0.00000000001.
3. Write 10^4 as an integer.
4. Write 10^{-5} as a decimal number.

1. 10^{10} 2. 10^{-11} 3. 10,000 4. 0.00001

The above two rules are natural consequences of the fact that, in multiplying any number by 10, we just move the decimal point one place to the right. This is the same as adding a zero to the right (e.g., $6 \times 10 = 60$; $443 \times 10 = 4430$). On the other hand, in dividing any number by 10, we just move the decimal point one place to the left (e.g., $30 \div 10 = 3$; $6280 \div 10 = 628$).

We have, therefore, a standard way of expressing any integer or decimal number in exponential form, whether or not it is a multiple or submultiple of 10 and whether or not it is a simple power of 10. Called **exponential notation** (or **scientific notation**), this facility brings welcome relief from having to write out the very large and very small numbers so common in science and technology. We use the following two rules for converting numbers into exponential notation.

1. *To express any number greater than 1 in exponential notation*, move the decimal to the left until the number has a value between 1 and 10. Then, append "$\times\ 10^b$," where b is the number of places you moved the decimal. For example, when expressed in exponential notation, the number 1,280,000,000 becomes 1.28×10^9. Realize what this notation means: simply that multiplication of 1.28 by 10^9 gives 1,280,000,000. Thus, these are just two different ways of expressing the same value, but one of them has seven zeros whereas the other has only one. Another example is 766,000,000,000, which in exponential notation becomes 7.66×10^{11}.
2. *To express any number less than 1 in exponential notation*, move the decimal to the right until the number has a value between 1 and 10. Then, append "$\times\ 10^{-b}$," where b is the number of places you moved the decimal. Therefore, when expressed in exponential notation, the number 0.0000035 becomes 3.5×10^{-6}, and the number 0.0000000000044 becomes 4.4×10^{-12}.

Thus, the standard format for exponential notation comprises two parts. One is the **significand** and the other is the **exponential term:**

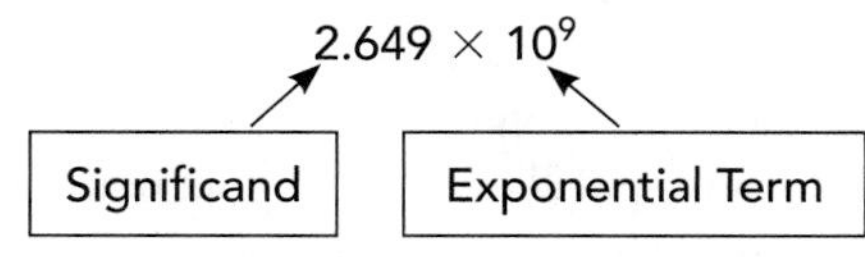

☑ CHECKPOINT 2-3

1. Write each of these numbers in exponential notation:
   (a) 4,500,000 (b) 887,000,000,000 (c) 500,100,000,000,000
2. Write each of these numbers in exponential notation:
   (a) 0.00000223 (b) 0.00019 (c) 0.00000000007002

1. (a) 4.5×10^6 (b) 8.87×10^{11} (c) 5.001×10^{14}
2. (a) 2.23×10^{-6} (b) 1.9×10^{-4} (c) 7.002×10^{-11}

ALGEBRAIC RULES FOR EXPONENTS

There are several algebraic rules that simplify calculations involving exponents and logarithms. Let us examine those for exponents first.

$$b^m b^n = b^{(m+n)}$$ ← "Product Rule" for Exponents

$$\frac{b^m}{b^n} = b^{(m-n)}$$

$$(bc)^n = b^n c^n$$

$$\left(\frac{b}{c}\right)^n = \frac{b^n}{c^n}$$

$$(b^m)^n = b^{mn}$$ ← "Power Rule"

$$b^{m/n} = (b^m)^{1/n} = (b^{1/n})^m$$

The usefulness of these rules becomes clear in an example. Suppose you had to calculate the product of 10^3 and 10^5. The direct approach, of course, is to multiply 1000 by 100,000, giving 100,000,000; effective though it is, this method is inconvenient because of the eight zeros. A simpler approach, given that the two bases are the same, is to use the "product rule" in the list above: $10^3 \times 10^5 = 10^{(3+5)} = 10^8$.

Similarly, evaluating $(3^3)^3$ may be accomplished by either (a) raising 27 to the 3rd power, or (b) invoking the "power rule" in the list above and raising 3 to the 9th power, that is, $3^{(3\times3)}$. Either approach gives an answer of 19,683.

ALGEBRAIC RULES FOR LOGARITHMS

We now turn our attention to the rules for logarithms.

$$\log xy = \log x + \log y$$ ← "Product Rule" for Logarithms

$$\log\left(\frac{x}{y}\right) = \log x - \log y$$

$$\log x^n = n \log x$$

We define any base raised to the power of zero as "1":

$$b^0 = 1$$

Therefore, the logarithm of 1 for any base is 0:

$$\log_b 1 = 0$$

Note that, whereas a logarithm can have the value "0," the number "0" itself does not have a logarithm; the logarithm for 0 is said to be *undefined* because there is no value of n that satisfies this equation:

$$b^n = 0$$

Any base raised to the power of 1 is defined as the base itself:

$$b^1 = b$$

For any base, therefore, the logarithm of the base itself is 1:

$$\log_b b = 1$$

Finally, there is the rule that captures the very essence of logarithms:

$$\log_b b^x = x$$

In words, this equation states that x is the exponent to which the base b must be raised to give b^x.

Neither the base nor the exponent has to be a whole number. Consider these expressions: $(4.2)^3 = 4.2 \times 4.2 \times 4.2 = 74.088$ and $(2.93)^2 = 2.93 \times 2.93 = 8.5849$. In these two cases, solving the problem is straightforward because the exponent is a whole number even though the base is not. But what does one do when the exponent is not a whole number?

First, consider decimal exponents that we may express as fractions ("rational" exponents). Take, for example, the number $10^{3.5}$. Although this notation tells you to multiply 10 by itself three and a half times, what does that mean? Clearly, $10^3 = 10 \times 10 \times 10 = 1000$ and $10^4 = 10 \times 10 \times 10 \times 10 = 10{,}000$. So, $10^{3.5}$ must fall between 1000 and 10,000. But is it halfway between? Does this mean to multiply 10 by itself three times and then once by half of 10 (5)? The answer to that question is "no."

$$10 \times 10 \times 10 \times 5 \neq 10^{3.5} \neq 5000$$

To understand this, realize that we can express the decimal exponent of 3.5 as the fraction "7/2." Next, recall the rule that $b^{m/n} = (b^m)^{1/n} = (b^{1/m})^n$. Therefore,

$$10^{7/2} = (10^7)^{1/2} = (10^{1/2})^7 = 3162$$

Rather than saying the notation "$10^{3.5}$" instructs us to multiply 10 by itself three and a half times, we can interpret it in one of two other ways: (1) multiply 10 by itself seven times and then take the square root, or (2) take the square root of 10 and then multiply the result by itself seven times. Using either approach gives the same result of 3162 (after rounding). Clearly, this number is between 1000 and 10,000, albeit far from halfway.

In exponential form, then, we have

$$10^{3.5} = 3162$$

In logarithmic form, the relationship is

$$\log_{10} 3162 = 3.5$$

How do we handle a decimal exponent that we cannot express as a fraction, that is, an "irrational" exponent? Two famous irrational numbers are $\sqrt{2}$ (1.41421 . . .) and π (3.14159 . . .), neither of which can be written as the ratio of two integers. We can carry out the evaluation of a number like $4^{\sqrt{2}}$ or 3^{π} using the method of approximation, in which rational exponents are used to approximate the irrational one. Nevertheless, when an exponent is irrational, a calculator is the practical resort.

☑ CHECKPOINT 2-4

1. Evaluate each of these exponential expressions:
   (a) 2.9^6 (b) 1290^3 (c) 0.663^7
2. Using the product rule, evaluate each of these exponential expressions:
   (a) $10^{1.5}$ (b) $10^{1.8}$
3. Using the product rule, evaluate each of these logarithmic expressions:
   (a) log 10 (b) log 21

1. (a) 594.8 (b) 2,146,689,000 (c) 0.0563112
2. (a) $10^{3/2} = (10^3)^{1/2} = (10^{1/2})^3 = 31.623$ (b) $10^{9/5} = (10^9)^{1/5} = (10^{1/5})^9 = 63.096$
3. (a) $\log 10 = \log 5 \times \log 2 = 0.69897 + 0.30103 = 1$
   (b) $\log 21 = \log 7 \times \log 3 = 0.84510 + 0.47712 = 1.32222$

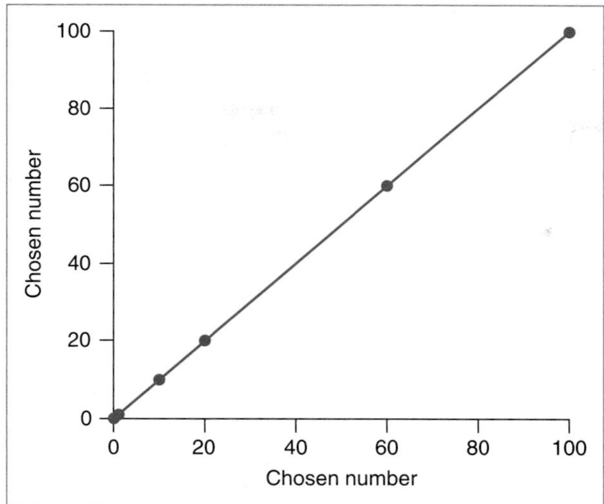

FIGURE 2-1 Seven chosen numbers plotted on both axes: 0.01, 0.1, 1, 10, 20, 60, and 100. The three lowest points are tightly clustered.

THE LOGARITHMIC SCALE

Let us choose seven numbers and plot them on both the x- and y-axes of a graph: 0.01, 0.1, 1, 10, 20, 60, and 100. The resulting straight line appears in Figure 2-1.

Notice that the three lowest points on the graph are tightly clustered and are therefore hard, if not impossible, to distinguish from each other. Fortunately, there are other ways to plot these numbers—alternatives that expand the space among the three crowded points and show their relationships clearly.

Using the same x-axis, for example, we can plot on the y-axis not the chosen number itself, but its logarithm. The result is the curve that appears in Figure 2-2A. The number 100 on the x-axis corresponds to 2, which is its logarithm, on the y-axis; the number 0.01 on the x-axis corresponds to -2, which is its logarithm, on the y-axis.

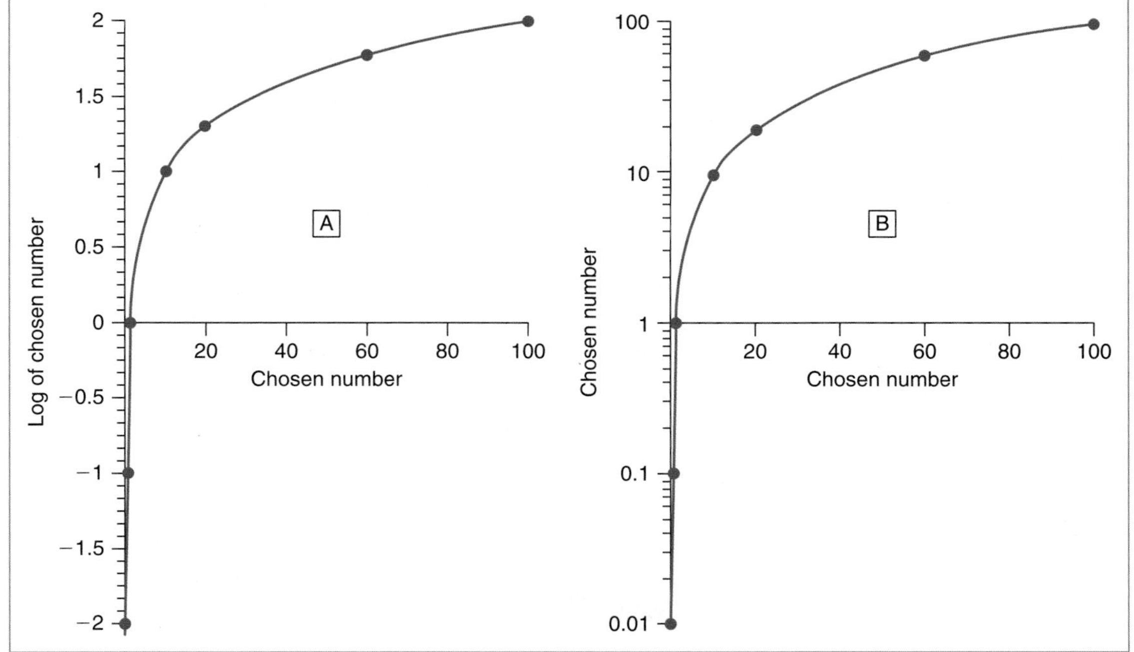

FIGURE 2-2 Alternatives to the direct plot in Figure 2-1. The same seven numbers as in Figure 2-1 are plotted on the x-axes. Panel A: On the y-axis are the logarithms of the x values, plotted on an arithmetic scale. Panel B: On the y-axis are the x values themselves, but the scale is logarithmic. Unlike Figure 2-1, these two graphs clearly separate the three lowest points.

In this graph (Figure 2-2A), a difference of 1 on the y-axis represents a 10-fold difference between the chosen numbers. For example, going from 2 to 1 on the y-axis corresponds to a change on the x-axis from 100 to 10, a 10-fold decrease. Notice that all the tick marks on the y-axis are equally spaced, each one representing either an increase or a decrease of 0.1 units from an adjacent mark. This scale on the y-axis is called an **arithmetic scale** (pronounced "arith-MET-ik") because equal distances between tick marks represent equal amounts. The distance between any two adjacent tick marks is the same as the distance between any other two adjacent tick marks.

There is yet another alternative to the plot in Figure 2-1. As Figure 2-2B shows, we can plot the seven chosen numbers themselves along the y-axis but on a **logarithmic scale**. Plotting the chosen numbers on a logarithmic scale gives the same curve as plotting the logarithms of those numbers on an arithmetic scale (Figure 2-2A). The advantage in using the logarithmic scale (Figure 2-2B) is that we can plot the chosen numbers directly on a graph without having to calculate their logarithms.

Notice in Figure 2-2B that the tick marks on the y-axis are not uniformly spaced, as they are on the arithmetic scales in Figures 2-1 and 2-2A. On a logarithmic scale, equal distances represent equal ratios; that is, the distance between 1 and 2 is the same as the distance between 5 and 10, or between 50 and 100. Every value on the y-axis of the logarithmic scale (Figure 2-2B) corresponds to its own logarithm on the y-axis of the arithmetic scale (Figure 2-2A). Figure 2-3 ■ clarifies this.

Do logarithmic scales offer an advantage over arithmetic scales? Figures 2-1 and 2-2 have already suggested an answer to this question. In our example, plotting the chosen numbers on a logarithmic scale (Figure 2-2B) or plotting their logarithms on an arithmetic scale (Figure 2-2A) put space between points that were otherwise too close together (Figure 2-1), thereby distinguishing them from each other.

In general, original data sometimes cover such a wide range of values that arithmetic scales become unmanageably long, and fitting those scales to a printed page or a computer screen compresses the data points so much that important information is obscured. The judicious use of logarithmic scales or of logarithms can solve this problem.

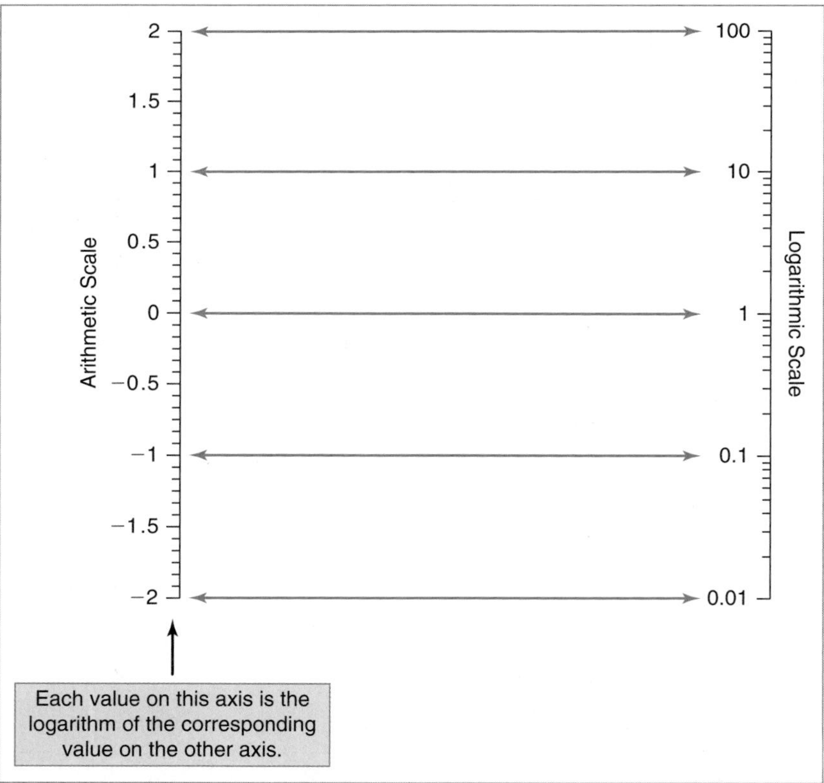

■ **FIGURE 2-3** The y-axes of Figures 2-2A and 2-2B are juxtaposed to show correspondence between their scales. Each pink double-headed arrow links a number on the logarithmic scale (the scale on the right) to its logarithm on the arithmetic scale (the scale on the left).

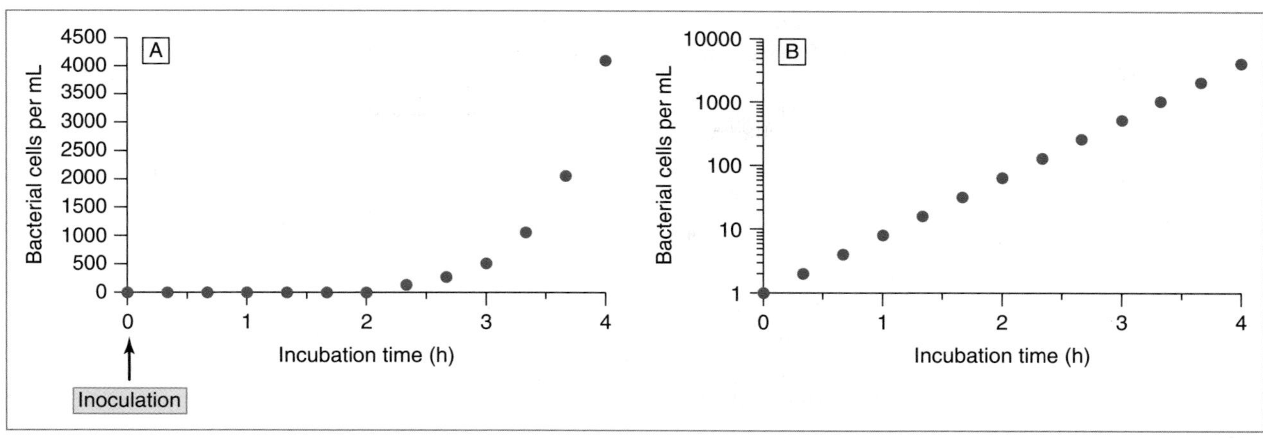

FIGURE 2-4 Growth data for a culture of *E. coli* in liquid medium. Panel *A:* Data plotted on arithmetic scales. Panel *B:* Same data but with *y* values plotted on logarithmic scale.

Consider a practical example from the microbiology laboratory. Suppose you are growing a culture of *E. coli* in liquid medium. You inoculate the medium, start the incubation, and then take samplings periodically to count the viable bacterial cells in a milliliter of your culture. From these counts you can find the growth rate and the generation time.

About every 20 minutes (three times per hour), each bacterium divides into two daughter cells (a process known as *binary fission*). Thus, the growth of your *E. coli* is exponential: one cell becomes 2 cells, 2 become 4, 4 become 8, 8 become 16, and so on. Needless to say, therefore, the equation describing this growth involves an exponent:

$$2^n = \text{number of cells after } n \text{ doublings}$$

Consequently, after 2 hours, six doublings have occurred, giving 2^6, or 64, bacterial cells in each milliliter of your culture. After 4 hours, there have been 12 doublings, generating 2^{12}, or 4096, cells per mL. And after only 8 hours, there would theoretically be 2^{24}, or 16,777,216, cells in every milliliter of the culture ("theoretically" because in reality nutrient depletion and other factors would prevent the culture from becoming this dense).

Now, imagine a graph of your data on arithmetic scales (Figure 2-4A ■), up to an incubation time of 4 hours. If you plot the number of bacterial cells per mL on the *y*-axis and the incubation time on the *x*-axis, then the *y*-axis must cover a very large range, from 1 to 4096 because in 4 hours there are 12 doublings and, therefore, 2^{12} cells.

As Figure 2-4A shows, fitting the very long *y*-axis to the page compresses the data points so much that, up to about 3 hours of incubation, it is impossible to see how much the cell number changes from one sampling to the next and whether that change is steady. This is where a logarithmic scale becomes helpful.

Figure 2-4B shows the result of plotting the same *y*-axis data on a logarithmic scale, against the same *x*-axis. Note that a **semilogarithmic plot** is one in which one of the scales is arithmetic and the other is logarithmic. The logarithmic *y*-axis in Figure 2-4B covers the range of the arithmetic *y*-axis in Figure 2-4A, but it does so without compressing the data points. As a result, it is clear in Figure 2-4B that the cell number increases by a factor of two from one sampling to the next and that the growth of the culture is steady up to an incubation time of 4 hours.

LOGARITHMIC TRANSFORMATION OF RATIOS

Data are sometimes reported in the form of ratios. Suppose, for example, that you are reporting the effects of two drugs on the concentration of circulating vitamin E. If the group of patients receiving drug **A** had a vitamin E level of 20 mg/L, whereas the group of patients receiving drug **B** had a level of 5 mg/L, then the ratio **A/B** is 20 mg/L ÷ 5 mg/L, or 4. In other words, the vitamin E level was four times higher in patients on drug **A** than in those on drug **B**:

Group	Serum Vitamin E (mg/L)	A/B
Drug **A**	20	4
Drug **B**	5	

If we had reversed the results, however, then drug **A** would have given a vitamin E level of 5 mg/L and drug **B** 20 mg/L. The corresponding ratio **A/B** would have been 0.25:

Group	Serum Vitamin E (mg/L)	A/B
Drug **A**	5	0.25
Drug **B**	20	

This illustrates the asymmetry inherent to ratios: whenever **A** > **B**, the ratio **A/B** is greater than 1, but whenever **A** < **B**, the ratio **A/B** is between 0 and 1. Of course, when **A** = **B**, the ratio is 1. This asymmetry conveniently disappears when we transform the ratios into logarithms.

In the first example above, log (**A/B**) is log (4), or 0.60206. In the second example, log (**A/B**) is log (0.25), or −0.60206. Thus, the two values have equal magnitudes but opposite signs:

A/B	log (A/B)
4	0.60206
0.25	−0.60206

By restoring symmetry, logarithmic transformation of a ratio causes the value to be positive whenever **A** > **B**, negative whenever **A** < **B**, and zero when **A** = **B**:

Relationship	A/B	log (A/B)
A > B	> 1	> 0
A = B	1	0
A < B	< 1	< 0

It is sometimes preferable, then, to report the logarithms of ratios than to report the ratios themselves.

THE NATURAL LOGARITHM

There is a curious constant in mathematics, denoted "*e*," which repeatedly leaps out of many theoretical and practical contexts. The value of *e* is 2.7182817 . . . In short, *e* represents the fundamental amount of change shared by all systems that grow or shrink exponentially and continuously. Consequently, it is useful in the calculations of compound interest, population growth, drug elimination, radioactive decay, and the spread of epidemics. It shows up in scores of seemingly disparate fields of human endeavor, a few examples being climatology, electronics, rocketry, gambling, economics, and ecology.

The value of *e* is the number that the following expression approaches as *n* increases:

$$\left(1 + \frac{1}{n}\right)^n$$

The table below shows how the value of this expression behaves as *n* keeps rising.

n	$\left(1 + \frac{1}{n}\right)^n$
1	2
10	2.59374246
100	2.70481382
1000	2.71692393
10,000	2.71814593
100,000	2.71826824
1,000,000	2.71828047
10,000,000	2.71828169
100,000,000	2.71828179

A natural logarithm, symbolized as "ln" (or as "ℓn") is the logarithm of a number to the base *e*:

$$\ln x = \log_e x = \log_{(2.7182818)} x$$

For example, the natural logarithm of 100 is 4.6052:

$$\ln 100 = \log_{(2.7182818)} 100 = 4.6052$$

which means, in turn, that *e* raised to the power of 4.6052 is 100:

$$e^{4.6052} = (2.7182818)^{4.6052} = 100$$

Be aware that "exp(x)" is another way of writing "e^x":

$$\exp(x) = e^x$$

Some reference sources present equations in terms of natural logarithms, whereas other sources use base-10 logarithms. Fortunately, converting between them is straightforward:

$$\ln x = 2.303 \log x$$

and

$$\frac{\ln x}{2.303} = \log x$$

☑ CHECKPOINT 2-5

1. Evaluate each of these expressions:
   (a) ln 1000 (b) e^4 (c) exp(3.6)
2. If the base-10 logarithm of x is q, then what is the natural logarithm of x?
3. If the natural logarithm of x is w, then what is the base-10 logarithm of x?

1. (a) 6.9078 (b) 54.5981 (c) 36.5982
2. $\ln x = 2.303q$
3. $\log x = w/2.303$

THE USEFULNESS OF LOGARITHMS

Clearly, logarithms have properties that make them quite useful in science and technology—properties that explain the importance of logarithms in the situations listed in the introduction to this chapter. At this point, let us summarize the reasons for laboratory professionals to develop a working understanding of logarithms.

1. **Because logarithms can accelerate calculations.** Before the advent of calculators, logarithms often shortened the time required for a multiplication or division problem, though admittedly we rarely use them for this purpose anymore. For example, consider Figure 2-5 ■. To multiply two numbers, say, q and r, we can carry out the calculation directly (black arrow) to get the

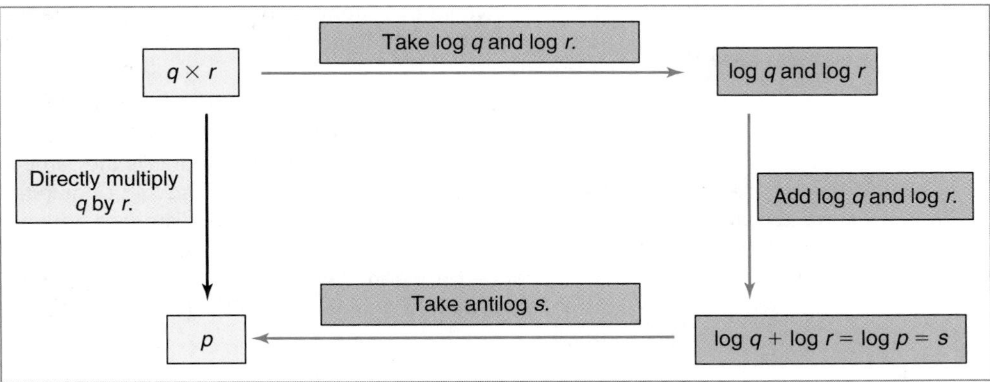

■ FIGURE 2-5 Two routes to the product of q and r. Black route: direct multiplication of q by r to give p. Pink route: finding p by means of the logarithms of q and r.

product, p. Alternatively (pink arrows), we can apply the "product rule" for logarithms: find the logarithm for each number (in a table), add the two logarithms together, and then take the antilogarithm of the sum (s). The antilogarithm of s is the product, p, of the two original numbers. Without a calculator, believe it or not, the logarithmic route is sometimes faster than the direct route.

2. **Because they simplify the expression of very large and very small numbers.** The cumbersome value of 66,500,000 is simpler when expressed as its logarithm, 7.823. Likewise, the value 0.000003394 is easier to write as its logarithm, −5.4693.
3. **Because they can make graphs more revealing.** Plotting data on a logarithmic scale or plotting the logarithms of those data on an arithmetic scale can put space between points—space that often reveals important information that is otherwise very difficult to discern.
4. **Because they restore symmetry to ratios.** Transforming a ratio into its logarithm makes the value "0" when the numerator and denominator are equal, positive when the numerator is greater than the denominator, and negative when the numerator is less than the denominator.
5. **Because blind reliance on calculators creates a risky dependency.** There will be times when no calculator is available. More importantly, however, any technologist, scientist, or engineer should be able to carry out rough logarithmic computations quickly in his or her head—or on paper—to detect errors, data anomalies, and instrument malfunctions.

Summary

1. We use *exponents* and *logarithms* widely in the clinical laboratory in, for example, the calculations of spectroscopy, first-order processes, bacterial growth, acidity, and data reporting.
2. In the following equation, b is the *base* and n is the exponent:

$$b^n = x$$

3. We call the variable n the "logarithm of x to the base b." The equation for this relationship is

$$\log_b x = n$$

in which x is called the *argument* of the logarithm.

4. We call the variable x the "*antilogarithm* of n to the base b." The equation for this relationship is

$$\text{antilog}_b\, n = x$$

5. When the base is 10, the notation is either "$\log_{10} x$" or "log x." We sometimes call base-10 logarithms *common logarithms*.
6. A negative exponent symbolizes the reciprocal of the base that has been raised to the *positive* exponent:

$$b^{-n} = \frac{1}{b^n}$$

7. *Exponential notation* is a standard way of expressing any integer or decimal number in exponential form, in order to make very large or very small values more convenient to write and read.
8. The standard format for exponential notation comprises two parts: the *significand* and the *exponential term:*

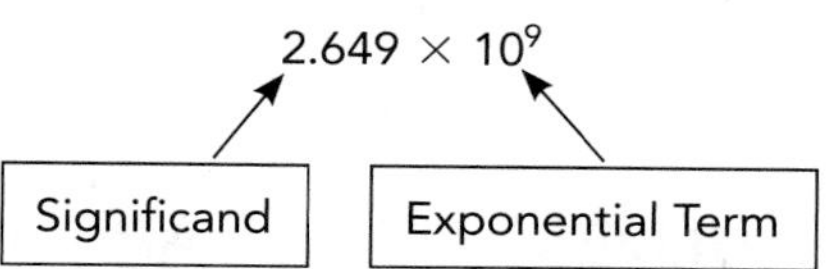

9. To express any number greater than 1 in exponential notation, move the decimal to the left until the number has a value between 1 and 10. Then, append "$\times 10^b$," where b is the number of places you moved the decimal. To express any number less than 1 in exponential notation, move the decimal to the right until the number has a value between 1 and 10. Then, append "$\times 10^{-b}$," where b is the number of places you moved the decimal.
10. There are algebraic rules for simplifying various calculations that involve exponents and logarithms. These equations are particularly handy for manipulating fractional exponents.
11. An *arithmetic scale* is one in which equal distances between tick marks represent equal amounts. The distance between any two adjacent tick marks is the same as the distance between any other two adjacent tick marks. A *logarithmic scale* is one in which equal distances between tick marks represent not equal amounts, but equal ratios. The distance between, say, 1 and 2, is the same as the distance between 5 and 10, or between 50 and 100.

12. Plotting data on a logarithmic scale or plotting their logarithms on an arithmetic scale can put space between points that are otherwise too close together for reliable interpretation.

13. When data are reported as ratios, transformation into logarithms can restore symmetry such that the value is positive whenever $A > B$, negative whenever $A < B$, and zero when $A = B$.

14. A *natural logarithm* ("ln") is the logarithm of a number to the base *e*, which is a frequently encountered mathematical constant whose value, to seven decimal places, is 2.7182818:

$$\ln x = \log_e x = \log_{(2.7182818)} x$$

15. Natural logarithms and base-10 logarithms are related to each other:

$$\ln x = 2.303 \log x$$

16. There are sound reasons for developing a working understanding of logarithms. Logarithms can accelerate calculations, they can simplify very large or very small numbers, they can make graphs more revealing, and they can restore symmetry to ratios. Furthermore, relying blindly on calculators creates dependency.

Practice Problems

1. (LO 2, 3) Write each of the following relationships in exponential form.

(a) $\log_{10}(66{,}590) = 4.8234$

(b) $\log_{10}(30{,}000{,}000) = 7.4771$

(c) $\log_{10}(206.5) = 2.3149$

(d) $\log_2(16) = 4$

(e) $\log_5(15{,}625) = 6$

(f) $\log_3(59{,}049) = 10$

(g) $\log(8) = 0.903$

(h) $\log(0.8) = -0.0969$

(i) $\log(0.0023) = -2.64$

2. (LO 2, 3) Write each of the following relationships in logarithmic form.

(a) $6^{2.3} = 67.193$ (b) $10^{-0.27} = 0.537$

(c) $10^6 = 1{,}000{,}000$ (d) $2^{14} = 16{,}384$

(e) $10^{-4} = 0.0001$ (f) $5.1^2 = 26.01$

(g) $10^{3.33} = 2137.96$ (h) $10^{-2.6} = 0.00251$

(i) $4.9^{0.67} = 2.90$

3. (LO 2, 3, 9) Evaluate each of the following expressions.

(a) $\log 300$ (b) $\log(11{,}000)$

(c) $\log_3 243$ (d) $\ln 10$

(e) $\log_2 128$ (f) $\ln 668$

(g) $\log_e 147$ (h) antilog 8.8

(i) $\ln(\log 10{,}000)$ (j) $\text{antilog}_2\ 7$

(k) $\log(\ln 8401)$ (l) antilog -0.2

(m) $\log 0.0443$ (n) $\ln 0.7$

(o) antilog -7.3

4. (LO 3, 10) Write each of the following numbers in exponential notation.

(a) 0.000655 (b) 9,030,000

(c) 101,200 (d) 400

(e) 0.165 (f) 3,700,000,000,000

(g) 0.00000092 (h) 3775

(i) 16,020

5. (LO 3, 10) Write each of the following exponential expressions as an integer or decimal number.

(a) 1.9×10^6 (b) 4.722×10^{-4}

(c) 9.0×10^{-3} (d) 5.510×10^5

(e) 6.08×10^9 (f) -2.6×10^4

(g) 7.4553×10^7 (h) -8.83×10^{-3}

(i) 2.05×10^2

6. (LO 4) Using an appropriate algebraic rule for exponents or logarithms, propose values for the variables that satisfy each of the following equations. The first problem has been worked to serve as an example.

(a) $(3^m)(3^n) = 2187$

For this equation, the product rule for exponents is suitable:

$$b^m b^n = b^{(m+n)}$$

Therefore,

$$(3^m)(3^n) = 3^{(m+n)} = 2187$$

Because $3^7 = 2187$,

$$m + n = 7$$

Any pair of numbers whose sum is 7 satisfies the equation. An example is

$$m = 2 \quad \text{and} \quad n = 5$$

(b) $(2^m)/(2^n) = 4$ (c) $\log x + \log y = 5$

(d) $10^n 5^n = 2500$ (e) $\log x^{6.2} = -12.5581$

7. (LO 2, 10) Convert each of the following numbers into its logarithm.

(a) 1,229,000 (b) 8.37×10^{-6}

(c) 0.011 (d) 1.99890×10^{-3}

(e) 0.000340 (f) 9.70023×10^{9}

8. (LO 2, 10) Calculate the antilogarithm of each of the following logarithms.

(a) −0.9655 (b) 4.9 (c) 3.6627

(d) 2.080 (e) −5.113 (f) 10.5669

9. (LO 2) By what factor is 10^8 greater than 10^4?

10. (LO 2) Which of the following numbers is (or are) twice as large as 3.8×10^4?

(a) 3.8×10^8 (b) 0.76×10^5 (c) 76×10^5

11. (LO 2) Which of the following numbers is (or are) 10 times smaller than 9.7×10^{-5}?

(a) 9.7×10^{-6} (b) 0.0000097 (c) 0.97×10^{-5}

12. (LO 2) Which of the following, when multiplied by 1000, give (or gives) 10^{-2}?

(a) 0.00001 (b) 1×10^{-5} (c) 0.01×10^{-4}

13. (LO 2) Consider two numbers, x and y. If $\log x = 1 + \log y$, then how much greater is x than y?

14. (LO 2) Consider two numbers, q and r. If

$$\log (q) - 3 = \log r,$$

then how much smaller is r than q?

15. (LO 2) Consider three numbers: a, b, and c. If

$$\log a = 2 + \log b$$

and

$$\log b = (\log c) - 3,$$

then which number is the largest?

16. (LO 2, 10) Calculate each of the following expressions.

(a) $(2.4 \times 10^{-5})(4.6 \times 10^3)$

(b) $(7.08 \times 10^6)(0.113)$

(c) $(3.55 \times 10^{-7})/3.8$

(d) $(3.0 \times 10^5)/(-3.0 \times 10^5)$

(e) $(-4.04 \times 10^8)(3.66 \times 10^{-8})$

(f) $144/(6.67 \times 10^3)$

17. (LO 2, 4) Complete the following table.

	log *a*	log *b*	*b*/*a*
(a)	2	5	
(b)	2		100
(c)		6	100
(d)	4		10
(e)	−1	2	
(f)	−8		100,000
(g)		3.17	10
(h)	4.9	6.9	
(i)	−3.5		10,000,000

18. (LO 2, 4) Explain whether each of the following assertions is true.

(a) If $\log x = \log y$, then $x = y$.

(b) If $\log x = 2 \log y$, then $x = y^2$.

(c) If $x = 28{,}446$, then $\log x$ is between 4 and 5.

(d) If $\log y = 6.39$, then y is between 1,000,000 and 10,000,000.

(e) If $\log x = -4$ and $y = 0.00025$, then $x > y$.

(f) If $\log x = -7.3$ and $y = 10^{-8}$, then $x > y$.

(g) If y is 10 times larger than x, then $\log y$ is larger than $\log x$ by 1.

(h) If x is 1/1000 of y, then $\log x$ is less than $\log y$ by 3.

Contextual Problems

1. (LO 1, 2, 3, 8) The physicians in your hospital have set a general goal of achieving a "1-logarithm drop" in the viral load for patients who have recently begun treatment for hepatitis C. We express viral load as copies of viral RNA present in a particular volume, usually 1 mL, of blood. For each of the following patients undergoing treatment for hepatitis C, determine whether the physicians achieved a 1-log drop in the viral load.

	Viral Load (copies/mL blood)	
Patient	**Previous**	**Present**
W	13,200,000	1.2×10^6
X	2.4 million	230,000
Y	990,000	120,000
Z	1.9×10^6	1.8×10^5

2. (LO 1, 2, 3, 8) For each of the following patients undergoing treatment for hepatitis C, determine the largest whole number of logarithms that the drop in viral load has spanned.

Patient	Viral Load (copies/mL blood)	
	Previous	Present
N	4.4 million	380,000
O	9.6×10^6	75,000
P	22,500,000	2.24×10^5
Q	5,600,000	3000

3. (LO 1, 2, 8) Some laboratories report viral loads as logarithms rather than counts. For example, rather than "2,560,000 copies/mL," they may report simply "6.408."

   (a) Explain whether this practice has an advantage for the physician.

   (b) If patient **G**'s viral load is reported as the logarithm "6.933," what is her count?

   (c) You determine the viral load of patient **J** to be 18,450,000 copies/mL. Express this result as a logarithm.

   (d) Expressed as a logarithm, patient **L**'s viral load (counts/mL) before treatment was 7.223; a few weeks after treatment began, it was 4.187. By what factor did the load decrease? By how many logarithms did the load decrease?

4. (LO 1, 2, 3, 8) There is another system for expressing viral load: the International Unit (IU). At this writing, there is no universal formula for interconverting "copies/mL" and "IU/mL." Currently, the ratio ranges from about 1 copy to about 5 copies of viral RNA per IU. In other words, whereas one laboratory may equate 1 copy to 1 IU, another may use a different ratio, say, of 4 copies to 1 IU.

   (a) For a laboratory that uses the ratio of 2.6 copies per IU, convert a result of 884,000 IU/mL into "copies/mL."

   (b) For a laboratory that uses the ratio of 1.5 copies per IU, convert 1.45×10^7 copies/mL into "IU/mL."

   (c) At a ratio of 3.8 copies per IU, convert 5.4 million copies/mL into "IU/mL."

   (d) At a ratio of 3.1 copies per IU, convert the logarithm of the copies/mL, 6.223, into "IU/mL."

   (e) At a ratio of 2.7 copies per IU, convert 1.2 million IU/mL into the logarithm of the copies/mL.

5. (LO 1, 2, 3, 8) (Refer to problems 3 and 4) An accrediting agency conducted a comparison of three laboratories' methods for quantifying hepatitis C virus in blood. All three laboratories analyzed the same sample, and each reported the result in its own standard format. The table below shows those results. Which laboratory reported the highest amount of viral RNA? (Laboratory 1 reports the log of the copies/mL. Laboratory 3 uses a ratio of 2.2 copies per IU.)

Laboratory	Viral Load
1	7.548
2	38.3 million copies/mL
3	1.45×10^7 IU/mL

6. (LO 1, 2, 8) Your microbiology laboratory is helping evaluate a new topical antiseptic for irrigation before eye surgery. A swab of a specified surface of the patient's eye was taken immediately before irrigation with the antiseptic and another immediately afterward. The table below summarizes the results for three patients.

Patient	Log of Number of Viable Bacterial Cells	
	Preirrigation	Postirrigation
A	4.13	2.36
B	3.01	1.02
C	2.64	1.17

   (a) Did any of the patients show a reduction of 1000-fold or greater? If so, which one?

   (b) Which patient showed a 100-fold reduction?

   (c) For patient **C**, calculate the percentage reduction in the number of cells.

7. (LO 1, 2) Analytical spectroscopy is one of the most important techniques in the clinical laboratory. It is based on the absorption of light of a particular wavelength by chemical substances. A beam of light of known intensity (I_0) is directed into a solution, and the intensity (I) of the light emerging from the solution is then measured. The fraction of light transmitted (I/I_0) is called the *transmittance* (T):

$$T = \frac{I}{I_0}$$

Being a fraction, T ranges in value from 0 to 1. The light that did not pass through the sample was *absorbed*. For example, if $T = 0.80$, then 80% of the light passing through the sample was transmitted and 20% was absorbed.

Although transmittance goes down as concentration goes up, the relationship is exponential, not linear. A plot, therefore, of T against concentration is difficult to use as a standard curve. But the logarithm of T as a function of concentration is a straight line and, as a result, a useful standard curve. For this purpose, *absorbance* (A) is defined as

$$A = -\log\frac{I}{I_0} = -\log T$$

Thus, if $T = 0.648$, then 64.8% of the light passing through the sample is transmitted and 35.2% is absorbed. The absorbance, then, or A, is

$$A = -\log T = -\log 0.648 = 0.188$$

(a) When 61% of the light passing through the sample is transmitted, what is the value of *T*?

(b) When 29/100 of the light passing through the sample is transmitted, what is the value of *T*?

(c) When 34% of the light passing through the sample is absorbed, what is the value of *T*?

(d) When 18% of the light passing through the sample is absorbed, what is the value of *A*?

(e) If half the light passing through a sample is transmitted, what is the absorbance?

(f) If 95% of the light passing through a sample is transmitted, what is the absorbance?

8. (LO 1, 2, 5, 6, 7, 10) Synthesized by the kidney, erythropoietin (EPO) is a hormone that regulates blood cell production in the bone marrow. In the following table appear data for a standard curve from an assay for serum EPO. The assay measures absorbance of light at a wavelength of 450 nm. The EPO concentration is expressed as milli-international units (mIU) per mL of serum.

(a) Complete the following data table.

Concentration of Standard (mIU/mL)	A_{450}	Log of Concentration	Log(A_{450})
2.50	0.042		
5.00	0.081		
20.0	0.319		
50.0	0.773		
100.	1.459		
200.	2.586		

(b) Construct the following four graphs of the data.

(1) A_{450} as *y* and concentration as *x*, with each variable on an arithmetic scale

(2) Log(A_{450}) as *y* and log(concentration) as *x*, with each variable on an arithmetic scale

(3) A_{450} as *y* and concentration as *x*, with concentration on a logarithmic scale

(4) A_{450} as *y* and concentration as *x*, with each variable on a logarithmic scale

(c) In what way is graph **2** superior to graph **1**?

(d) In what way is graph **4** superior to graph **3**?

(e) What is the practical advantage of graph **4** over graph **2**?

9. (LO 1, 2, 5, 6, 7, 10) Inhibin-A is a protein hormone whose serum concentration in pregnant women correlates with the risk of Down syndrome. In the following table appear data for a standard curve from an assay for serum inhibin-A. The assay measures absorbance of light at a wavelength of 450 nm. The inhibin-A concentration is expressed as pg per mL of serum.

(a) Complete the following data table.

Concentration of Standard (pg/mL)	A_{450}	Log of Concentration	Log(A_{450})
12.0	0.019		
32.0	0.056		
97.0	0.171		
249	0.448		
495	0.814		
890.0	1.507		

(b) Construct the following four graphs of the data.

(1) A_{450} as *y* and concentration as *x*, with each variable on an arithmetic scale

(2) Log(A_{450}) as *y* and log(concentration) as *x*, with each variable on an arithmetic scale

(3) A_{450} as *y* and concentration as *x*, with concentration on a logarithmic scale

(4) A_{450} as *y* and concentration as *x*, with each variable on a logarithmic scale

(c) In what way is graph **2** superior to graph **1**?

(d) In what way is graph **4** superior to graph **3**?

(e) What is the practical advantage of graph **4** over graph **2**?

10. (LO 1, 2, 5, 6, 7, 10) In your laboratory's radioimmunoassay for vitamin D, the sample to be analyzed is mixed with (a) radiolabeled vitamin D in a known amount and (b) an antibody specific for vitamin D. As incubation proceeds, the endogenous vitamin D and the exogenous radiolabeled vitamin D compete with each other for the same binding sites on the antibody. Consequently, as the concentration of endogenous vitamin D rises, the probability of its binding to the antibody goes up, whereas the probability of radiolabeled vitamin D's binding goes down. Thus, the concentration of endogenous vitamin D present in the sample and the amount of radiolabeled vitamin D bound to antibody move in opposite directions.

In the following table appear data for a standard curve from an assay for vitamin D. The assay determines how much radiolabeled vitamin D is bound to the antibody and reports that amount as a percentage of the total radiolabeled vitamin D added.

(a) Complete the following data table.

Concentration of Endogenous Vitamin D (ng/mL)	% of Added Radiolabeled Vitamin D Bound to Antibody (%Bound)	Log of Concentration	Log (%Bound)
0.5	96.00		
5	82.36		
12	61.57		
20	44.25		
40	28.05		
100	16.68		

(b) Construct the following three graphs of the data.

(1) %Bound as *y* and concentration as *x*, with each variable on an arithmetic scale

(2) Log(%Bound) as *y* and log(concentration) as *x*, with each variable on an arithmetic scale

(3) %Bound as *y* and concentration as *x*, with concentration on a logarithmic scale

(c) On graph **2**, which is a plot of one logarithm versus another logarithm, the values of 0, 1, and 1.8 on the *x*-axis correspond to which vitamin D concentrations?

(d) In what way is graph **3** superior to graph **1**?

(e) In what way is graph **1** superior to graph **3**?

(f) What unique difficulty does graph **2** pose?

11. (LO 1, 2, 8) You're working for a manufacturer of a diagnostic test for protein Q in human serum. Your task is to run the test in the presence and absence of known chemical substances that sometimes occur in serum in order to determine whether those substances interfere with the assay and affect the results. According to the table below, you select one serum sample, divide it among five tubes, add the specified chemical substance in a known amount, and then run the test on the contents of each tube.

Tube	Chemical Substance	Result for Protein Q (pg/mL)	Relative Result for Protein Q
1	none	3.4	
2	caffeine	3.5	
3	vancomycin	6.7	
4	acetaminophen	4.0	
5	lead	1.7	

(a) Complete the fourth column of the table by calculating the ratio of the found concentration in the presence of each chemical substance to the found concentration with no substance present.

(b) What is true about the extent to which vancomycin and lead affect the results of this assay method?

(c) Transform the relative results for tubes **1**, **3**, and **5** into logarithms.

(d) How do the logarithmic values for vancomycin and lead show more clearly how these two substances affect the results?

PEARSON

myhealthprofessionskit™

Go to www.myhealthprofessionskit.com <http://www.myhealthprofessionskit.com/> to access the Companion Website created for this textbook. Simply select "Clinical Laboratory Science" from the choice of disciplines. Find this book and log in using your username and password to access additional practice problems, answers to the practice and contextual problems, additional information, and more.

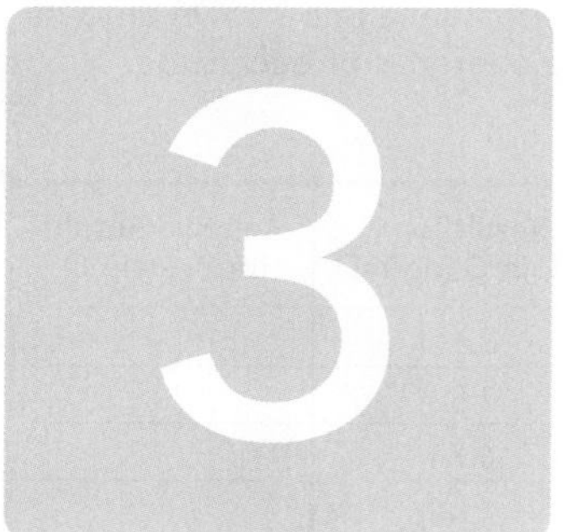

Rounding and the Significance of Figures

Learning Objectives

At the end of this chapter, the student should be able to do the following:

1. Round whole numbers, decimal numbers, and exponential expressions
2. Predict the effect of rounding on the average of a set of numbers
3. Explain the nature of figure significance
4. Relate figure significance to precision
5. Identify, count, and report the significant figures, whether nonzeros or zeros, in any measurement
6. Round, to the correct number of significant figures, a numerical result from any arithmetic operation or combination of operations
7. Round a calculated average to the correct number of significant figures
8. Identify, count, and report the significant figures in an exponential expression or logarithm
9. Calculate and interpret absolute uncertainty, relative uncertainty, and implied relative uncertainty
10. Calculate bias introduced by rounding
11. Round meaningfully when the rules of figure significance give unacceptable results

Key Terms

absolute uncertainty
accuracy
bias
characteristic
embedded zero
implied relative uncertainty
leading zero
mantissa
precision
relative uncertainty
rounding digit
significant figure
trailing zero

Chapter Outline

Numbers are either exact or inexact. Exact numbers are those that result from counting things, whereas inexact numbers result from measuring things. Even though we sometimes round exact numbers, such as the population of a city to the nearest 1000, we always round inexact numbers because of the uncertainty inherent to making measurements. Rounding numbers is a simple mathematical practice that should become automatic for anyone who works in a laboratory. Although everyone approximates numbers in daily life, the need for precision and consistency in the technical setting calls for a particular set of rules for rounding. Through it all, however, remember that *rounding is about keeping a number consistent with the level of our certainty in it.*

SIMPLE ROUNDING

Consider the number "263." Suppose someone in the laboratory reports this number to us as a measurement of, say, a length in "mm" or a volume in "μL." If we want the measurement only to the nearest hundred, then we recognize 263 to be closer to 300 than it is to 200; so, we round 263 up to 300.

If, instead, we want the measurement to the nearest 10, then we recognize 263 to be closer to 260 than it is to 270; so, we round the number to 260.

Clearly, the raw measurement of "263" was actually some number that rounds to 263. It may have been, for example, 263.42 or 262.88. If we want the measurement only to the nearest whole number, then either of these possibilities rounds to 263. If we want the measurement to the nearest tenth, however, then we recognize 263.42 as being closer to 263.4 than it is to 263.5; likewise, 262.88 is closer to 262.9 than it is to 262.8.

Here are the step-by-step procedures for rounding numbers.

Rounding Whole Numbers

1. Identify the place (ones, tens, hundreds, etc.) to which the number is to be rounded. The **rounding digit** stands in that place.
2. If the first digit to the right is less than 5, then do not change the rounding digit but do change to "0" all digits to the right of it.

EXAMPLE

87,329 —rounds to→ 87,300

(↑ *Rounding Digit*: the 3)

3. If the first digit to the right is 5 or greater, then add 1 to the rounding digit and change to "0" all digits to the right of it.

EXAMPLE

87,362 —rounds to→ 87,400

(↑ *Rounding Digit*: the 3)

Rounding Decimal Numbers

1. Identify the decimal place (tenths, hundredths, thousandths, etc.) to which the number is to be rounded. The rounding digit stands in that place.
2. If the first digit to the right is less than 5, then do not change the rounding digit but do drop all digits to the right of it.

EXAMPLE

87.329 —rounds to→ 87.3

(↑ *Rounding Digit*: the 3)

★ TABLE 3-1 How the Average is Affected by Different Rules on the Rounding of Numbers with a Final Digit of "5"

		Average
Raw numbers	63.5, 61.6, 65.5, 67.2, 62.5, 62.1, 60.5, 64.5	**63** (63.4)
Rounded up when final digit is "5"	64, 62, 66, 67, 63, 62, 61, 65	**64** (63.75)
Rounded up or down to even number when final digit is "5"	64, 62, 66, 67, 62, 62, 60, 64	**63** (63.4)

3. If the first digit to the right is 5 or greater, then add 1 to the rounding digit and drop all digits to the right of it.

EXAMPLE 87.362 rounds to → 87.4
↑ *Rounding Digit*

Rounding Fives

As the rules state, when the final digit is "5," round up. For example, 262.5 rounds up to 263, not down to 262. Similarly, 7.095 rounds up to 7.10, not down to 7.09. Be aware, however, that some authorities disapprove of this practice because it creates a different number of chances to round down than it does to round up (a number is rounded down when the final digit is 1, 2, 3, or 4, but up when the final digit is 5, 6, 7, 8, or 9). Consequently, we will round down four out of every nine times, but round up five out of every nine times. This introduces bias (discussed below), which is defined as a constant error in a series of observations or calculations. Why does this matter?

Under these rules, as Table 3-1 ★ shows, the average of a set of numbers is higher *after* rounding than it is *before* rounding because more numbers are rounded up than down. There is, however, a way to prevent this unintended consequence: whenever the final digit is "5," simply round to an even number, whether doing so amounts to a rounding up or a rounding down. In this approach, there are about as many roundings down as there are roundings up, and the average of the rounded numbers should, therefore, be closer to the average of the raw numbers (Table 3-1).

☑ CHECKPOINT 3-1

1. Using the standard rules, round each number to the nearest whole.
   (a) 29.6 (b) 11,803.1 (c) 8.70 (d) 1.5
2. Using the standard rules, round each number to the nearest hundredth.
   (a) 0.233 (b) 2.009 (c) 17.102 (d) 6.996
3. Using the standard rules, round each number to the nearest 10.
   (a) 119 (b) 6044 (c) 703 (d) 241,558

1. (a) 30 (b) 11,803 (c) 9 (d) 2
2. (a) 0.23 (b) 2.01 (c) 17.10 (d) 7.00
3. (a) 120 (b) 6040 (c) 700 (d) 241,560

FIGURE SIGNIFICANCE

What Significant Figures Are

In any number arising from a measurement, a **significant figure** is one that either is known with certainty or has been estimated. *In a properly reported measurement, therefore, any nonzero digit is significant* (zeros are discussed below). Suppose you measure, in "mL," the volume of a liquid in a graduated cylinder, as in Figure 3-1 ■.

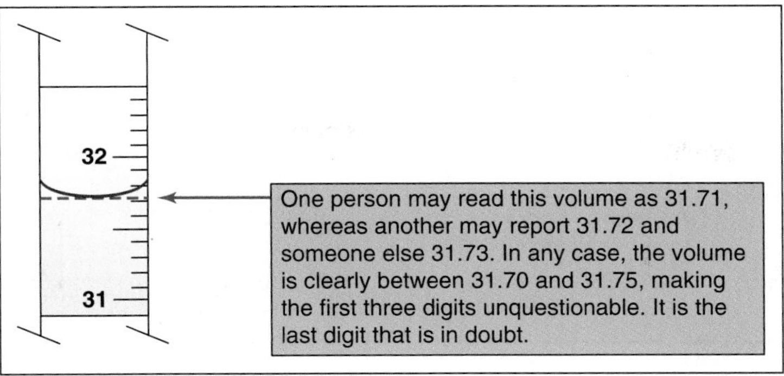

FIGURE 3-1 Typical uncertainty in volume measurements.

Different technologists will estimate the final digit slightly differently; reported values, for example, may range from 31.71 mL to 31.73 mL. If the volume is reported as "31.72," we can conclude that it is undoubtedly greater than 31.70, less than 31.80, and less than halfway between those two limits. Where exactly it lies between them, however, is questionable. Thus, there are four significant figures in the measurement "31.72," but the last one is the least reliable. *It is customary in science to report a measurement such that only the last digit is uncertain.*

Figure Significance and Precision

Whoever measures the volume may choose to round the result to "32" or "31.7," or may report it as "31.72." The value "32" is accurate to the nearest whole number, which means that the raw measurement was between 31.5 and 32.5. The number "31.7," however, is accurate to the nearest tenth, the measurement being between 31.65 and 31.75. The number "31.72," of course, is accurate to the nearest hundredth, lying between 31.715 and 31.725. In these three values, notice that the measurement becomes more precise as the number of decimal places increases.

The degree of that precision lies in the number of significant figures the value has within it. The value "32" has two significant figures, "31.7" has three, and "31.72" has four. Thus, as the number of significant figures increases, the precision in the value also goes up. But what does this mean?

Suppose four technologists measured the volume in Figure 3-1 and reported the results (in "mL") to be 31.72, 31.71, 31.72, and 31.73. The lowest value, 31.71, comes from a measurement that was between 31.705 and 31.715, whereas the highest value, 31.73, corresponds to a measurement between 31.725 and 31.735. Therefore, the possible range for all four measurements reported by the technologists starts at 31.705 and ends at 31.735. The difference is only 0.030 mL, or 0.09% of 31.720, which is the middle of that range.

Now suppose the technologists had merely read the volume to the nearest whole number, each of them reporting it to be "32." Although it seems at first glance that their agreement is perfect, realize that the number "32" could have arisen from any volume between 31.5 and 32.5, a difference of 1.0 mL, or 3.1% of 32.0, which is the middle of that range. As a percentage, therefore, this difference is much higher (33 times higher) than the difference in the previous example.

The upshot of this comparison is the fact that, when more significant figures are present, the agreement among repeated measurements is tighter (unless, of course, someone makes a gross error). Agreement among repeated measurements is called **precision**, which Chapter 8 discusses in more depth. By contrast, the number of significant figures has no bearing on whether a value is correct or incorrect, that is, the **accuracy**, because, even if the manufacturer of the cylinder in Figure 3-1 had accidentally mislabeled the mark "32" instead of "31," the four technologists would still have read the volume as they did. Their readings would have been incorrect, of course, but still close to each other.

The Significance of Zeros

Numbers that contain zeros pose questions that require more thought. Let us focus on the three categories of zero, classified by location within numbers. Table 3-2 ★ summarizes the significance of zeros.

★ TABLE 3-2 The Significance of Zeros

Category	Definition	Examples	Rule
Trailing zero	Any zero that follows the last nonzero digit	40, 8900, 60., 5.7700	Significant only if there is a decimal point in the number
Leading zero	Any zero that precedes the first nonzero digit	0.119, 0.000083	Never significant
Embedded zero	A zero that occurs anywhere between two nonzero digits	2096, 101, 47.8006	Always significant

Trailing Zero

A trailing zero is any zero that follows the last nonzero digit in a number. A multiple of 10, such as the number "80," is ambiguous because we do not know whether it represents rounding to the nearest whole number or to the nearest 10. In other words, the raw measurement in this case may have been 79.8 rounded to the nearest whole number, or it may have been 83 rounded to the nearest 10. Because the number "80" itself does not distinguish between these two possibilities, the zero is uncertain, and it has not been estimated in the measurement. Therefore, it is not significant and "80" has only one significant figure; the zero serves only to indicate the scale.

There is, however, a way to eliminate the ambiguity and give meaning to the zero. If the measurement was indeed 79.8 rounded to the nearest whole number, then a decimal point would remove all doubt. Instead of "80," we could write "80.", indicating that the raw measurement was between 79.5 and 80.5. In the number "80.", the zero is significant because it has some certainty; thus, there are now two significant figures in the number. We can say, then, that a trailing zero is significant only if there is a decimal point in the number.

Likewise, the number "6700" does not distinguish among its three possible origins. The raw measurement may have been 6700.2 rounded to the nearest whole number. Perhaps it was 6704 rounded to the nearest 10 or 6681 rounded to the nearest 100. Therefore, only the "6" and "7" in "6700" are significant. However, writing "6700." would tell us that the measurement had been rounded to the nearest whole number; all four figures, therefore, would become significant.

Another way to eliminate the ambiguity is to specify the number of significant figures, such as "5000 (3 s.f.)," or to underline the last significant zero, such as "50$\underline{0}$0." These conventions, however, are not universally used. A better approach is to declare the uncertainty outright, an example being "5000 $\pm$ 10" (the chapter discusses this practice later).

As seen above, trailing zeros followed by a decimal point are significant. However, *any trailing zero in a number containing a decimal point is significant.* The number "80.0," for example, is not at all ambiguous; it tells us clearly that the raw measurement was between 79.95 and 80.05, rounded to the nearest tenth. Thus, each zero in "80.0" is significant. Likewise, "6700.000" tells us without a doubt that the raw measurement was between 6699.9995 and 6700.0005, rounded to the nearest thousandth. Consequently, every zero is significant.

Leading Zero

A leading zero is any zero that precedes the first nonzero digit in a number. Consider the number "0.0062." It resulted from the rounding of a measurement between 0.00615 and 0.00625, to the nearest ten-thousandth. The leading zeros contribute nothing to the precision of the number itself; they only indicate the scale. To prove this, consider the following line of thinking.

The difference between the top and bottom of the range, 0.00625 and 0.00615, is 0.00010; this is 1.6% of 0.00620, the middle of the range. Now remove the leading zeros (and the decimal point) to make the range run from 615 up to 625. The difference between the top and bottom is now 10, but 10 is still 1.6% of 620, the middle of the range. Clearly, whether or not the leading zeros are present, the difference between the top and bottom of the range is 1.6% of the middle of the range. Thus, *leading zeros are never significant.* In this example, the number "0.0062" has only two significant figures.

Embedded Zero

An embedded zero is a zero that occurs anywhere between two nonzero digits in a number. Because its value is certain, *a zero that falls between two nonzero significant figures is itself significant.* The number "706," for example, is the result of rounding a measurement that fell between 705.5 and 706.5; the zero has meaning and is not even involved in the rounding. Similarly, the number "1.0025" is the result of rounding a measurement that fell between 1.00245 and 1.00255. Again, the zeros are unambiguous in this number and are, therefore, significant.

☑ CHECKPOINT 3-2

How many significant figures are present in each number?

(a) 42	(b) 1693	(c) 302	(d) 0.225	(e) 1.004
(f) 0.077	(g) 44,000	(h) 20.	(i) 2.000	
(j) 628.01	(k) 0.90	(l) 80.80	(m) 100	

(a) 2	(b) 4	(c) 3	(d) 3	(e) 4
(f) 2	(g) 2	(h) 2	(i) 4	
(j) 5	(k) 2	(l) 4	(m) 1	

SIGNIFICANT FIGURES IN THE RESULTS OF CALCULATIONS

It is logical that only figures that are certain or that have been estimated should be treated as significant. The complication arises in deciding how many significant figures to include in the final result of a process that comprises several measurements or calculations.

Suppose, for example, that you prepare a glucose solution by (1) dissolving 5 g of glucose in water, and (2) bringing the volume up to 100. mL. It would be ridiculous to report the concentration as 5.0000 g/mL. That implies certainty in the concentration out to the nearest ten-thousandth of a gram, even though the mass of glucose was known only to the nearest whole number of grams. *The result cannot be more certain than the least-reliable measurement that went into the calculation.*

Consider an assay for an analyte in serum that requires you to add 220 μL of reagent **A** to 11 mL of reagent **B**; results are in "pg/mL." Such a method might be an ELISA (enzyme-linked immunosorbent assay) that uses a 96-well microplate. Because each volume has only two significant figures, it would be absurd (and dishonest) to report the final concentration of the analyte in a sample to be 386.714 pg/mL. There is no justification for asserting that six figures can be reliable in the concentration when only two were significant in each of the volumes that went into the calculations.

How, then, does one decide how many significant figures to include in the result of a calculation or a series of calculations? As you learn the rules for figure significance in the following sections, remember that the word *rules* is too strong. They are actually guidelines that serve as shortcuts to the correct number of significant figures by making it unnecessary to carry out a detailed error analysis for every calculation you face.

Multiplication and Division

The result of a calculation involving only multiplication and/or division can have no more significant figures than there are in the measured quantity with the fewest. Consider the following two examples.

EXAMPLE 1

While carrying out a diagnostic test, you dispense 2.0 mL of a glucose solution at a concentration of 0.629 g/mL. How many grams of the glucose are in this volume?

$$2.0 \text{ mL} \times 0.629 \text{ g/mL} = 1.258 \text{ g}$$

The measured quantity with the fewest significant figures is "2.0"; therefore, the product of this equation may have no more than two. The correct answer is **1.3 g**.

EXAMPLE 2

You are preparing an aqueous solution of 0.272 g of sodium chloride in a final volume of 300. mL. What is the concentration of the resulting solution?

$$0.272 \text{ g} \div 300. \text{ mL} = 0.00090667 \text{ g/mL}$$

Each measured quantity has three significant figures (note the decimal point in the volume). Therefore, the quotient of this equation may have no more than three, and the correct answer is **0.000907 g/mL**.

Addition and Subtraction

In addition or subtraction operations, the last significant figure in the final result must occupy the same place as the last significant figure in the measurement that has the greatest uncertainty. The measurement with the greatest uncertainty is the one whose last significant figure is farthest to the left among all the numbers going into the calculation. A consequence of this, of course, is that the number of significant figures can change in the course of addition or subtraction, in contrast to multiplication or division. Consider the following three examples.

EXAMPLE 1

Add the following three measurements together.

$$\begin{array}{r} 33 \\ 109 \\ +\ \underline{20} \\ 162 \end{array}$$

The sum must have its last significant figure in the same place as the least-certain quantity does. That number is "20," in which the last significant figure (also the only one) is in the tens place; therefore, the last significant figure in the sum must also be in the tens place. The correct answer is **160**, not 162.

EXAMPLE 2

Add the three measurements below together.

$$\begin{array}{r} 33.77 \\ 109.61 \\ +\ \underline{2.07918} \\ 144.91018 \end{array}$$

The least-certain number is "33.77," in which the last significant figure occupies the hundredths place. Therefore, the last significant figure in the sum must also occupy the hundredths place. The correct answer is **144.91**, not 144.91018.

EXAMPLE 3

Consider the following subtraction.

$$\begin{array}{r} 668.94 \\ -\ \underline{72} \\ 596.94 \end{array}$$

The least-certain number is "72," in which the last significant figure is in the ones place. Therefore, the last significant figure in the difference must also be in the ones place. The correct answer is **597**, not 596.94.

Combined Operations

When a calculation combines operations (multiplication, division, addition, and subtraction), *apply the rules for figure significance before and after every step involving addition or subtraction.* Table 3-3 ★ shows how these rules affect rounding.

Examples 1 and 2 in Table 3-3 are straightforward. The operations involve only addition or subtraction, and the values of *x* and *y* force the final result to stop in the third decimal place. In examples 3 and 4, the operations involve only multiplication and division, which means that the final result can have no more significant figures than does *x*, which has only two.

Example 5, however, combines the operations of multiplication and addition. The first step is multiplication of *x* by *y*, giving 0.314578. Because *x* has only two significant figures, this product must be rounded to 0.31 before the next step. It is then added to *z* to give 92.1142, which must be rounded to 92.11 because "0.31" has only two decimal places.

Example 6 is similar to 5. The first step is multiplication of *y* by *z*, giving 365.56432, which must be rounded to 365.6 because the value of *y* has four significant figures. This number is then added to *x* to give 365.7, which has only one decimal place because "365.6" has only one.

Examples 7 and 8 follow logic similar to that of examples 5 and 6.

The Exception of Repeated Measurements

Suppose that you quantify the drug methotrexate in the same patient specimen five times. The results, in "μmol/L," are 62.33, 62.69, 61.56, 63.02, and 61.79. The average of these five values is

$$\frac{62.33 + 62.69 + 61.56 + 63.02 + 61.79}{5} = 62.278$$

But remember that, in the addition step, the last significant figure in the sum must occupy the same place as the last significant figure in the measurement that has the greatest uncertainty, which in this case is the hundredths place:

$$\begin{array}{r} 62.33 \\ 62.69 \\ 61.56 \\ 63.02 \\ +61.79 \\ \hline 311.39 \end{array}$$

Next, we divide the sum by 5 to get the average:

$$\frac{311.39}{5} = 62.278$$

The number "5" in the denominator is an exact count—not an estimation or a measurement; therefore, it does not bear on the number of significant figures in the final answer. But the sum in the

★ **TABLE 3-3** Examples of Figure Significance in Combined Operations

x	y	z	Operations	Raw Result from Calculator (without rounding at any step)	Final Result (after proper rounding at each step)
0.079	3.982	91.8042	1 $x + y + z$	95.8652	95.865
			2 $x + y - z$	−87.7432	−87.743
			3 $x \cdot y \cdot z$	28.879581	29
			4 $x \div (y \cdot z)$	0.000216104	0.00022
			5 $(x \cdot y) + z$	92.118778	92.11
			6 $x + (y \cdot z)$	365.64332	365.7
			7 $(x \div y) + z$	91.824039	91.824
			8 $x + (y \div z)$	0.1223749	0.122

numerator has five significant figures, and the rule for multiplication and division requires, in this case, that the result of the calculation also have five significant figures. If we obey this rule, then the average is 62.278. However, because each concentration has only four significant figures, the average itself should have no more than four; it cannot be more certain than any of the measurements that went into it. It would *seem*, then, that the correctly reported average is 62.28 μmol/L. But is it really?

Notice that the five concentrations, which range from 61.79 to 63.02, vary not only in the tenths and hundredths places but also in the ones place. It is not defensible to claim certainty to the hundredths place (62.28 μmol/L) when the first uncertain digit in the concentration is in the ones place. The value "62.28" means that the real concentration lies between 62.275 and 62.284, but there is no way to justify this conclusion with such a wide range of individual concentrations. As stated earlier in this chapter, we customarily report measurements such that only the last digit is uncertain. Therefore, the correctly reported average for our five concentrations must terminate in the ones place: **62 μmol/L.**

This exception for repeated measurements reflects a flaw in the rules of figure significance. The final section of this chapter addresses this issue.

☑ CHECKPOINT 3-3

1. Specify the number of significant figures that should be present in the result of each calculation.

   (a) 2.445×0.921 (b) $451 \div 9.3$ (c) 0.0022435×66.2778 (d) $2378 \div 1.09880$

2. With the correct number of significant figures, give the result of each calculation.

   (a) $101 + 33.5$ (b) $0.02775 - 0.0104$ (c) $2.0046 + 0.11708$ (d) $55.66 - 2.189$

3. With the correct number of significant figures, give the result of each calculation.

   (a) $(2.33 + 0.988) \times 66$ (b) $\dfrac{119 + 83}{0.7558}$ (c) $(18 \times 0.500) - 2.3$

   (d) $3445.9 + \dfrac{0.885}{0.919}$ (e) $0.08475 + 0.40(106)$

   (f) $1.0556 - 0.00664 - 0.802$ (g) $0.033000(1.229845 + 0.0009443 - 0.0730721)$

1. (a) 3 (b) 2 (c) 5 (d) 4
2. (a) 135 (b) 0.0174 (c) 2.1217 (d) 53.47
3. (a) 220 (b) 267 (c) 6.7 (d) 3446.9
   (e) 40 (f) 0.247 (g) 0.038205

SIGNIFICANT FIGURES IN EXPONENTIAL EXPRESSIONS AND LOGARITHMS

As Chapter 2 explains, an exponential expression, such as 8.332×10^6, has two parts: the significand (8.332) and the exponential term (10^6). *All the significant figures in an exponential expression are in the significand; there are none in the exponential term.*

The expression above is the same as 8,332,000, a number that consists of four significant figures. Thus, when written exponentially, all four of those figures appear in the significand.

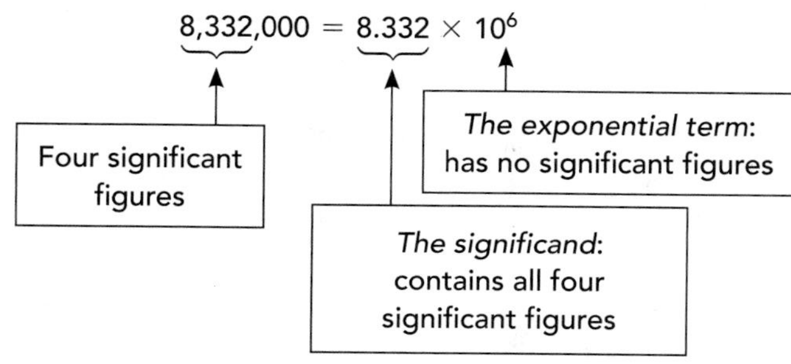

The exponential term tells us nothing about the number of significant figures; it only specifies the order of magnitude. After all, if the expression were 8.332×10^{13}, there would still be four significant figures, even though the value has seven more zeros: 83,320,000,000,000.

How does one identify the significant figures in a logarithm? A logarithm comprises two parts: the **characteristic**, which is the set of numbers to the left of the decimal point, and the **mantissa**, which is the set of numbers to the right of the decimal point. Consider, for example, the logarithm of 150,000, or 1.5×10^5:

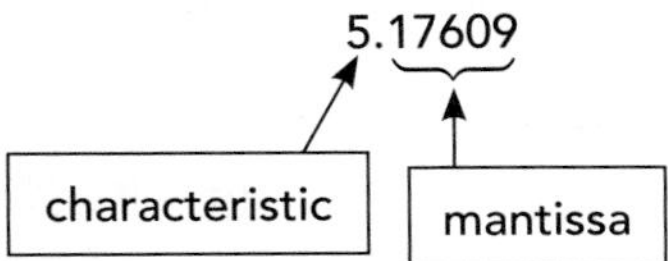

The characteristic merely locates the decimal point, telling us only the power of 10, which in this case is 5. It is *not* a significant figure. The mantissa, however, does contain significant figures and must contain the same number of them as does the argument. In this case, because there are two significant figures in the argument (150,000), there must also be two in the mantissa. Calculated to two significant figures, therefore, the logarithm of 150,000 is 5.18. To convince yourself of this rule, consider the following table.

Argument	$\log_{10}$
1.5	0.17609
15	1.17609
150	2.17609
1500	3.17609
15,000	4.17609
150,000	5.17609
1,500,000	6.17609

Regardless of the power of 10, every argument in this table has two significant figures. In fact, they are the same two: "1" and "5." Clearly, the characteristic of the logarithm changes from one argument to the next, whereas the mantissa stays the same. Thus, the characteristic says nothing about the two significant figures, instead showing only the location of the decimal point. The mantissa is what captures the "1" and "5," no matter how many zeros follow them in the argument.

Therefore, *in counting significant figures in a logarithm, ignore the characteristic. Only the mantissa contains significant figures*, and it contains the same number of them as does the argument. For example, if the argument is 365, there are three significant figures, and the logarithm is reported as 2.562. If the argument is 2.3374×10^9, there are five significant figures, and the logarithm is reported as 9.36873.

☑ CHECKPOINT 3-4

1. Count the significant figures in each of these expressions:
   (a) 3.772×10^{-5} (b) 0.110×10^5 (c) 9.6×10^{17} (d) 3.09400×10^5
2. For each number, write its base-10 logarithm with the correct number of significant figures.
   (a) 1.22760×10^9 (b) 0.00330 (c) 600 (d) 10,460
3. Write each number in exponential notation with the correct number of significant figures.
   (a) 5,003,000,000 (b) 25,010 (c) 0.0000116 (d) 0.00070070

1. (a) 4 (b) 3 (c) 2 (d) 6
2. (a) 9.089057 (b) −2.481 (c) 2.8 (d) 4.0195
3. (a) 5.003×10^9 (b) 2.501×10^4 (c) 1.16×10^{-5} (d) 7.0070×10^{-4}

ABSOLUTE AND RELATIVE UNCERTAINTY

There are more-rigorous ways to quantify uncertainty than relying on the number of significant figures. Practicing scientists usually express measurements in the form "$x \pm y$," where x is the value of the measurement and y is the uncertainty. The volume in Figure 3-1, for example, might be reported as "31.72 mL ± 0.02 mL."

Suppose you weigh a substance on an analytical balance and it gives a mass of 4.38 g; the balance's stated uncertainty is 0.05 g. You record the mass as "4.38 g ± 0.05 g," which implies that the true mass is between 4.33 and 4.43 g. The "0.05 g" is the **absolute uncertainty**, which simply represents the raw amount of uncertainty in the measurement.

The importance of that uncertainty, however, is captured in the **relative uncertainty**, which is the fraction of the measurement's value represented by the absolute uncertainty:

$$\text{relative uncertainty} = \frac{\text{absolute uncertainty}}{\text{measurement's value}}$$

In other words, it tells us how large the uncertainty is in relation to the measurement. It is usually expressed as a percentage. In our example, the relative uncertainty is

$$\frac{0.05\text{ g}}{4.38\text{ g}} = 0.011 = 1.1\%$$

Note that the relative uncertainty has no units because the ratio cancels them out. Therefore, the measurement may be expressed as "4.38 ± 1.1%."

If someone reports to you the measurement "22 mg," you have no indication of uncertainty apart from the number of significant figures. Because the measurement was rounded to the nearest whole number, the true value is presumably between 21.5 and 22.5, making the uncertainty "± 0.5." Therefore, the **implied relative uncertainty** is 0.5 out of 22:

$$\frac{0.5}{22} = 0.023 = 2.3\%$$

Consequently, the result of any calculation involving this value (22 mg) can have an implied relative uncertainty no smaller than 2.3%.

☑ CHECKPOINT 3-5

1. Calculate the relative uncertainty for each of the following measurements.
   (a) 23.66 g ± 0.03 g
   (b) 0.00557 moles ± 0.00005 moles
   (c) 469 mL ± 10 mL
2. Calculate the implied relative uncertainty for each of the following measurements.
   (a) 0.571 g/L (b) 145 mg (c) 4 g

1. (a) 0.1% (b) 0.9% (c) 2%
2. (a) 0.09% (b) 0.3% (c) 13%

ROUNDING ERROR

Rounding introduces bias. As mentioned earlier in the chapter, bias is an error that remains constant in a series of observations or calculations. To understand this point, consider a mass of 1.629 g, measured on a balance that the manufacturer claims has an uncertainty of 0.005 g. The true mass, then, is probably between 1.624 and 1.634 g.

If we round the measurement to "1.63 g," the next person to read it will infer that the true measurement is between 1.625 and 1.635 g. The new range is higher than the original by 0.001; this difference is a positive bias—a constant error—that will accompany this value into any subsequent calculations, affecting the outcomes accordingly.

Rounding also sacrifices information about precision. For example, the value "3.8" implies a range of 3.75 to 3.85, which represents an uncertainty of 0.05. However, rounding "3.8" up to "4" changes the implied range to 3.5–4.5, an uncertainty of 0.5. The new uncertainty is 10 times greater than the previous uncertainty.

KEEPING FIGURE SIGNIFICANCE IN PERSPECTIVE

Illusory precision is something we want to avert. The rules of figure significance were developed to prevent misunderstandings about the level of uncertainty in the measurements we share with each other. They keep us from implying more precision in our measurements than exists in the devices with which we make those measurements. Even so, the rules only approximate the uncertainty in our numbers, and sometimes that approximation is unacceptable. What follows are three examples of problems that illustrate why this chapter earlier described the rules as "guidelines." In each example, we must check the rules against solid reasoning in order to find a trustworthy solution.

EXAMPLE 1

Consider the following addition of four measured masses (in "grams").

$$100 + 23 + 40 + 31$$

The reasonable answer is 194 grams ("190" if rounded to the nearest 10, or even "200" if rounded to the nearest 100). However, applying the rule of figure significance for addition gives the preposterous total of 100. In this case, reasonableness trumps the rules.

EXAMPLE 2

Consider the following 10 measured volumes (in "mL"). If we choose to report only the average of these volumes, and not the individual volumes themselves, what is the proper value?

89 95 102 93 97 100. 96 92 100. 95

The unrounded average is "95.9 mL." The exception of repeated measurements, presented earlier, would remind us to write the average of these values such that only the last digit is uncertain. Unfortunately, there is no unquestionable digit in either the ones, tens, or hundreds place. Therefore, we might round the average up to "100" in order to report only one significant figure, but this would be grossly misleading for the following two reasons.

1. As the reported average, "100" is too far from most of the values and from the unrounded average. There is no justification for declaring the average to be so near the upper end of these measurements.
2. The value "100" has only one significant figure, implying that the average may be as high as 149 (which becomes "100" when rounded to one significant figure). That range, however, would be silly for the values given. So, we might try to circumvent this absurdity by making two digits significant, that is, by writing "100 (2 s.f.)" or "1$\underline{0}$0." But if we do, then the implied range for the average becomes 95-105, which is also indefensible because the highest measured volume is only 102. If we make all three digits significant by writing "100." or "100 (3 s.f.)," then the implied range is 99.5-100.5, which is still too high and which carries more precision than exists in any of the measurements.

Like "100 (3 s.f.)" above, reporting the unrounded average of 95.9 would also imply too much precision. The best option, then, is to round the average to the nearest whole number, 96. Even though it implies that the uncertain "9" is certain, this value is a rational compromise between inflating the average (by choosing "100") and overstating the precision (by choosing "95.9").

EXAMPLE 3

Suppose we measure the volume of a liquid to be 6.97 mL in a cylinder that has a stated uncertainty of 0.05 mL. We properly record the volume as "6.97 mL ± 0.05 mL," realizing that the true volume falls between 6.92 and 7.02 mL. Rounding this number, therefore, presents a puzzle in that the digit in the ones place is questionable. Because only the last digit in our measurement should be uncertain, is it reasonable to round off to one decimal place, or must we stop at a whole number?

We have two options. First, we could simply round the volume to "7 mL." It would be correct for the entire range from 6.92 to 7.02, although it has only one significant figure and, thus, less precision than the measurement itself. Second, we could round the reading to "7.0," which has a precision closer to that of the original, but which assumes the true reading to be at least 6.95. We can settle the issue by comparing the implied relative uncertainties of the two rounded values to the relative uncertainty of the original measurement.

Value (mL)	Absolute Uncertainty (mL)	Implied Minimum (mL)	Implied Maximum (mL)	Relative Uncertainty
6.97	**0.05**	**6.92**	**7.02**	**0.7%**
7	0.5	6.5	7.5	7%
7. 0	0.05	6.95	7.05	0.7%

As the above table shows, rounding to one decimal place (two significant figures) gives the same relative uncertainty as there is in the original measurement. Thus, if we round off, our choice should be "7.0 mL." Generally, a raw measurement should be rounded to the number of digits most consistent with the measurement's uncertainty.

The Upshot

Although the rules of figure significance keep us mindful about overestimating precision, they do not always yield a good answer. Never apply them uncritically. They do not substitute for mathematical common sense, in the same way that calculators do not substitute for fast arithmetic skills nor statistics for sound scientific judgment.

Summary

1. Rounding is about keeping a number consistent with the level of our certainty in it.
2. Rounding whole numbers. (*a*) Identify the *rounding digit.* (*b*) If the first digit to the right is less than 5, then do not change the rounding digit but do change to "0" all digits to the right of it. (*c*) If the first digit to the right is 5 or greater, then add 1 to the rounding digit and change to "0" all digits to the right of it.
3. Rounding decimal numbers. (*a*) Identify the rounding digit. (*b*) If the first digit to the right is less than 5, then do not change the rounding digit but do drop all digits to the right of it. (*c*) If the first digit to the right is 5 or greater, then add 1 to the rounding digit and drop all digits to the right of it.
4. Under the standard rules for rounding, the average of a set of numbers is higher after rounding than it is before rounding. One way to prevent this is to round to an even number whenever the final digit is "5," whether doing so amounts to a rounding up or a rounding down.
5. A *significant figure* is one that either is known with certainty or has been estimated.
6. In a properly reported measurement, any nonzero digit is significant.
7. A measurement is typically reported such that only the last digit is uncertain.
8. Figure significance is related to *precision*, or the agreement among repeated measurements, rather than to *accuracy*, or the degree to which the value is correct.
9. A *trailing zero*, which is any zero that follows the last nonzero digit in a number, is significant only if there is a decimal point somewhere in the number.

10. A *leading zero,* which is any zero that precedes the first nonzero digit in a number, is never significant.
11. An *embedded zero,* which is any zero that occurs between two nonzero significant figures, is significant.
12. The result of a calculation involving only multiplication and/or division can have no more significant figures than there are in the measured quantity with the fewest.
13. In addition or subtraction operations, the last significant figure in the final result must occupy the same place as the last significant figure in the measurement that has the greatest uncertainty.
14. When a calculation combines operations (multiplication, division, addition, and subtraction), apply the rules for figure significance before and after every step involving addition or subtraction.
15. Averaging can be an exception to the rules for figure significance. An average should be reported such that only the last digit is uncertain, even if the individual measurements have more significant figures.
16. All the significant figures in an exponential expression are in the significand; there are none in the exponential term.
17. In a logarithm, the *characteristic* is the set of digits to the left of the decimal point, and the *mantissa* is the set of digits to the right of the decimal point.
18. In a logarithm, only the mantissa contains significant figures.
19. *Absolute uncertainty* is the raw amount of uncertainty in a measurement. *Relative uncertainty* is the ratio of the absolute uncertainty to the value of the measurement (usually expressed as a percentage):

$$\text{relative uncertainty} = \frac{\text{absolute uncertainty}}{\text{measurement's value}}$$

Implied relative uncertainty is relative uncertainty that has been calculated from an absolute uncertainty assumed from the number of significant figures in a value.

20. Rounding sacrifices information about precision and introduces *bias,* which is error that remains constant in a series of observations or calculations.
21. Because the rules of figure significance do not always yield a good answer, results arising from the application of those rules should be checked for reasonableness.

Practice Problems

1. (LO 1) Round each number to the nearest tenth.

(a) 42.77	(b) 0.24	(c) 106.03
(d) 8.95	(e) 0.83	(f) 50.09
(g) 2866.04	(h) 17.08	(i) 7.042
(j) 33.566	(k) 0.705	(l) 91.229

2. (LO 1) Round each number to the nearest 10.

(a) 13,406	(b) 19	(c) 505
(d) 65	(e) 377	(f) 4601
(g) 1007	(h) 221	(i) 48.3
(j) 9.074×10^3	(k) 2.2855×10^4	(l) 603

3. (LO 1) Round each number to the nearest whole.

(a) 2.5	(b) 27.8	(c) 103.2
(d) 99.6	(e) 18,404.7	(f) 4.03
(g) 55.19	(h) 600.0	(i) 1003.3
(j) 8.22	(k) 9090.9	(l) 13.7

4. (LO 1) Round each number to the nearest thousandth.

(a) 4.1336	(b) 0.9315	(c) 12.0020
(d) 8.4×10^{-3}	(e) 20.0092	(f) 20.0096
(g) 7.15×10^{-2}	(h) 0.20335	(i) 61.7743
(j) 15.0005	(k) 2.49128	(l) 185.2366

5. (LO 1) Round each number to the nearest hundredth.

(a) 5.022	(b) 199.755	(c) 0.691
(d) 1.8×10^{-2}	(e) 2.505	(f) 35.384
(g) 0.027	(h) 0.996	(i) 40.531
(j) 0.016	(k) 9.080	(l) 58.111

6. (LO 5) The following numbers represent measurements (without units). Count the significant figures in each.

(a) 44.73	(b) 100	(c) 0.227
(d) 83.602	(e) 6912	(f) 200.
(g) 17.0093	(h) 466	(i) 0.0065
(j) 40.0	(k) 1.882660	(l) 3
(m) 144,000	(n) 0.0000010	(o) 4050
(p) 513.05	(q) 2.00000	(r) 5088
(s) 6.2	(t) 70.	

7. (LO 8) The following exponential expressions represent measurements. Count the significant figures in each.

(a) 3.66×10^{-4}	(b) 1.067×10^5
(c) 7.1×10^3	(d) 9.8080×10^{-3}
(e) 2.000×10^6	(f) 4.0061×10^{-9}
(g) 5.0×10^{13}	(h) 1.7300×10^{-8}

(i) 6×10^5 (j) 7.702×10^2

(k) 8×10^{-12} (l) 3.0001×10^4

8. (LO 5, 8) With the correct number of significant figures, write the logarithm of each exponential expression in problem 7 above.

9. (LO 7) Honoring figure significance, write the average of each set of measurements.

(a) 0.0881, 0.0892, 0.0886, 0.0865, 0.0873

(b) 2.66, 2.54, 2.64, 2.70, 2.61

(c) 64, 58, 59, 61, 60, 59

(d) 1.24, 1.25, 1.24, 1.23, 1.24, 1.23

(e) 7.55×10^4, 7.70×10^4, 7.64×10^4, 7.59×10^4, 7.57×10^4

10. (LO 8) Count the significant figures in each of the following exponential expressions.

(a) 1.775×10^{-8} (b) 5.20×10^5

(c) 9.0010×10^{-4} (d) 6.0000×10^6

(e) 4.097×10^{11} (f) 2.3×10^{-3}

11. (LO 8) Count the significant figures in each of the following logarithms.

(a) 0.663 (b) 8.7100

(c) −2.090 (d) 4.2239

(e) −9.0 (f) −6.77881

12. (LO 2) Round the values in each of the following data sets to the nearest whole (round up values ending in "5"). For which of the data sets would the average change if we rounded values ending in "5" to even numbers rather than rounding them up? Try to answer this question without calculating the averages outright.

(a) 13.3, 13.5, 13.2, 13.6, 13.9, 13.5

(b) 139.7, 137.5, 136.5, 136.1, 134.5, 136.6

(c) 45.0, 42.4, 46.5, 43.5, 46.6, 42.5

(d) 1.8, 1.9, 1.5, 1.8, 1.9, 1.7

13. (LO 9) Calculate the relative uncertainty of each measurement.

(a) 4.667 ± 0.005

(b) 0.00293 ± 0.00002

(c) 172 ± 5

14. (LO 9) Calculate the implied relative uncertainty of each measurement.

(a) 0.48 (b) 260 (c) 16.3 (d) 30.

(e) 5.14 (f) 200 (2 s.f.) (g) 300 (h) 0.075

15. (LO 6) Obeying the rules of figure significance, write the solution to each of the following problems.

(a) $(19.2 + 8.66) \times 1.3$

(b) 6.01×2.033

(c) $0.03365 \div 4.480$

(d) $13.62 - (7.9 \times 1.44)$

(e) $7.307 - 6.224 + 10.000$

(f) $5667 + (8.1 \times 0.9) - 140.6$

(g) $\frac{70.9}{3.662}\left(\frac{13.8}{2.0005}\right)$

(h) $\frac{0.8883}{7.2}(3.4 + 5.55)$

(i) $(3.445 \times 10^5) + 100{,}000$

(j) $(1.9077 \times 10^{-3}) \times 2.0$

16. (LO 1) Round each of the following values to the nearest whole number.

(a) 39.01 (b) 25.48 (c) 19.66 (d) 89.47

(e) 60.80 (f) 7.51 (g) 32.11 (h) 103.62

(i) 2.39 (j) 50.09 (k) 29.99 (l) 122.46

(m) 1.49 (n) 76.50 (o) 10.32 (p) 99.52

17. (LO 1, 10) Round each of the values above (*a* through *p*) to one decimal place and then round that value to the nearest whole number. Is there bias relative to the corresponding averages in problem 16? If so, what is the magnitude of the bias?

18. (LO 3, 4, 5, 9) Complete the following table. What rule of figure significance does the completed table confirm? Explain.

Row	Mass of an Object (g)	Implied Range (g)	Implied Relative Uncertainty
1	480		
2	480.		
3	480.0		
4	48		

Contextual Problems

1. Answer the following questions in terms of figure significance or uncertainty.

   (a) You must replace the ultraviolet lamp in your automated analyzer periodically. Manufacturer *A* touts its lamp as having an average life expectancy of 2118.6 hours. Why is this claim suspect?

   (b) Suppose the manufacturer in part *a* above claims 2100 hours for its own lamp and 2060 hours for its competitor's lamp. Is this comparison meaningful? Explain.

   (c) Your method for quantifying acetaminophen in serum has given a concentration of 9.66 μg/mL for one patient and 102.17 μg/mL for another. What do these particular values imply about the method's precision, whether or not that implication is true?

   (d) For patient *X*, your analyzer returns a concentration for retinol-binding protein of 2.2 mg/dL. The concentration 3 months later is 6.1 mg/dL. Is the physician correct in saying that the concentration rose 2.77-fold during that period? Explain.

2. (LO 9, 11) An analyzer returns a result for a hormone in urine as 8.94 ± 0.05 pg/mL. Determine whether it would be better to round this result to one decimal place or to a whole number.

3. (LO 2, 4, 9, 10, 11) Sirolimus (Rapamune®) is an immunosuppressant drug used to inhibit the rejection of a transplanted kidney. Your laboratory is monitoring the concentration of sirolimus in the blood in a cohort of research patients. The analyzer gives the concentration with two decimal places, but your laboratory information system accepts the result with only one decimal place. The researcher who uses the result with one decimal place rounds it to the nearest whole number. Ten concentrations appear below.

4.48	4.99	3.46	6.82	7.74	
9.16	4.90	5.72	3.27	4.85	(ng/mL)

   (a) Calculate the best value for the average of the raw data.

   (b) Calculate the best value for the average of the data that have been rounded to one decimal place.

   (c) Calculate the bias introduced by rounding the raw data from two decimal places to one.

   (d) Calculate the best value for the average of the data after the researcher has rounded them.

4. The RBCs in a particular whole-blood specimen are counted three times: first by an automated analyzer, second by a technologist, and third by a physician. These three counts are treated as inexact because (a) they represent estimations based on a small sampling of the blood specimen, and (b) neither a person nor a machine would ever count 4 million individual cells. Furthermore, during the counting procedure, some cells might be accidentally overlooked, misidentified, or counted more than once. Calculate the average of the three counts and discuss the rounding options, including the strengths and weaknesses of each.

	Count (RBCs/μL)
Analyzer	4,661,000
Technologist	4,715,000
Physician	4,809,000

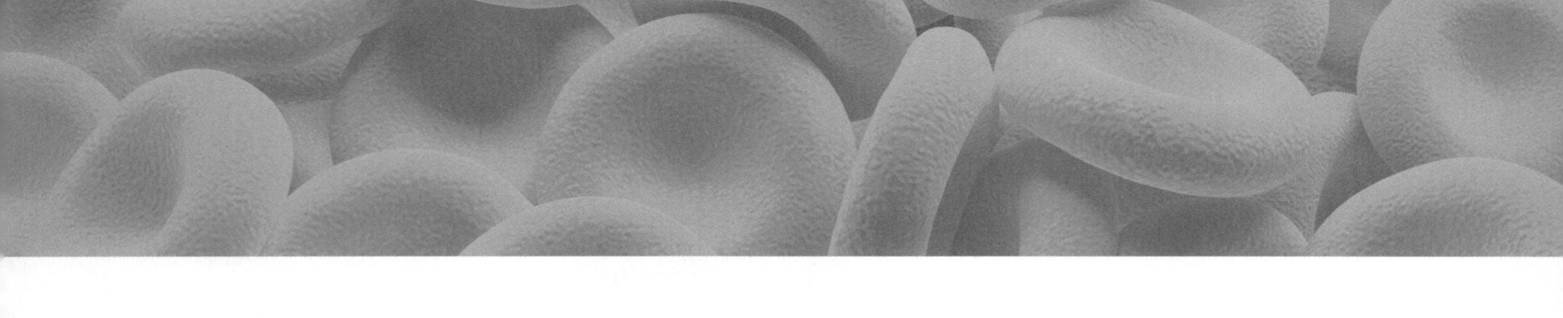

4 Systems of Measurement

Learning Objectives

At the end of this chapter, the student should be able to do the following:

1. Use metric units and their prefixes properly
2. Convert between metric prefixes
3. Convert between U.S. customary units and metric units
4. Use dimensional analysis as a technique for unit conversions
5. Use the ratio method as a technique for unit conversions
6. Calculate formula weight and molar mass
7. Convert between mass and number of moles
8. Interconvert values in the Fahrenheit, Celsius, and Kelvin temperature scales

Key Terms

Avogadro's number
Celsius
dimensional analysis
Fahrenheit
formula weight
International System of Units (SI)
Kelvin
metric system
molar mass
mole
ratio method
United States Customary System of Units

Chapter Outline

This chapter presents systems of measurement, their units and symbols, and strategies and procedures for converting among them.

UNITED STATES CUSTOMARY SYSTEM OF UNITS

The **United States Customary System of Units** is also called the "English Imperial" or "American" system. The most commonly used units in this system appear below.

Length	inch (in)	
	foot (ft)	= 12 inches
	yard (yd)	= 3 feet
	mile (mi)	= 1760 yards = 5280 feet
Volume	cup (c)	
	pint (pt)	= 2 cups
	quart (qt)	= 2 pints
	gallon (gal)	= 4 quarts
Weight	ounce (oz)	
	pound (lb)	= 16 ounces
	(short) ton	= 2000 pounds

THE METRIC SYSTEM

In contrast to the U.S. system, the **metric system** has only one basic unit for length, one for volume, and one for weight.

Length	meter (m)
Volume	liter (L)*
Weight**	gram (g)

* The symbol for "liter" is usually a capital "L" because in some typefaces the lowercase letter "l" is confusingly similar to the number "1" and to the letter "I."
** Although we use the terms "weight" and "mass" interchangeably, mass is the amount of matter in a substance, whereas weight is the gravitational force on that matter. Under ordinary circumstances in the laboratory, we use the two terms as though they had the same meaning. In some other contexts, however, they are not interchangeable.

Prefixes and How to Interpret Them

The metric system exploits the convenience of the number "10." As Table 4-1 ★ shows, we attach a prefix to the basic unit of measure to create a decimal multiple or submultiple. The purpose of prefixes is to reduce the number of zeros in the value; it is much easier to write "μg" than it is to write "0.000001 g" or "1×10^{-6} g."

Let us consider some examples, starting with the basic unit of "gram" (g), which is about the weight of a typical paper clip. If we have an object that weighs 1000 g, we can report the weight as such, or we can call it "1 kilogram" (1 kg). As Table 4-1 shows, 1 kg is the same as 1000 of its basic unit, the gram:

$$1 \text{ kg} = 1000 \text{ g}$$

If we have an object that weighs 0.001 g, we can report the weight as such, or we can call it "1 milligram" (1 mg). As Table 4-1 shows, 1 mg is the same as $\frac{1}{1000}$, or one-thousandth, of its basic unit, the gram:

$$1 \text{ mg} = 0.001 \text{ g}$$

★ **TABLE 4-1** Metric Prefixes and the Arithmetic Relationships They Indicate

Prefix	Symbol	Factor (How many, or how much, of the basic unit)	Power of 10 (10^x)	American Term
giga	G	1,000,000,000	9	billion
mega	M	1,000,000	6	million
kilo	k	1000	3	thousand
hecto	h	100	2	hundred
deka (or deca)	da	10	1	ten
No prefix. This is the level of the *basic unit* (meter, liter, gram)		1	0	one
deci	d	1/10 (0.1)	−1	one-tenth
centi	c	1/100 (0.01)	−2	one-hundredth
milli	m	1/1000 (0.001)	−3	one-thousandth
micro	μ*	1/1,000,000 (0.000001)	−6	one-millionth
nano	n	1/1,000,000,000 (0.000000001)	−9	one-billionth
pico	p	1/1,000,000,000,000 (0.000000000001)	−12	one-trillionth
femto	f	1/1,000,000,000,000,000 (0.000000000000001)	−15	one-quadrillionth
atto	a	1/1,000,000,000,000,000,000 (0.000000000000000001)	−18	one-quintillionth

*This is the proper symbol for "micro," although some clinics and hospitals prefer the abbreviation "mc" because the handwritten letter "μ" can be mistaken for "M" or "m".

Likewise, a microliter (μL) is a millionth of a liter:

$$1\ \mu L = \frac{1}{1{,}000{,}000} L = 0.000001\ L = 10^{-6}\ L$$

A kilometer (km) is 1000 meters:

$$1\ km = 1000\ m = 10^3\ m$$

Converting Between Units

It is often necessary to convert one unit into another, whether within one system or between systems. Always remember that *in moving to a larger unit, we divide;* we do not multiply. Conversely, *in moving to a smaller unit, we multiply;* we do not divide. This is true in all unit conversions, regardless of the system. For example, in moving from "minutes" to "hours," the number goes down, not up:

60 minutes → 1 hour

In moving to the larger unit ("hours"), we have divided by "60."

However, in moving from "hours" to "minutes," the number goes up, not down; we multiply by "60" in moving to the smaller unit:

1 hour → 60 minutes

In the metric system, there are several equally effective ways to think through a conversion involving prefixes. We present two approaches now and two more later.

APPROACH 1

This approach comprises two steps.

Step 1 In Table 4-1, locate the starting prefix and the target prefix and note their corresponding powers of 10. Subtract the target power of 10 from the starting power of 10:

$$\text{starting power of 10} - \text{target power of 10} = \Delta x$$

Step 2 Multiply the starting value by $10^{\Delta x}$, where Δx is the difference between the powers of 10.

Consider, for example, the conversion of "100 g" to "kg."

Step 1

	Prefix	Unit	Power of 10
Starting	None	gram	0
Target	Kilo	kilogram	3

$$\Delta x = \text{Starting power of 10} - \text{Target power of 10} = 0 - 3 = \underline{-3}$$

Step 2

$$(\text{Starting value}) \times 10^{\Delta x} = 100 \times 10^{-3} = 100 \div 1000 = 0.1$$

Therefore, 100 g = 0.1 kg

Notice that, in moving to the larger unit (g → kg), the value went down, not up; the procedure was the same as *division* by 1000. Here is a way to visualize the conversion:

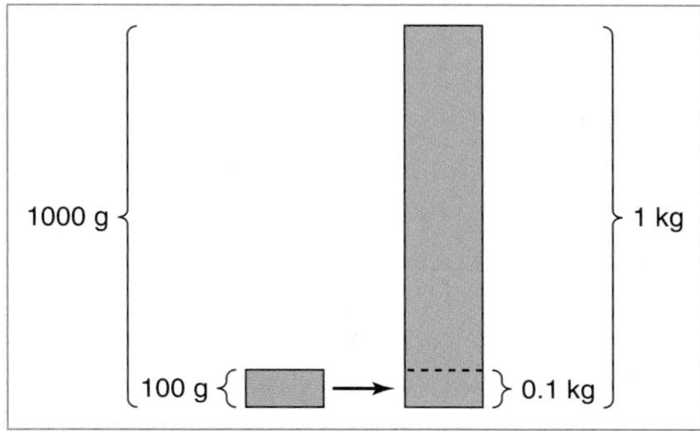

Now let us take an example that converts in the opposite direction, say, from "0.1 mg" to "µg."

Step 1

	Prefix	Unit	Power of 10
Starting	Milli	milligram	−3
Target	Micro	microgram	−6

$$\Delta x = \text{Starting power of 10} - \text{Target power of 10} = (-3) - (-6) = \underline{3}$$

Step 2

$$(\text{Starting value}) \times 10^{\Delta x} = 0.1 \times 10^{3} = 0.1 \times 1000 = 100$$

Therefore, 0.1 mg = 100 µg

Notice that, in moving to the smaller unit (mg → µg), the value went up, not down; the procedure was the same as *multiplication* by 1000. Here is a way to visualize the conversion:

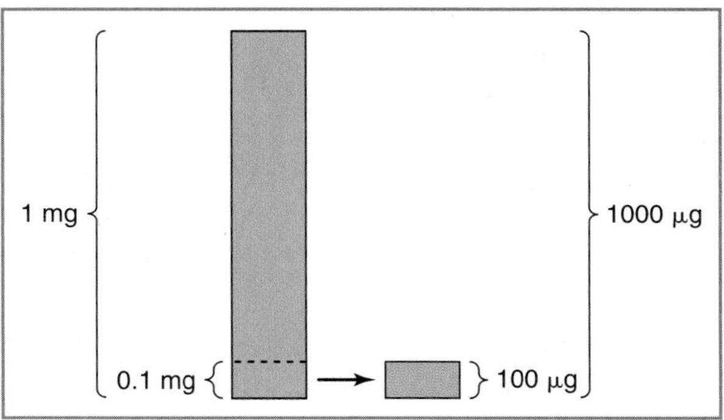

APPROACH 2

This approach also comprises two steps.

Step 1 In Table 4-1, locate the starting prefix and the target prefix and note their corresponding factors. Calculate the ratio of the larger to the smaller.

$$\frac{\text{larger factor}}{\text{smaller factor}}$$

Step 2 If the conversion is going toward the larger unit, then *divide* the value by the above ratio. If it is going toward the smaller unit, then *multiply*.

Let us turn to the same two examples we saw in the first approach. In the conversion of "100 g" into "kg," the larger factor is 1000 (for "kilo"), and the smaller is 1 (for "gram," a basic unit). Therefore, the ratio of the larger to the smaller is

$$\frac{1000}{1} = 1000$$

Because the conversion is going toward the larger unit, we *divide* the original value by the ratio, which is 1000:

$$\frac{100}{1000} = 0.1 \text{ kg}$$

In the second example, we carry out a conversion toward the smaller unit, that is, from "0.1 mg" to "μg". The larger factor is 0.001 (for "milli"), and the smaller is 0.000001 (for "micro"). Therefore, the ratio of the larger to the smaller is

$$\frac{0.001}{0.000001} = 1000$$

Because the conversion is going toward the smaller unit, we *multiply* the original value by the ratio, which is 1000:

$$0.1 \times 1000 = 100\ \mu\text{g}$$

APPROACHES 3 AND 4

Dimensional analysis and the *ratio method* are two more approaches to solving problems of this type, but because their usefulness extends far beyond the conversion of metric prefixes, we treat them in their own later sections of this chapter.

Let us consider a final example that has a numeral other than "0" or "1," say, the conversion of 0.382 mg into "μg."

Using approach 1:

Step 1.

$$\text{Starting power of 10} - \text{target power of 10} = \Delta x$$

$$(-3) - (-6) = 3$$

Step 2.

$$0.382 \text{ mg} \times 10^3 = 382\ \mu\text{g}$$

Using approach 2:

Step 1.

$$\frac{\text{larger factor}}{\text{smaller factor}} = \frac{0.001}{0.000001} = 1000$$

Step 2. Conversion is toward the smaller unit. Therefore, we multiply:

$$0.382 \text{ mg} \times 1000 = 382\ \mu\text{g}$$

INTERNATIONAL SYSTEM OF UNITS

The **International System of Units**, abbreviated "SI" for the French *Système International d'Unités*, is a modern version of the metric system. Established in 1960, the SI has become the most widely used system of measurement in the world, although the United States still employs customary units alongside it.

There are seven basic units of measurement in the SI.

Length	meter (m)
Weight (Mass)	kilogram (kg)
Amount of Substance	mole (mol)
Time	second (s)
Electric Current	ampere (A)
Temperature	kelvin (K)
Luminous Intensity	candela (cd)

Some non-SI units are acceptable for use within the SI. In the clinical laboratory, the most important of these units is the "liter." Furthermore, it is acceptable to use metric prefixes with SI units, although there is one exception. Because the basic unit "kilogram" already has a multiplying prefix, we may not attach another prefix to it. For example, we may *not* report a "microkilogram" (μkg). Instead, we attach a prefix to the unit "gram" (that prefix would be "milli").

☑ CHECKPOINT 4-1

Carry out the following conversions.

(a) 1 dL → mL (b) 100 μL → L (c) 4 cg → mg
(d) 150 cm → m (e) 2.0×10^4 ng → kg (f) 6.7×10^{-3} L → mL

(a) Using approach 1:

$$\Delta x = (-1) - (-3) = 2 \qquad 1\text{ dL} \times 10^2 = 100\text{ mL}$$

Using approach 2:

$$\frac{\text{larger factor}}{\text{smaller factor}} = \frac{0.1}{0.001} = 100 \qquad 1\text{ dL} \times 100 = 100\text{ mL}$$

(b) 0.0001 L (c) 40 mg (d) 1.5 m (e) 2.0×10^{-8} kg (f) 6.7 mL

EQUIVALENCIES BETWEEN SYSTEMS

It is possible to interconvert U.S. customary units and metric units. The following table lists the most common equivalencies used in the clinical laboratory.

Length	Volume	Weight
1 in = 2.54 cm	1 c = 236.6 mL	1 oz = 28.35 g
1 yd = 0.914 m	1 gal = 3.785 L	1 lb = 0.454 kg
1 mi = 1.609 km		
1 cm = 0.394 in	1 mL = 0.00423 c	1 g = 0.0353 oz
1 m = 1.094 yd	1 L = 0.264 gal	1 kg = 2.20 lb
1 km = 0.622 mi		

THE MOLE

A **mole**, which we symbolize as "mol," is the amount of a substance that consists of as many entities (molecules, ions, particles, etc.) as there are atoms in exactly 12 grams of the element ^{12}C (carbon-12). Although that definition is just a bit convoluted, the number in question is

$$6.022137 \times 10^{23} \text{ or } 602{,}213{,}700{,}000{,}000{,}000{,}000{,}000$$

We call this **Avogadro's number**.[1] In other words, 12 grams of ^{12}C consists of 602,213,700,000,000,000,000,000 atoms. The classic illustration of this number's unimaginable enormity is to try to appreciate an Avogadro's number of dollars. If a person started with 6.022137×10^{23} dollars, and spent a billion dollars every second for 75 years, more than 99.99% of the starting balance would still be available.

Like the prefixes on basic units of measurement, the term "mole" simplifies quantities by deleting zeros. After all, it is much easier to talk about frequent-flyer "miles" than it is to talk about frequent-flyer "inches." To erase even more zeros, we can affix those same metric prefixes to "mole" or "mol." For example,

$$0.001 \text{ mol} = 1 \text{ millimole} = 1 \text{ mmol}$$

$$0.000001 \text{ mol} = 1 \text{ micromole} = 1\ \mu\text{mol}$$

$$0.000000001 \text{ mol} = 1 \text{ nanomole} = 1 \text{ nmol}$$

$$0.000000000001 \text{ mol} = 1 \text{ picomole} = 1 \text{ pmol}$$

If the masses of two atoms differ, then a mole of one substance weighs more than a mole of the other. Consequently, a mole of ^{12}C atoms weighs 12.0 grams, and a mole of Fe (iron) atoms weighs 55.8 grams.

The **formula weight** of a substance is the sum of all the atomic weights in the formula. For example, the formula weight of water (H_2O) is 18.0 g:

$$\underbrace{2 \times 1.0 \text{ g}}_{\text{H atoms}} + \underbrace{1 \times 16.0 \text{ g}}_{\text{O atom}}$$

Therefore, one mole of water molecules weighs 18.0 grams. Likewise, a mole of glucose ($C_6H_{12}O_6$) weighs 180 grams:

$$\underbrace{6 \times 12.0 \text{ g}}_{\text{C atoms}} + \underbrace{12 \times 1.0 \text{ g}}_{\text{H atoms}} + \underbrace{6 \times 16.0 \text{ g}}_{\text{O atoms}}$$

The **molar mass** of a substance is numerically equal to the formula weight and is defined as the mass of one mole of the substance. Table 4-2 ★ lists several selected elements and their average atomic weights.

★ **TABLE 4-2** Selected Elements and Their Atomic Weights

Element	Average Atomic Weight (g/mol)
Hydrogen (H)	1.01
Calcium (Ca)	40.08
Carbon (C)	12.01
Chlorine (Cl)	35.45
Cobalt (Co)	58.93
Magnesium (Mg)	24.31
Nitrogen (N)	14.01
Oxygen (O)	16.00
Phosphorus (P)	30.97
Potassium (K)	39.10
Sodium (Na)	22.99
Sulfur (S)	32.07

[1]The value of 6.023 is also used widely as the significand. Because the difference between 6.023 and 6.022 is only 0.02%, this book uses both values.

☑ CHECKPOINT 4-2

Compute the formula weight of each of the following chemical compounds.

(a) CO_2 (b) H_2S (c) $MgSO_4$ (d) Na_2O

(a) (1 × 12.01 g/mol) + (2 × 16.00 g/mol) = 44.01 g/mol
(b) 34.09 g/mol (c) 120.38 g/mol (d) 61.98 g/mol

DIMENSIONAL ANALYSIS

Mentioned earlier, **dimensional analysis** is a unit-conversion technique based on the fact that any quantity can be multiplied by "1" without its value being changed. We use this technique to convert one unit into another by multiplying by what we call "unit factors." Let us consider four examples.

EXAMPLE 1

To convert "3.0 in" to "cm," we employ the equivalence of

$$1 \text{ in} = 2.54 \text{ cm}$$

From this equivalence, we can create two unit factors:

$$\frac{1 \text{ in}}{2.54 \text{ cm}} \quad \text{and} \quad \frac{2.54 \text{ cm}}{1 \text{ in}}$$

Next, we multiply our original value, "3.0 in," by the unit factor that gives us our target unit, "cm":

$$3.0 \text{ in} \times \frac{2.54 \text{ cm}}{1 \text{ in}} = 7.6 \text{ cm}$$

The units of "in" cancel, leaving the units of "cm", and we conclude that 3.0 inches is the same as 7.6 centimeters.

To convert in the reverse direction, say, from "9.1 cm" to "in," we follow the same procedure by multiplying our original value by the unit factor that gives us our target unit:

$$9.1 \text{ cm} \times \frac{1 \text{ in}}{2.54 \text{ cm}} = 3.6 \text{ in}$$

The units of "cm" cancel, leaving the units of "in."

EXAMPLE 2

It is sometimes necessary to string several unit factors together. For example, let us calculate the number of ounces in one ton. We start with "1 ton," identify our target as "ounces", and then note any unit factors that link "tons" to "ounces."

Conversion: 1 ton → ? oz

Relevant Unit Factors:

$$\frac{2000 \text{ lb}}{\text{ton}} \quad \frac{\text{ton}}{2000 \text{ lb}} \qquad\qquad \frac{16 \text{ oz}}{\text{lb}} \quad \frac{\text{lb}}{16 \text{ oz}}$$

Solution: $1 \text{ ton} \times \dfrac{2000 \text{ lb}}{\text{ton}} \times \dfrac{16 \text{ oz}}{\text{lb}} = 32{,}000 \text{ oz}$

We solve the problem by multiplying the original value ("1 ton" in this case) by unit factors in such a way that only the target units emerge at the end of the calculation. The units of "ton" cancel, as do the units of "lb." We conclude that there are 32,000 ounces in one ton.

EXAMPLE 3

Let us now try a slightly longer conversion, one that is more germane to laboratory work. How many micromoles are there in 6.0 milligrams of glucose (molar mass = 180 g/mol)?

Conversion: 6.0 mg → ? μmol

Relevant Unit Factors:

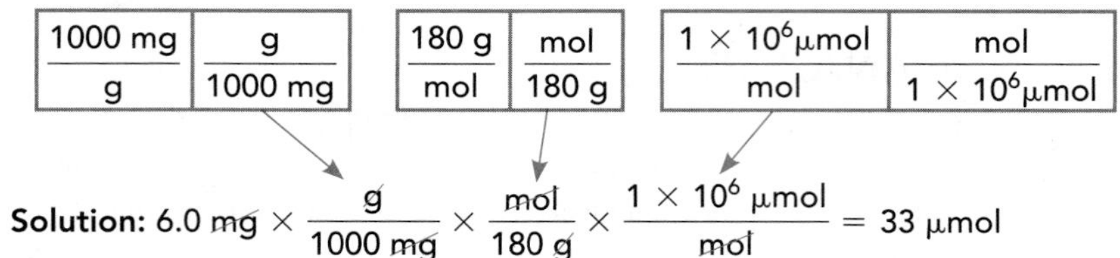

$$\frac{1000\ \text{mg}}{\text{g}} \quad \frac{\text{g}}{1000\ \text{mg}} \qquad \frac{180\ \text{g}}{\text{mol}} \quad \frac{\text{mol}}{180\ \text{g}} \qquad \frac{1 \times 10^6 \mu\text{mol}}{\text{mol}} \quad \frac{\text{mol}}{1 \times 10^6 \mu\text{mol}}$$

Solution: $6.0\ \text{mg} \times \frac{\text{g}}{1000\ \text{mg}} \times \frac{\text{mol}}{180\ \text{g}} \times \frac{1 \times 10^6\ \mu\text{mol}}{\text{mol}} = 33\ \mu\text{mol}$

As in the earlier example, we solve this problem by multiplying the original value (6.0 mg) by unit factors in such a way that only the target units emerge at the end of the calculation. The units of "mg," "g," and "mol" cancel. For glucose, then, we conclude that 6.0 mg is the equivalent of 33 μmol.

EXAMPLE 4

This example of dimensional analysis involves a concentration. Suppose we must convert a test result of 0.739 mmol/L to "nmol/mL." Although the strategy is the same as in the preceding two examples, we now have *two* units to convert.

Conversion: 0.739 mmol/L → ? nmol/mL

Relevant Unit Factors:

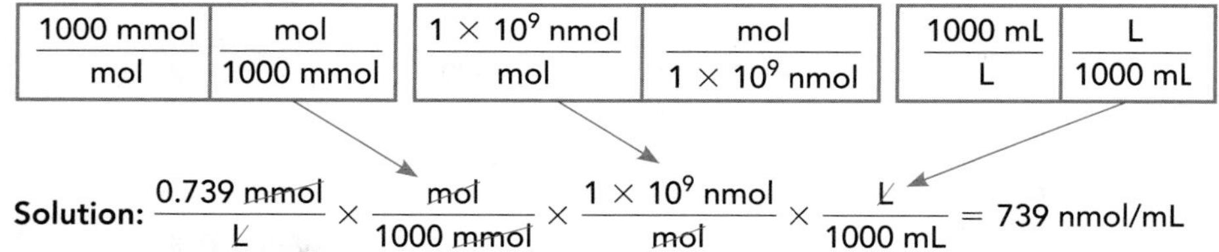

$$\frac{1000\ \text{mmol}}{\text{mol}} \quad \frac{\text{mol}}{1000\ \text{mmol}} \qquad \frac{1 \times 10^9\ \text{nmol}}{\text{mol}} \quad \frac{\text{mol}}{1 \times 10^9\ \text{nmol}} \qquad \frac{1000\ \text{mL}}{\text{L}} \quad \frac{\text{L}}{1000\ \text{mL}}$$

Solution: $\frac{0.739\ \text{mmol}}{\text{L}} \times \frac{\text{mol}}{1000\ \text{mmol}} \times \frac{1 \times 10^9\ \text{nmol}}{\text{mol}} \times \frac{\text{L}}{1000\ \text{mL}} = 739\ \text{nmol/mL}$

☑ CHECKPOINT 4-3

1. Using dimensional analysis, convert "890 nmol/L" to "μmol/dL."

$$\frac{890\ \text{nmol}}{\text{L}} \times \frac{\text{mol}}{1 \times 10^9\ \text{nmol}} \times \frac{1 \times 10^6\ \mu\text{mol}}{\text{mol}} \times \frac{\text{L}}{10\ \text{dL}} = 0.089\ \mu\text{mol/dL}$$

2. Using dimensional analysis, convert "0.864 g of CO_2" to "mmol of CO_2."

$$0.864\ \text{g}\ CO_2 \times \frac{\text{mol}\ CO_2}{44.01\ \text{g}\ CO_2} \times \frac{1000\ \text{mmol}\ CO_2}{\text{mol}\ CO_2} = 19.6\ \text{mmol}\ CO_2$$

THE RATIO METHOD

The **ratio method** is another way to convert between units. For example, if we want to convert "13 yards" to "feet," we can set up an equation of ratios and then cross-multiply:

$$\frac{3\text{ ft}}{\text{yd}} = \frac{x}{13\text{ yd}}$$

$$(3\text{ ft})(13\text{ yd}) = (1\text{ yd})x$$

$$\frac{(3\text{ ft})(13\text{ yd})}{\text{yd}} = x$$

$$39\text{ ft} = x$$

For longer conversions, a sequence of ratio calculations can substitute for dimensional analysis. Consider example 3 above, the conversion of "6.0 mg" of glucose to "micromoles." The order in which we convert the units is

$$\text{mg} \rightarrow \text{g} \rightarrow \text{mol} \rightarrow \mu\text{mol}$$

This is the same order in which we converted them using dimensional analysis above.

Conversion 1 (mg → g) $$\frac{1000\text{ mg}}{\text{g}} = \frac{6.0\text{ mg}}{x}$$

$$x = 0.0060\text{ g}$$

Conversion 2 (g → mol) $$\frac{180\text{ g}}{\text{mol}} = \frac{0.0060\text{ g}}{x}$$

$$x = 3.3 \times 10^{-5}\text{ mol}$$

Conversion 3 (mol → μmol) $$\frac{1 \times 10^{6}\ \mu\text{mol}}{\text{mol}} = \frac{x}{3.3 \times 10^{-5}\text{ mol}}$$

$$x = 33\ \mu\text{mol}$$

☑ CHECKPOINT 4-4

Using the ratio method, carry out the following conversions.

(a) 6.2 m → yd (b) 535 μL → mL (c) 0.5844 g NaCl → μmol NaCl

(a) $\frac{1.094\text{ yd}}{\text{m}} = \frac{x}{6.2\text{ m}}$ $x = 6.8$ yd

(b) 0.535 mL (c) 10,000 μmol = 1.0×10^{4} μmol

TEMPERATURE SCALES

There are three temperature scales, each with its own history and utility. On the **Fahrenheit** scale, the freezing point of water (at sea level) is 32 degrees (°F) and the boiling point is 212°F, setting these two temperatures 180F° apart. On the **Celsius** scale, however, water freezes at 0°C and boils at 100°C, the interval being 100C°.

Thus, 180 Fahrenheit degrees covers the same range as 100 Celsius degrees, making each Celsius degree 1.8 times a Fahrenheit degree:

$$\frac{180\text{ F}^\circ}{100\text{ C}^\circ} = 1.8\text{ F}^\circ/\text{C}^\circ$$

There are two formulas for converting between Fahrenheit and Celsius temperatures:

$$°F = \left(°C \times \frac{9}{5}\right) + 32°$$

$$°C = \frac{5}{9}(°F - 32°)$$

The third temperature scale bears the name of its developer, Lord Kelvin. On the **Kelvin** scale, the zero-degree point corresponds to the theoretical absence of all thermal energy, "absolute zero." A temperature on the Kelvin scale is represented by "K," *with no degree symbol.*

Each degree, or increment, on the Kelvin scale is a "kelvin" (all lowercase). Each increment on the Kelvin scale is the same as an increment on the Celsius scale. Therefore, the two scales have a simple relationship, and the formula for interconverting them is

$$K = °C + 273.15$$

Summary

1. The *metric system* has only one basic unit for length, one for volume, and one for weight. The *United States Customary System of Units* has several units for each quantity.
2. The metric system is built on the number "10." Prefixes create decimal multiples and submultiples of basic units.
3. The *International System of Units (SI)* has seven basic units but permits the use of some non-SI units.
4. U.S. customary units and metric units are interconvertible.
5. The *mole* ("mol") is the amount of a substance that consists of as many entities (molecules, ions, particles, etc.) as there are atoms in exactly 12 grams of the element ^{12}C (carbon-12). The number is 6.022137×10^{23} or 602,213,700,000,000,000,000,000. It is called *Avogadro's number*. We can affix metric prefixes to "mole" or "mol."
6. The *formula weight* of a substance is the sum of all the atomic weights in the formula. The *molar mass* of a substance is numerically equal to the formula weight and is defined as the mass of one mole of the substance.
7. *Dimensional analysis* is a problem-solving technique based on the fact that any quantity can be multiplied by "1" without its value being changed. We use this technique to convert one unit into another by multiplying by "unit factors."
8. The *ratio method* is useful in the conversion of units. An equation of ratios is established, and then cross-multiplication gives the value of the unknown quantity. For longer conversions, a sequence of ratio calculations can substitute for dimensional analysis.
9. There are three temperature scales: *Fahrenheit*, *Celsius*, and *Kelvin*. Their values are interconvertible by these equations:

$$°F = \left(°C \times \frac{9}{5}\right) + 32°$$

$$°C = \frac{5}{9}(°F - 32°)$$

$$K = °C + 273.15$$

Practice Problems

1. (LO 1, 2, 4, 5) Carry out each of the following unit conversions.

(a) 3.1 mL → μL (b) 420 ng → mg
(c) 0.002 mL → μL (d) 0.78 μg → ng
(e) 8.5 dL → L (f) 1445 mg → g
(g) 0.0364 L → mL (h) 13 pg → ng
(i) 620 nmol → μmol (j) 9.7×10^{-5} mol → mmol
(k) 4.0 dL → mL (l) 73 μg → mg
(m) 400 μL → mL (n) 2.5×10^{-4} μg → pg
(o) 6.09×10^{4} μmol → mol (p) 0.62 L → dL
(q) 705 μmol → pmol (r) 2 ng → pg

2. (LO 6) Calculate the molar mass of each of the following substances.

(a) KCl (b) NH_3 (c) K_3PO_4 (d) Na_2S (e) $MgCl_2$

3. (LO 4, 5, 7) For each of the following substances, suppose you have either the actual mass or the actual number of moles specified. Complete the table by supplying the missing information.

Substance	Molar Mass (g/mol)	Actual Mass (g)	Actual Moles
sodium chloride ($NaCl$)	58.44	3.50	**(a)**
sucrose ($C_{12}H_{22}O_{11}$)	342.3	**(b)**	0.0004
urea (CH_4N_2O)	60.06	0.70	**(c)**
potassium hydrogen phosphate ($KHPO_4$)	174.18	**(d)**	0.062
glucose ($C_6H_{12}O_6$)	180.2	5.66	**(e)**

4. (LO 8) Convert each of the following Celsius temperatures to its Fahrenheit equivalent.

   (a) 37°C (b) 82°C (c) 140°C (d) −20°C (e) 4°C

5. (LO 8) Convert each of the following Fahrenheit temperatures to its Celsius equivalent.

   (a) 72°F (b) 230°F (c) −7°F (d) 45°F (e) 10°F

6. (LO 8) Convert each of the following Celsius temperatures to its Kelvin equivalent.

   (a) 0°C (b) 100°C (c) −273.15°C

7. (LO 3, 4, 5) Carry out the following conversions.

   (a) 53 km → mi (b) 5.6 in → cm (c) 128 lb → kg
   (d) 2 kg → oz (e) 31 ft → m (f) 3500 yd → km
   (g) 8.9 L → gal (h) 0.20 cups → mL (i) 6.2 qt → L

Contextual Problems

1. (LO 1, 2, 4) If the typical red blood cell has a volume of 90 fL, then how many such cells could theoretically occupy a volume of 1 mL?

2. (LO 1, 2, 4, 5) One of the automated instruments in your laboratory requires the preparation of a special cleaning solution, made by mixing 30 mL of concentrate with enough water to bring the final volume to 250 mL. How much concentrate do you use to make 1 L of the cleaning solution?

3. (LO 2, 4, 5) On a balance that reads in "grams," you must weight out 450 mg of a substance. How many grams does this represent?

4. (LO 2, 4, 5) Using a pipet that reads in "microliters," you must deliver 0.080 mL of a solution. How many microliters does this represent?

5. (LO 2, 4, 5) Some of your laboratory's instruments return test results in units that must be converted into other units before being released into the hospital information system. Convert each of the following results into the units specified.

   (a) 628 pg/mL → ng/L

   (b) 0.0198 μmol/L → pmol/mL

   (c) 1.74 μg/dL → mg/mL

   (d) 0.49 mmol/L → μmol/dL

PEARSON
myhealthprofessionskit™

Go to www.myhealthprofessionskit.com <http://www.myhealthprofessionskit.com/> to access the Companion Website created for this textbook. Simply select "Clinical Laboratory Science" from the choice of disciplines. Find this book and log in using your username and password to access additional practice problems, answers to the practice and contextual problems, additional information, and more.

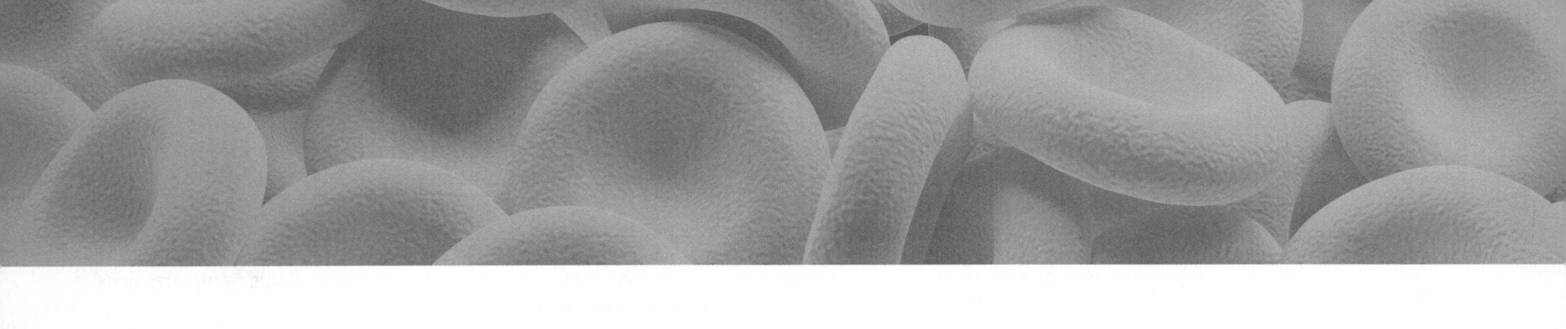

5 Solutions and Concentrations

Learning Objectives

At the end of this chapter, the student should be able to do the following:

1. Explain the nature of solutions and distinguish between the solute and solvent
2. Explain the various expressions of concentration
3. Calculate and interpret concentrations expressed in any of these four systems: percentage, molarity, molality, and normality
4. Use specific gravity in diluting concentrated solutions
5. Describe the relative convenience of the *p*H scale
6. Calculate *p*H values and interconvert them with molarity
7. Interconvert expressions of concentration

Key Terms

aqueous
concentration
dissolve
equivalent
equivalent weight
immiscible
insoluble
miscible
molality
molarity
normality
*p*H
ppb
ppm
ppt
soluble
solute
solution
solvent
sparingly soluble
specific gravity
(v/v)
(w/v)
(w/w)

Chapter Outline

A **solution** is a homogeneous mixture of two or more substances that do not chemically react with each other. Because the distribution of substances is uniform throughout a homogeneous mixture, a solution's composition, appearance, and properties are the same in any one portion as they are in any other portion. The substance present in the largest amount is called the **solvent**, whereas every other component of the solution is referred to as a **solute**. As a mixture forms, the solute is said to **dissolve** in the solvent. In the clinical laboratory, the most common solvent is water, and a solution of anything in water is referred to as **aqueous**.

A solution may consist of a solid and a liquid, a common example being hot tea sweetened with sugar. An example from the clinical laboratory is normal saline, which is a well-defined solution of sodium chloride in water. The solids in these cases are **soluble**, meaning they dissolve in water. **Insoluble** solids do not dissolve in water, whereas **sparingly soluble** solids dissolve only to a small degree.

A solution may be composed of two liquids, common examples of which are (1) rubbing alcohol, which is a mixture of isopropyl alcohol and water, and (2) vinegar, which is a mixture of acetic acid and water. In such cases, the liquids are **miscible** with each other, meaning that they are capable of being mixed in any ratio without separating. Two **immiscible** liquids, such as gasoline and water, do not form solutions but instead separate on standing, with the less dense liquid rising to the top.

A solution may comprise a gas dissolved in a liquid. Two common examples are (1) sparkling water, which is just an aqueous solution of carbon dioxide gas, and (2) household ammonia, which is an aqueous solution of ammonia gas.

Depending on the test we are conducting, serum and other body fluids can be regarded as any or all of the three kinds of solution outlined above. For example, when we quantify alcohol in blood, the serum is a liquid-in-liquid solution. However, we can view it as a solid-in-liquid solution when glucose is the analyte of interest or as a gas-in-liquid solution when the partial pressure of oxygen is being determined.

This chapter focuses on the calculation and expression of **concentration**, which is a measure of how much solute and solvent are present in a solution. It is difficult to exaggerate the importance of mastering this material because the consequences of reporting an incorrect concentration on a patient sample can be grave, as, for example, when it leads to the misdiagnosis of an illness or the administration of an inappropriate drug. Nearly every liquid in a clinical laboratory—from reagents to control solutions, from serum to spinal fluid, from disinfectants to cleaning agents—has a concentration that we must specify correctly and unambiguously.

Quantifying an analyte in a patient sample requires that the concentration of every reagent used in the assay be accurate to an acceptable degree. Although some reagents do come ready to use from the manufacturer, others must be prepared in the laboratory directly before use. Erroneous concentrations can even have repercussions not directly related to patient results. Consider two examples. First, the concentration of an unconsumed reagent that has expired may determine whether the solution is poured down the drain or consigned to hazardous waste—a decision that affects both the environment and the laboratory's budget. Second, there is the issue of laboratory hygiene. We commonly use bleach as a general disinfectant for surfaces in the laboratory. The required concentration, however, depends on the purpose; it may be as high as 10% for surface disinfection or as low as 0.5% for decontaminating the tubing in an automated instrument. If the concentration is too low, the bleach will fail to disinfect thoroughly; if too high, it might damage expensive parts. When bleach is an unsuitable disinfectant, alcohol serves as an alternative, most effective when its concentration is 70%; it is markedly less bactericidal at higher or lower concentrations. Thus, a solution labeled "70%" that was improperly prepared will lack the expected disinfecting power, possibly creating a risk to laboratory personnel.

EXPRESSING CONCENTRATION

There are many ways to express concentration, some deriving from convenience and others from tradition; it can be based on mass, volume, or number of moles.

Percentage

The following are the three common systems for expressing concentration as a mass or volume percentage.

- **Weight of solute per volume of solution (w/v).** In this system, the value is the number of grams of solute in 100 mL of solution. For example, "10% NaCl (w/v)" describes an aqueous solution of 10 grams of sodium chloride in every 100 mL of solution. Understand that this is *not* the same as 10 grams of NaCl in 100 mL of water (see "Molality"). Preparation of 10% NaCl entails dissolving 10 g NaCl in a small volume of water in a volumetric flask and then adding water until the volume is 100 mL.

- **Weight of solute per weight of solution (w/w).** In this system, the value is the number of grams of solute in 100 grams of solution. Thus, 6% KOH (w/w) is a solution of 6 grams of sodium hydroxide in 100 grams of solution. In simple terms, it is prepared by dissolving 6 g KOH in a small volume of water in a suitable vessel resting on a balance and then adding water until the weight of the solution is 100 g.
- **Volume of solute per volume of solution (v/v).** Used for liquid solutes, this system gives the number of milliliters of solute in 100 mL of solution. Therefore, 70% ethanol (v/v) is a solution of 70 mL of ethanol in 100 mL of solution, prepared by transferring 70 mL of ethanol into a volumetric flask and then adding water until the volume is 100 mL. Because we can weigh liquids, of course, we may also express the concentration of a liquid-in-liquid solution in the other two systems (w/v, w/w).

At this point, it should be clear that expressing concentration just as a percentage (e.g., "10% $C_6H_{12}O_6$") is inadequate because it does not give the basis for the ratio. Therefore, it is necessary to specify the system in a suffix: "10% $C_6H_{12}O_6$ (w/w)."

Parts-Per Notation

For very dilute solutions, when the value of the percentage is inconveniently small, we can express the concentration as "parts per million" (**ppm**), "parts per billion" (**ppb**), or "parts per trillion" (**ppt**). Strictly speaking, "1 ppm" means "one part in one million parts," such as 1 gram of solute in 1,000,000 grams of solution. Because the units in the numerator and denominator are the same, they cancel each other and the value turns out dimensionless. Thus, this system is similar to that of expressing concentrations as weight-per-weight percentages, or "% (w/w)." Consider this example:

$$\begin{aligned} 10 \text{ ppm} &= 10 \text{ g solute/1,000,000 g solution} \\ &= 0.001 \text{ g solute/100 g solution} \\ &= 0.001\% \text{ (w/w)} \end{aligned}$$

For aqueous solutions, however, parts-per notation is sometimes used as an alternative to weight-per-volume (w/v) percentages, even though this practice can cause confusion by mixing units. Because the scientific community knows that 1000 grams of water has a volume of 1 liter, and because a very dilute aqueous solution has the same mass as an equal volume of water, exchanging mass for volume in the parts-per expression does not appreciably change the information it gives us. For example,

$$\begin{aligned} 6 \text{ ppm} &= 6 \text{ g of solute/1,000,000 g of solution} \\ &= 0.006 \text{ g of solute/1000 g of solution} \\ &= 0.006 \text{ g of solute/liter of solution} \end{aligned}$$

Therefore, we can use "ppm" to mean 1 mg of solute in 1 L of very dilute solution:

$$\begin{aligned} 1 \text{ ppm} &= 1 \text{ g/1,000,000 mL} \\ &= 0.001 \text{ g/1000 mL} \\ &= 1 \text{ mg/L} \end{aligned}$$

Expressing this concentration as "1 ppm" is clearly easier than writing it out as a percentage, "0.0001% (w/v)":

$$\begin{aligned} 1 \text{ ppm} &= 0.001 \text{ g/1000 mL} \\ &= 0.0001 \text{ g/100 mL} \\ &= 0.0001\% \text{ (w/v)} \end{aligned}$$

☑ CHECKPOINT 5-1

1. What is the % (w/v) of a solution that comprises 8.2 g of NaOH per 100 mL?
2. How many grams of KCl are present in 200 mL of 10% KCl (w/v)?

1. 8.2%
2. Each 100 mL contains 10 g of KCl. Thus, 200 mL contains 20 g.

Molarity

Whereas percentage expresses concentration in terms of a measurable quantity (weight or volume), molarity does not. Rather, **molarity** refers to something that we can neither measure nor count: the molecules, ions, or atoms of a substance.

Molarity is the number of moles of a substance in 1 liter of solution (Equation 1). Thus, if 1 mole of glucose is dissolved in water and the volume is brought to 1 liter, the resulting solution is said to be "1 molar in glucose," and its concentration is written as "1 M." Often, we write the molarity of a substance as the name or chemical symbol in brackets: [glucose] or [Na^+].

$$\text{molarity} = \frac{\text{moles of solute}}{\text{liters of solution}}$$

EQUATION 1

Preparing a solution with its concentration expressed as molarity requires the ability to interconvert grams and moles. Remember that 1 mole equals 6.023×10^{23} particles, in the same way that a dozen is equal to 12 particles and a gross equals 144 particles. Remember also that the formula mass (or formula weight) is the sum of the masses of all the atoms and/or ions in a formula unit, and that the mass of 1 mole of a substance is its molar mass.

A 1.0 M solution of glucose ($C_6H_{12}O_6$), then, comprises 1.0 mole of glucose, or 180 grams, in a volume of 1.0 liter. Of course, the solution should be at room temperature and at atmospheric pressure, or its concentration may not be exactly 1 M.

There are variations on the molarity theme intended to simplify the expression of low concentrations. For example, if the concentration is 0.001 M, there is 1 millimole in every liter of solution. A simpler representation of this solution is "1 mM," or "1 millimolar." Likewise, if the concentration is 0.000001 M, there is 1 micromole per liter of solution; this is more easily expressed as "1 μM," or "1 micromolar." Another unit commonly used in the laboratory, especially in research, is "nM," or "nanomolar."

Because molarity is a function of volume, its value changes with temperature. Therefore, a cold solution may have a different molarity than it does when warm.

☑ CHECKPOINT 5-2

1. What is the molarity of a solution comprising 2 moles of sucrose (table sugar) in 4 liters?
2. How many moles of sucrose are in 0.500 L of the above solution?

1. 0.50 M. The ratio is 2 mol per 4 L:

$$\frac{2\text{ mol}}{4\text{L}} = 0.50\text{ mol/L} = 0.50\text{ M}$$

2. 0.25 mol. The quantity 0.500 L is, of course, half a liter, and a liter contains 0.5 moles:

$$0.500\text{ L} \times \frac{0.50\text{ mol}}{\text{L}} = 0.25\text{ mol}$$

Molality

Molality denotes the amount of solute in solution per kilogram of *solvent*—not per kilogram of *solution*. The symbol is "*m*," pronounced "molal." For example, dissolving 1 mole of molecules in 2 kilograms of solvent constitutes a 0.5 *m* solution.

$$\text{molality} = \frac{\text{moles of solute}}{\text{kilograms of solvent}}$$

EQUATION 2

Unlike molarity, molality is not a function of volume, and its value, therefore, does not depend on temperature. Thus, a cold solution has the same molality as it does when warm.

Normality

Normality, symbolized by "*N*," is similar to molarity except that it expresses concentration in terms of **equivalent weight** rather than formula mass. The equivalent weight of a substance is the amount that contains, theoretically combines with, or theoretically replaces 1 mole of hydrogen ions (H^+).

Consider, for example, a 1 *N* (pronounced "one-normal") HCl solution. By definition, this solution comprises 1 equivalent weight of HCl, or 36.5 g, in a volume of 1 L. The amount of HCl that contains 1 mole of hydrogen ions is, of course, 1 mole; the molar mass of HCl is 36.5 g, which is, therefore, the equivalent weight. Thus, for HCl the normality and molarity are equal.

By contrast, consider a 1 *N* H_2SO_4 solution. Although this solution, like 1 *N* HCl, comprises 1 equivalent weight of H_2SO_4 in 1 L, only one-half a mole of H_2SO_4 contains 1 mole of hydrogen ions. Because the molar mass of H_2SO_4 is 98.1 g, the equivalent weight is half that value, or 49.0 g. Thus, for H_2SO_4, a 1 *N* solution is the same as a 0.5 M solution.

For an acid, then, an **equivalent** is one hydrogen ion in the formula. Thus, 1 mole of HCl is 1 equivalent, whereas 1 mole of H_2SO_4 is 2 equivalents and 1 mole of H_3PO_4 is 3 equivalents.

For a base or a salt, an equivalent is the number of hydrogen ions with which it can theoretically combine; however, we can just as easily regard it as 1 mole of ionic charges. For example, because the bicarbonate ion (HCO_3^-) carries a single charge and can combine with 1 hydrogen ion, then obviously 1 mole of bicarbonate ions carries 1 mole of charges and can combine with 1 mole of hydrogen ions. Therefore, 1 equivalent of HCO_3^- ions is 1 mole.

The magnesium ion (Mg^{2+}), by contrast, carries two charges and can theoretically replace two hydrogen ions. Thus, 1 mole of Mg^{2+} ions is the same as 2 equivalents.

In general, then, the number of equivalents is the product of the number of moles and the number of charges:

EQUATION 3

$$\text{equivalents} = \text{moles} \times \text{charges}$$

In fact, we can express concentration in terms of equivalents ("Eq"), a system widely used in medicine because it directly reports the concentration of positive or negative charges. For example, the concentration of potassium ion in serum typically can be about 5 mEq/L, which is the same as 5 mmol/L (or 5 mM). However, calcium ion (Ca^{2+}) can also typically be present in serum at about 5 mEq/L, which is *not* 5 mmol/L, but half of that, or 2.5 mmol/L. Clearly, a mole of potassium ions gives the same concentration of positive charges as does half a mole of calcium ions, but expressing that concentration in terms of equivalents makes it necessary to convert from moles to charges.

☑ CHECKPOINT 5-3

1. What is the normality of a solution consisting of 2 mol NaCl in 1 liter?
2. A 2 *N* H_2SO_4 solution has how many grams of H_2SO_4?

1. 2 *N*. One mole of NaCl is 1 equivalent.
2. An equivalent weight for sulfuric acid is half a mole, 49 g. Therefore, 2 equivalent weights is 98 g, the molar mass.

Preparing for Possible Changes

At this writing, the National Institute of Standards and Technology (NIST) considers obsolete the previously discussed three concentration terms "molarity," "molality," and "normality," along with their symbols, "M," "*m*," and "*N*," respectively. Nevertheless, the term "molarity" and its symbol remain very common in chemistry and probably will be so for a long time to come. The terms "molality" and "normality," despite being used less often than "molarity," are still common enough that it is necessary to understand them. Table 5-1 ★ summarizes the changes proposed by NIST.

SPECIFIC GRAVITY

Specific gravity is the ratio of the density of a solution to the density of water at 4°C (1 g/mL). A substance with a value greater than 1 is denser than water, and a substance with a value smaller than 1 is less dense. And, because specific gravity is a ratio of two densities, the units cancel each other, leaving only a magnitude.

Specific gravity is helpful in diluting concentrated commercial acids in the laboratory. Measuring the weight of a liquid is awkward and, when that liquid is a concentrated acid, dangerous. Measuring its volume, however, is markedly easier, although precautions are still necessary.

★ TABLE 5-1 Concentration Terms That NIST Considers Obsolete, and Their Proposed Replacements

Obsolete Quantity and Symbol	Proposed Term	Proposed Symbol	Proposed Units
Molarity (M)	Amount-of-substance concentration of *B*	c_B	mol/dm^3 mol/L kmol/m^3
Molality (*m*)	Molality of solute *B*	b_B	mol/kg
Normality (*N*)	Amount-of-substance concentration of H_nA	$c[(1/n)H_nA]$*	mol/dm^3 mol/L kmol/m^3

*In this notation, *n* represents the number of hydrogen ions an acid can release. For example, if the acid is sulfuric (H_2SO_4), then rather than writing "a 0.5 *N* solution of sulfuric acid," we would write "a solution of sulfuric acid with an amount-of-substance concentration of $c[(1/2)\ H_2SO_4]$ of 0.5 mol/L."

Suppose, for example, that you have a bottle of concentrated aqueous HCl, the label of which states the specific gravity to be 1.18 and the purity 36%. What these two values mean is that 1 mL of the liquid in the bottle weighs 1.18 g and that 36% of this weight is HCl (the rest is water). If your task is to dilute this acid to a concentration of 1 *N* in a final volume of 100 mL, then the final solution must have 1 equivalent weight of HCl in every liter.

To do this, you must first determine the equivalent weight of HCl in 100 mL of the dilute acid. Because HCl contains one hydrogen ion, the equivalent weight is the formula mass, or 36.5 g. Therefore,

$$100\text{ mL}\left(\frac{1\text{ L}}{1000\text{ mL}}\right)\left(\frac{36.5\text{ g}}{1\text{ L}}\right) = 3.65\text{ g}$$

What this means is that the diluted acid has 3.65 g of HCl in a final volume of 100 mL. Next, you must calculate the volume of concentrated aqueous HCl that contains 3.65 g—the volume that you will subsequently dilute to that final volume of 100 mL. You know that 36% of the weight of the concentrated aqueous acid is HCl; therefore,

$$0.36 \times \left(\frac{1.18\text{ g}}{1\text{ mL}}\right) = 0.425\text{ g/mL}$$

This means that every mL of the liquid contains 0.425 g of HCl. Now you can calculate the volume needed for dilution to 100 mL:

$$3.65\text{ g HCl} \times \left(\frac{1\text{ mL}}{0.425\text{ g HCl}}\right) = 8.6\text{ mL}$$

Thus, you pipet 8.6 mL (slowly and under a hood) of the concentrated aqueous HCl into water and then add enough water to bring the final volume to 100 mL. The result is a solution of 1 *N* HCl.

THE *p*H SCALE

The concentration of hydrogen ions profoundly affects many chemical reactions in the laboratory and nearly all physiological processes in the human body. Understanding the expression of hydrogen-ion concentrations, therefore, is critical both to the physician, who makes medical decisions, and to the laboratorian, who generates the test results that help guide those decisions.

Serum, urine, other biological fluids, and common laboratory solutions have H^+ concentrations that are ponderous to express in the units discussed previously. For example, the concentration of H^+ in the blood is 0.00000004 M (4×10^{-8} M). To simplify such inconvenient numbers, Danish biochemist Søren Sørenson proposed the quantity "*p*H" in 1909. He defined the term ***p*H** as the *puissance d'hydrogène*, which translates as the *power of hydrogen*, expressing $[H^+]$ as a negative logarithm of 10. In other words, $[H^+] = 10^{-pH}$.

Rearranging this equation gives

$$pH = -\log[H^+]$$

EQUATION 4

★ **TABLE 5-2 The *p*H Scale**

$[H^+]$ (mol/L)		*p*H	
0.1	10^{-1}	1	↑
0.01	10^{-2}	2	
0.001	10^{-3}	3	
0.0001	10^{-4}	4	
0.00001	10^{-5}	5	
0.000001	10^{-6}	6	**Acidic**
0.0000001	10^{-7}	7	**Neutral**
0.00000001	10^{-8}	8	**Alkaline**
0.000000001	10^{-9}	9	
0.0000000001	10^{-10}	10	
0.00000000001	10^{-11}	11	
0.000000000001	10^{-12}	12	
0.0000000000001	10^{-13}	13	
0.00000000000001	10^{-14}	14	↓

The *p*H of blood, then, is

$$pH = -\log(4 \times 10^{-8}\ \text{M})$$

$$pH = 7.4$$

Clearly, "7.4" is much simpler than "0.00000004" or "4×10^{-8}." Now, let us look at the *p*H scale (Table 5-2 ★) that emerges from Equation 4.

This scale has at least four salient features:

1. As *p*H increases, the concentration of H^+ decreases. Thus, their relationship is inverse.
2. A difference of 1 *p*H unit—for example, 8 to 9 or 5 to 4—represents a 10-fold change in the H^+ concentration. This is so because the scale is logarithmic and its base is 10. Thus, with respect to H^+, a solution at *p*H 6 is 100 times more concentrated than it is at *p*H 8.
3. The concentration of H^+ is in "mol/L." The *p*H convention is valid *only* for this unit of concentration.
4. By virtue of being a logarithm, the *p*H is dimensionless; that is, it has no units. Thus, we say "the *p*H is 7," not "the *p*H is 7 moles per liter."

A solution at *p*H 7 is "neutral." At *p*H < 7, it is acidic, and at *p*H > 7, it is alkaline, or basic. (Strictly speaking, this is true only at 25°C. At other temperatures, these guidelines vary somewhat.)

Although a whole *p*H unit corresponds to a factor of 10, every decrement of 0.30 *p*H units reflects a doubling of the H^+ concentration, and every increment reflects a halving of the H^+ concentration. This knowledge is helpful in a quick comparison of two *p*H values. If the H^+ concentration doubles, the *p*H goes down by 0.30, and if the H^+ concentration halves, the *p*H goes up by 0.30. For example, if the *p*H decreases from 4.50 to 4.20, the H^+ concentration has risen by a factor of ~2 from 3.16×10^{-5} M to 6.31×10^{-5} M. Likewise, if the *p*H increases from 7.10 to 7.40, the H^+ concentration has fallen by a factor of ~2 from 7.94×10^{-8} M to 3.98×10^{-8} M.

This relationship comes about because the logarithm of 2 is 0.30. Consider what happens when the H^+ concentration doubles:

$$pH = -\log([H^+] \times 2)$$

$$pH = -\log[H^+] - \log 2$$

$$= -\log[H^+] - 0.30$$

What the last equation in this sequence says is that when $[H^+]$ doubles, the original *p*H goes down by 0.30.

When the H^+ concentration halves, the original *p*H goes up by 0.30:

$$pH = -\log([H^+] \times {}^1\!/_2)$$

$$pH = -\log[H^+] - \log{}^1\!/_2$$

$$= -\log[H^+] + 0.30$$

☑ CHECKPOINT 5-4

1. What is the *p*H of a solution in which $[H^+]$ is 0.062 M?
2. What is $[H^+]$ of a solution whose *p*H is 8.5?

1. $pH = -\log(0.062\ \text{M}) = 1.21$
2. $10^{-pH} = [H^+] = 10^{-8.5} = 3 \times 10^{-9}\ \text{M}$

CONVERTING BETWEEN UNITS

We can convert between two sets of units in any of several ways. Let us consider three such ways, using the example of converting a result for serum glucose of 80 mg/dL to "mM" ("mmol/L").

APPROACH 1

Dimensional analysis, introduced in Chapter 4, is the most efficient approach. Setting up the factors correctly is the key to a successful calculation; this comes about by choosing numerators and denominators such that cancellations occur and the target units emerge at the end:

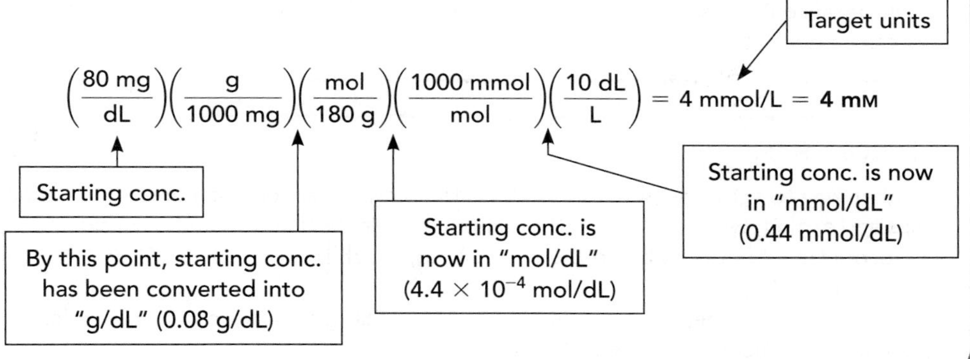

Notice that there is only one significant figure in the final result because the measured quantity with the fewest in the computation, "80 mg/dL," has only one.

APPROACH 2

An alternate approach to solving the above problem is the ratio method, also introduced in Chapter 4. Using this method, our first objective is to convert "80 mg" into "mmol," which requires taking it to "grams," then to "moles," and finally to "millimoles." In the first step, we set up equivalent ratios:

$$\frac{1000\text{ mg}}{1\text{ g}} = \frac{80\text{ mg}}{x}$$

Cross-multiplication gives

$$(1000\text{ mg})(x) = (80\text{ mg})(1\text{ g})$$

$$x = 0.08\text{ g}$$

(continued)

In the next step, we convert "0.08 g" into "moles" (the molar mass of glucose is 180 g/mol):

$$\frac{180\text{ g}}{1\text{ mol}} = \frac{0.08\text{ g}}{x}$$

$$x = 0.0004\text{ mol}$$

Finally, we convert "0.0004 mol" into "millimoles":

$$\frac{1\text{ mol}}{1000\text{ mmol}} = \frac{0.0004\text{ mol}}{x}$$

$$x = 0.4\text{ mmol}$$

Thus, this solution contains 0.4 mmol of glucose in each dL. To complete the conversion, we change "dL" into "liters":

$$\frac{10\text{ dL}}{1\text{ L}} = \frac{1\text{ dL}}{x}$$

$$x = 0.1\text{ L}$$

The solution, therefore, has 0.4 mmol of glucose in 0.1 L, giving a concentration of 4 mmol/L:

$$\frac{0.4\text{ mmol}}{0.1\text{ L}} = 4\text{ mmol/L} = \mathbf{4\text{ m}\textsc{m}}$$

As in the first approach above, notice that there is only one significant figure in the final result because the measured quantity with the fewest in the computation, "80 mg/dL," has only one.

APPROACH 3

Another way to solve the above problem is to recognize simple mathematical relationships and exploit them to speed up the computation. In the problem under consideration, we recognize "80 mg" as being 8% of 1000 mg, which is the same as 8% of 1 g. That amounts to 0.08 g.

Next, because the formula mass of glucose is 180 g/mol, we can quickly calculate that 0.08 g of glucose is 0.04% of 1 mol:

$$\frac{0.08\text{ g}}{180\text{ g}} \times 100\% = 0.04\%$$

And 0.04% of 1 mol is 0.0004 mol. Thus, at this point in the computation, we know that 1 dL of our glucose solution contains 0.0004 mol.

We recognize that 1 mol of anything—glucose molecules, golf balls, or votes—is the same as 1000 mmol. In other words, there are 1000 mmol per mol. Therefore, no matter the number of moles, we merely multiply it by 1000 mmol/mol to convert the units to "millimoles"; the number of millimoles is always 1000 times greater than the number of moles. In this case, we have 0.0004 mol:

$$0.0004\text{ mol} \times 1000\text{ mmol/mol} = 0.4\text{ mmol}$$

Now we know that our glucose solution has 0.4 mmol per dL. All that remains at this point is to convert "dL" to "L." We also know that 1 liter of any liquid—glucose solution, gasoline, or tea—occupies the same volume as 10 deciliters. In other words, there are 10 dL per L. Therefore, no matter the number of deciliters, we merely divide it by 10 dL/L to convert the units to "liters"; the number of liters is always 1/10 the number of deciliters. In this case, we have 1 dL:

$$1\text{ dL} \div 10\text{ dL/L} = 0.1\text{ L}$$

At the end of our computation, we see that there are 0.4 mmol of glucose in 0.1 L of our solution. Therefore, the concentration is

$$\frac{0.4\ \text{mmol}}{0.1\ \text{L}} = 4\ \text{mmol/L} = \mathbf{4\ mM}$$

As in the first and second approaches above, notice that there is only one significant figure in the final result because the measured quantity with the fewest in the computation, "80 mg/dL," has only one.

☑ CHECKPOINT 5-5

1. For a glucose solution, convert "2.3 mg/mL" to "mol/L" (honor figure significance).

Approach 1

$$\left(\frac{2.3\ \text{mg}}{\text{mL}}\right)\left(\frac{\text{g}}{1000\ \text{mg}}\right)\left(\frac{\text{mol}}{180\ \text{g}}\right)\left(\frac{1000\ \text{mL}}{\text{L}}\right) = 0.013\ \text{mol/L}$$

Approach 2

$$\frac{1000\ \text{mg}}{1\ \text{g}} = \frac{2.3\ \text{mg}}{x} \qquad x = 0.0023\ \text{g}$$

$$\frac{180\ \text{g}}{1\ \text{mol}} = \frac{0.0023\ \text{g}}{y} \qquad y = 1.27 \times 10^{-5}\ \text{mol}$$

$$\frac{1000\ \text{mL}}{1\ \text{L}} = \frac{1\ \text{mL}}{z} \qquad z = 0.001\ \text{L}$$

$$\frac{1.27 \times 10^{-5}\ \text{mol}}{0.001\ \text{L}} = 0.013\ \text{mol/L}$$

2. For a KOH solution, convert "5 μmol/mL" to "mg/L" (honor figure significance).

Approach 1

$$\left(\frac{5.0\ \mu\text{mol}}{\text{mL}}\right)\left(\frac{\text{mol}}{10^6\ \mu\text{mol}}\right)\left(\frac{56.1\ \text{g}}{\text{mol}}\right)\left(\frac{1000\ \text{mg}}{\text{g}}\right)\left(\frac{1000\ \text{ml}}{\text{L}}\right) = 280\ \text{mg/L}$$

Approach 2

$$\frac{1 \times 10^6\ \mu\text{mol}}{1\ \text{mol}} = \frac{5.0\ \mu\text{mol}}{w} \qquad w = 5.0 \times 10^{-6}\ \text{mol}$$

$$\frac{1\ \text{mol}}{56.1\ \text{g}} = \frac{5.0 \times 10^{-6}\ \text{mol}}{x} \qquad x = 0.00028\ \text{g} = 2.8 \times 10^{-4}\ \text{g}$$

$$\frac{1\ \text{g}}{1000\ \text{mg}} = \frac{2.8 \times 10^{-4}\ \text{g}}{y} \qquad y = 0.28\ \text{mg}$$

$$\frac{1000\ \text{mL}}{1\ \text{L}} = \frac{1\ \text{mL}}{z} \qquad z = 0.001\ \text{L}$$

$$\frac{0.28\ \text{mg}}{0.001\ \text{L}} = 280\ \text{mg/L}$$

Summary

1. A *solution* is a homogeneous mixture of substances. The *solvent* is the substance present in largest amount, whereas every other substance is a *solute*.
2. The *concentration* of a solution is a measure of the amounts of solute and solvent in the mixture.
3. The expression of concentration by percentage has three commonly used systems: (a) weight per volume (*w/v*), which gives the number of grams of solute in 100 mL of the solution; (b) weight per weight (*w/w*), which gives the number of grams of solute in 100 g of the solution; and (c) volume per volume (*v/v*), which gives the number of milliliters of solute in 100 mL of the solution.
4. *Molarity* expresses concentration as the number of moles of solute in 1 liter of solution. Its symbol is "M."
5. *Molality* expresses concentration as the number of moles of solute per kg of solvent. Its symbol is historically "*m*."
6. *Normality* expresses concentration as the number of equivalent weights in 1 liter of the solution. An *equivalent weight* is the amount of a substance that contains, theoretically combines with, or theoretically replaces 1 mole of hydrogen ions (H^+).
7. For an acid, an *equivalent* is one hydrogen ion in the formula. For a base or a salt, an equivalent is the number of hydrogen ions with which it can theoretically combine; however, it can just as easily be regarded as 1 mole of ionic charges.
8. *Specific gravity* is the ratio of the density of a solution to the density of water at 4°C (1 g/mL).
9. The *p*H system for expressing concentration simplifies the numbers involved. The *p*H value is the negative logarithm of the H^+ concentration:

$$pH = -\log[H^+]$$

10. The *p*H scale has four important properties: (a) the relationship between *p*H and $[H^+]$ is inverse, (b) a difference of 1 *p*H unit represents a 10-fold difference in $[H^+]$, (c) the *p*H is valid only for molarity, and (d) the *p*H value is dimensionless.
11. A *p*H difference of 0.30 reflects a two-fold difference in $[H^+]$.

Practice Problems

1. (LO 3) Calculate % (w/v) for each of the following solutions.

   (a) 400 g KOH in 1 L

   (b) 60 g KCl in 500 mL

   (c) 1.8 g NaCl in 200 mL

   (d) 0.5 g glucose in 1 dL

   (e) 250 mg $Pb(NO_3)$ in 300 mL

   (f) 3.08 g NaOCl in 50 mL

2. (LO 3) Calculate % (w/w) for each of the following solutions.

   (a) 9.2 g $CaCl_2$ dissolved in 800 g of water

   (b) 500 mg cholesterol dissolved in 5 g of ethyl acetate

   (c) 200 mg Na_2CO_3 dissolved in 25 g of water

3. (LO 3) If isopropyl alcohol is added to 50 mL of water until the volume of the solution is 150 mL, what is the % (v/v)?

4. (LO 3) Calculate the molarity of each of the following solutions.

   (a) 4 g KOH in 1 L of solution

   (b) 60 g NaCl in 400 mL of solution

   (c) 0.18 mmol Fe^{2+} in 200 mL of solution

   (d) 0.70 μmol HCl in 50 μL of solution

   (e) 164 mg $Ca(NO_3)_2$ in 10 mL of solution

   (f) 0.130 mg $Co(NO_3)_2$ in 300 μL of solution

5. (LO 3) Calculate the normality of each of the following solutions.

   (a) 14.9 g KCl in 200 mL of solution

   (b) 320 g NaOH in 2 L of solution

   (c) 24.53 g H_2SO_4 in 250 mL of solution

6. (LO 3, 7) Complete the following table for $MgCl_2$.

Molarity	% (w/v)
1.0	
	2.6
3.4×10^{-4}	
	29.1
0.0025	

7. (LO 3, 7) Complete the following table for NaCl.

Molarity	% (w/v)
2.0	
	0.90
1.7×10^{-3}	
	16.0
0.082	

8. (LO 3, 7) Complete the following table for glucose ($C_6H_{12}O_6$).

Molarity	% (w/v)
0.80	
	5.0
9.6×10^{-4}	
	0.83
0.066	

Contextual Problems

1. (LO 2, 3, 7) If the reference range for serum Ca^{2+} is 8.5–10.5 mg/dL, would a result of 2.3 mmol/L be within that range? A result of 4.8 mEq/L?

2. (LO 2, 3, 7) If the reference range for serum Mg^{2+} is 1.8–3.0 mg/dL, would a result of 2.6 mEq/L be within that range? A result of 0.8 mmol/L?

3. (LO 6) Complete the following table.

pH	$[H^+]$ (M)
3.90	
	1.9×10^{-6}
7.05	
	2.29×10^{-10}
11.38	
	8.71×10^{-14}

4. (LO 6, 7) Complete the following table. Note the units requested.

pH	$[H^+]$ (mM)
2.61	
	0.0200
7.00	
	7.10×10^{-8}
12.27	
	1.00×10^{-11}

5. (LO 3) Consider a 2.00 *m* glucose solution. In 2720 g of this solution, what is the total mass of the glucose?

6. (LO 2, 3, 7) Your laboratory analyzes samples that are part of the proficiency testing program being conducted by an oversight agency. For eight of the analytes, the agency requests units that happen to differ from those that your laboratory uses. Convert your results appropriately in the following table.

Analyte	Your Result	Result in Requested Units
creatinine (112.3 g/mol)	6.4 mg/L	μM
folic acid (441.6 g/mol)	14 ng/mL	nmol/L
phenobarbital (230.8 g/mol)	15 μg/mL	μM
lead	4.2 μM	μg/L
phosphorus	1.62 mM	mg/L
iron	22.9 μmol/L	μg/L
glucose	160 mg/dL	mmol/L
uric acid (168.1 g/mol)	77 mg/L	μM

7. (LO 2, 3, 7) Your laboratory's method for quantifying a particular drug in whole blood requires regular decontamination by running through the instrument a solution of bleach (sodium hypochlorite, NaOCl) at a concentration between 0.6% and 1% (w/v). A lower concentration fails to decontaminate the apparatus, and a higher concentration damages it. You have a NaOCl solution at 0.083 M. Does this concentration fall within the range specified?

8. (LO 2, 3, 7) You work in a private laboratory that is about to implement a new method for quantifying ionized calcium in serum. Your supervisor explains that the new method gives results in units of "mg/dL," whereas the physicians in the clinics want results in units of "mmol/L." Therefore, your supervisor instructs you to routinely multiply the first result by 0.2495 to get the second result, which you may then release to the physician. Is your supervisor correct?

9. (LO 2, 3, 7) Ethylene glycol is a toxic substance used in such products as brake fluid, inks, synthetic waxes, and antifreeze. In cases of accidental ingestion, the physicians in your hospital treat the patient with hemodialysis when the ethylene glycol concentration in the serum is greater than 50 mg/dL (molar mass = 62 g/mol). From the emergency room, you receive a serum sample for a suspected case of ethylene glycol poisoning. Your test for ethylene glycol in the sample returns a result of 9.2 mmol/L. Does this concentration make the patient a candidate for hemodialysis?

10. (LO 4) One of the assays your laboratory routinely carries out requires 1 *N* H_2SO_4. You have in stock a bottle of concentrated sulfuric acid with a specific gravity of 1.84 and a purity of 97%. To achieve the target concentration of 1 *N*, how many milliliters of this acid must be diluted to a final volume of 100 mL?

PEARSON

myhealthprofessionskit™

Go to www.myhealthprofessionskit.com <http://www.myhealthprofessionskit.com/> to access the Companion Website created for this textbook. Simply select "Clinical Laboratory Science" from the choice of disciplines. Find this book and log in using your username and password to access additional practice problems, answers to the practice and contextual problems, additional information, and more.

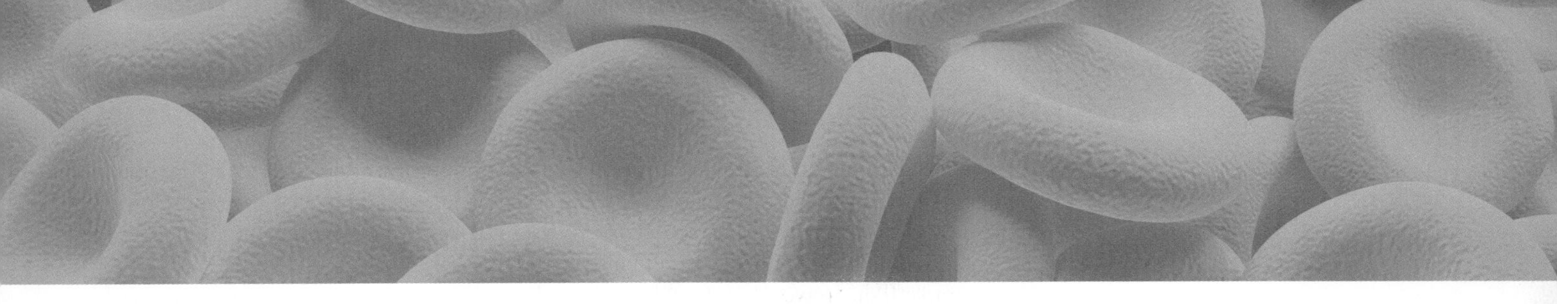

6 Dilutions

Learning Objectives

At the end of this chapter, the student should be able to do the following:

1. Explain the nature, purpose, and strategy of dilution, as well as the general procedure for executing it
2. Use the dilution ratio, factor, and equation; plan a dilution for a target volume or concentration; and correct a raw test result on a diluted sample
3. Distinguish between simple and serial dilution and know when to use one over the other
4. Calculate and use the tube and sample dilutions in planning or interpreting a serial procedure

Chapter Outline

Key Terms

antibody titer
diluent
dilution factor
dilution ratio
sample dilution
serial dilution
tube dilution

In the clinical laboratory, we often need to carry out dilutions. In clinical chemistry, we most often make dilutions when the concentration of a given analyte is higher than the upper limit of the method we are using and when we prepare solutions for constructing a standard curve. The quality of test results, and therefore the quality of patient care, depends on how well the technologist pipets the solutions and carries out the calculations. In microbiology, we make dilutions in order to prepare liquid cultures for plating on agar, whereas in serology, we need dilutions to determine antibody titers.

SIMPLE DILUTIONS

To begin, consider the following scenario from a clinical laboratory. A physician suspects that a patient in the emergency department took an accidental overdose of carbamazepine, a drug used to prevent epileptic seizures. Life-threatening toxic effects sometimes occur when the plasma concentration of this drug exceeds 15 μg/mL. A technologist in the laboratory runs the test for carbamazepine on a blood sample from this patient, using a method that is reliable for drug concentrations from 2 to 20 μg/mL. The result for this sample, however, is 22 μg/mL, an unreliably high value. Therefore, the technologist must lower the carbamazepine concentration into the acceptable range (2–20 μg/mL) by diluting the sample, running the test again, and then correcting the result for the dilution.

For example, if she[1] mixes 100 μL of the undiluted sample with 100 μL of saline solution (the **diluent**), the total final volume is now 200 μL (Figure 6-1 ■). The drug is present in twice as much volume as it was before dilution, and its concentration is now one-half of its real value. In other words, the ratio of the initial volume (100 μL) to the final volume (200 μL) is 1:2, the same as the ratio of the final concentration to the initial concentration. Therefore, the **dilution ratio** is 1:2, and the resulting solution is a "1:2 dilution" (pronounced "1-to-2"):

EQUATION 1

$$\text{dilution ratio} = \frac{V_{\text{initial}}}{V_{\text{final}}} = \frac{C_{\text{final}}}{C_{\text{initial}}}$$

where V is volume and C is concentration. The technologist could have prepared a 1:2 dilution from any initial volume, provided the final volume satisfied Equation 1. For example, she might have diluted 234 μL of the patient sample to 468 μL with saline solution, or 1.3 mL of the sample to 2.6 mL.

The technologist then runs the same analytical test on the 1:2 dilution of the original sample. The result is 12 μg/mL (Figure 6-1), a value that is clearly reliable because it falls between 2 and 20. Nevertheless, she must correct this result for the fact that the test was carried out on a 1:2 dilution, in which the drug's concentration is only one-half of its real value. Thus, she multiplies the result by 2, giving a final carbamazepine concentration of 24 μg/mL, which she then reports to the physician. The value of 2 by which the technologist multiplied the result of 12—the **dilution factor**—is simply the reciprocal of the dilution ratio.

However, she might well have chosen to mix 100 μL of the original sample with some other volume of saline solution, say, 300 μL, in which case the total volume would be 400 μL and the resulting dilution would be 1:4. The drug would then be present in four times as much volume as it was before dilution, which decreases its concentration to one-fourth of the real value. Substitution of these volumes into Equation 1 confirms this. The result of the test on a 1:4 dilution of the original sample would be 6, which, when multiplied by the dilution factor of 4, gives 24 μg/mL. This is the same final carbamazepine concentration as the 1:2 dilution yields.

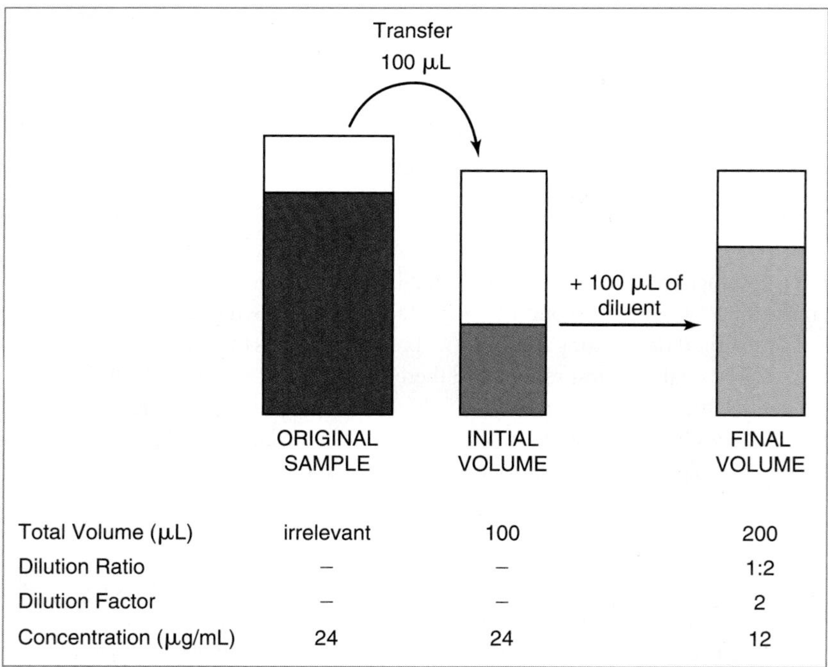

	ORIGINAL SAMPLE	INITIAL VOLUME	FINAL VOLUME
Total Volume (μL)	irrelevant	100	200
Dilution Ratio	–	–	1:2
Dilution Factor	–	–	2
Concentration (μg/mL)	24	24	12

■ **FIGURE 6-1** A simple dilution.

[1]Because English does not have a gender-neutral singular pronoun, this book alternates genders between scenarios.

For this patient, the consequences of a calculation mistake, of a pipetting error, or of simply forgetting to correct for the dilution, could be serious—even fatal. This is true for other analytes as well, underscoring the importance of making dilutions accurately and carrying out calculations correctly.

For the 1:2 dilution, the volume of sample before dilution (its "initial volume") was 100 μL, and the volume after dilution (its "final volume") was 200 μL. Furthermore, the carbamazepine concentration after dilution ("final concentration") was determined to be 12 μg/mL. The concentration before dilution ("initial concentration") was the target value—the result that the technologist calculated and reported to the physician: 24 μg/mL. Thus, the process of dilution increased the volume and decreased the concentration by the same factor of 2. This means, in turn, that the ratio of the final volume to the initial volume equals the ratio of the initial concentration to the final concentration:

$$\frac{V_{\text{final}}}{V_{\text{initial}}} = \frac{200\ \mu\text{L}}{100\ \mu\text{L}} = \frac{C_{\text{initial}}}{C_{\text{final}}} = \frac{24\ \mu\text{g/mL}}{12\ \mu\text{g/mL}} = 2$$

EQUATION 2

It is clear from this equation that, if three of the variables are known, we can calculate the fourth. In this example, the technologist knew V_{final}, V_{initial}, and C_{final}, and from these three values she calculated C_{initial}, which corresponds to the undiluted sample. Simple algebraic rearrangement of Equation 2 isolates the target variable:

$$\frac{V_{\text{final}} C_{\text{final}}}{V_{\text{initial}}} = C_{\text{initial}}$$

EQUATION 3

Substitution into Equation 3 gives

$$\frac{(200\ \mu\text{L})(12\ \mu\text{g/mL})}{100\ \mu\text{L}} = 24\ \mu\text{g/mL}$$

We can apply Equation 3 to the 1:4 dilution on the same patient sample, giving the same result:

$$\frac{(400\ \mu\text{L})(6\ \mu\text{g/mL})}{100\ \mu\text{L}} = 24\ \mu\text{g/mL}$$

The general mathematical expression of this relationship becomes a useful tool in the laboratory:

$$V_{\text{final}} C_{\text{final}} = V_{\text{initial}} C_{\text{initial}}$$

EQUATION 4

For example, consider the use of Equation 4 in the following scenario. Your laboratory uses an analytical instrument for lead (Pb) that requires calibration with four standard solutions of lead at 5, 10, 20, and 50 μg/mL in 5% HNO_3. The manufacturer supplies a stock lead solution of 1000 μg/mL, which must be diluted to those four concentrations.

A technologist in your laboratory prepares the standard solutions by using Equation 4. His task is to determine the volume of stock solution to be diluted to a certain final volume with the diluent (5% HNO_3) in order to achieve the target concentrations. He decides to set the final volume of each standard solution at 50 mL because it is convenient to prepare and because it will provide enough solution to last many weeks. Next, he arranges Equation 4 to isolate the target variable, V_{initial}, which represents the volume of stock solution that must be diluted:

$$\frac{V_{\text{final}} C_{\text{final}}}{C_{\text{initial}}} = V_{\text{initial}}$$

EQUATION 5

Thus, for the standard solution of 50 μg/mL,

$$\frac{(50\ \text{mL})(50\ \mu\text{g/mL})}{1000\ \mu\text{g/mL}} = 2.5\ \text{mL}$$

The technologist, therefore, will dilute 2.5 mL of the stock solution of lead to a final volume of 50 mL, using 5% HNO_3 as the diluent. The result is 50 mL of a lead solution at a concentration of 50 μg/mL; he can likewise use Equation 5 for each of the other three standard solutions.

☑ CHECKPOINT 6-1

1. If we dilute 10 μL of a sample up to 160 μL, what is the dilution ratio? What is the dilution factor?
2. A sample at 200 mM is diluted 1:6. What is the final concentration?
3. We mix 50 μL of a sample with 200 μL of diluent. If the concentration after dilution is 60 mg/dL, what was it before dilution?

1. Dilution ratio $= V_{initial}/V_{final} = 1{:}16$. Dilution factor $= (\text{dilution ratio})^{-1} = 16$
2. $C_{final} = C_{initial} \times (V_{initial}/V_{final}) = 200\ \text{mM} \times (1/6) = 33.3\ \text{mM}$
3. $C_{initial} = C_{final} \times (V_{final}/V_{initial}) = 60\ \text{mg/dL} \times (250\ \mu\text{L}/50\ \mu\text{L}) = 300\ \text{mg/dL}$

SERIAL DILUTIONS

The two preceding scenarios, one involving an out-of-range test result and the other a set of standard solutions, show the two most common reasons for carrying out dilutions in the clinical laboratory, as the first paragraph of this chapter states. However, some special cases require dilution in several steps, rather than the single step used above.

Consider, for example, the case in which a procedure calls for a 1:8000 dilution. Performing such a large dilution in one step is impractical to the extent that it requires a vessel big enough to hold the large final volume and because a vessel containing 8 L of an aqueous solution weighs about 20 pounds. Also, if the vessel is glass, the combination of weight and breakability creates unnecessary risk for the technologist.

To avoid this problem, perform **serial dilutions**, a series of small dilutions that ultimately gives the same target ratio of 1:8000. Figure 6-2 ■ depicts the procedure. In this example, first perform a 1:20 dilution of the original sample, which in this case is at 200 mM; transfer 1 mL of this sample into another tube

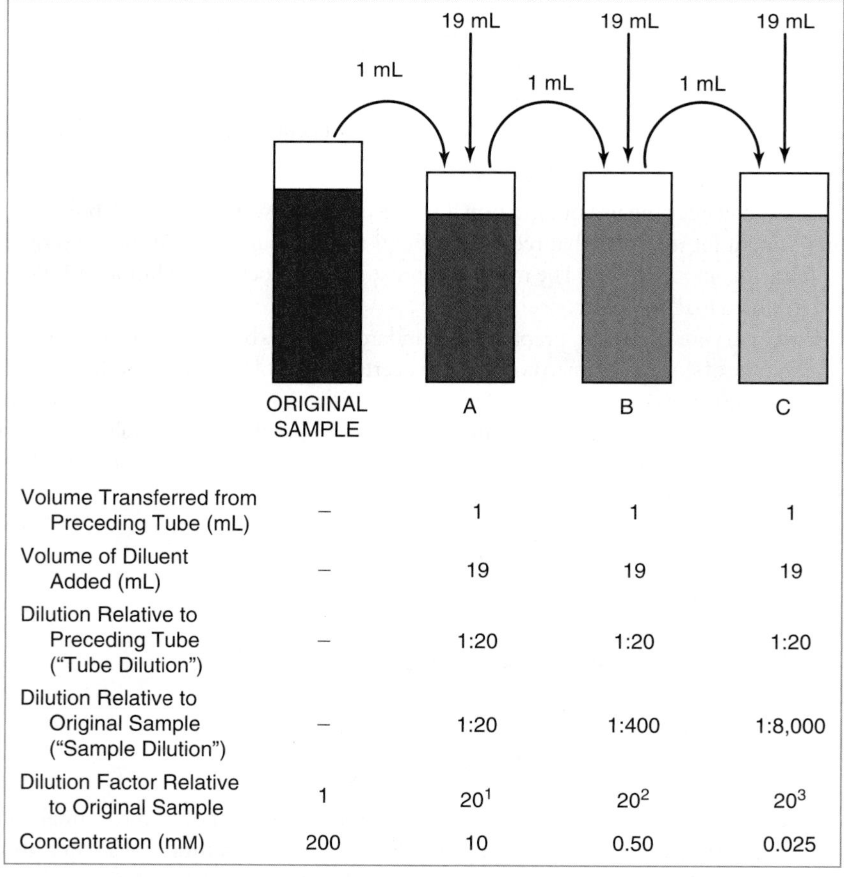

	ORIGINAL SAMPLE	A	B	C
Volume Transferred from Preceding Tube (mL)	–	1	1	1
Volume of Diluent Added (mL)	–	19	19	19
Dilution Relative to Preceding Tube ("Tube Dilution")	–	1:20	1:20	1:20
Dilution Relative to Original Sample ("Sample Dilution")	–	1:20	1:400	1:8,000
Dilution Factor Relative to Original Sample	1	20^1	20^2	20^3
Concentration (mM)	200	10	0.50	0.025

■ **FIGURE 6-2** A serial dilution.

("**A**") and dilute it to 20 mL. The resulting concentration is 10 mM. Then carry out a 1:20 dilution of solution **A** by transferring 1 mL into another tube ("**B**") and diluting it to 20 mL. The resulting concentration is 0.50 mM. Solution **B** is 20-fold less concentrated than solution **A**, which in turn is 20-fold less concentrated than the original sample. Therefore, solution **B** is 400-fold less concentrated than the original sample.

Lastly, dilute solution **B** 1:20 by transferring 1 mL into another tube ("**C**") and diluting it to 20 mL. Its concentration being only 0.025 mM, solution **C** proves to be a 1:8000 dilution of the original sample.

As Figure 6-2 shows, each of the solutions **A**, **B**, and **C** is 20 times less concentrated than the preceding solution; that is, the dilution factor of each tube is 20 times higher than that of the preceding tube. The corresponding dilution ratio is the **tube dilution**, which is usually constant from one tube to the next and which is calculated from this equation:

$$D_{tube} = \frac{V_{sample}}{V_{sample} + V_{diluent}}$$

where D_{tube} is the tube dilution, V_{sample} is the sample volume, and $V_{diluent}$ is the diluent volume. However, the dilution ratio of each tube relative to the starting solution is the **sample dilution**, and it reflects how much the original sample has been diluted up to that point in the sequence. In fact, because the tube dilution is the same for all tubes, the sample dilution forms a geometric series, which in this example is 1/20, 1/400, 1/8000, or $1/20^1$, $1/20^2$, $1/20^3$. Thus, we can calculate the sample dilution for a given tube from this equation:

$$D_{sample} = (D_{tube})^N$$

EQUATION 6

where N is the number of the tube in the sequence. For tube **C** in Figure 6-2, which is the third tube containing a dilution of the original sample, the sample dilution is $(1/20)^3$, or 1/8000; the concentration of the sample in tube **C** is 1/8000 of the original.

At this point, be sure to understand the difference between dilution ratio and dilution factor. As Equation 1 shows, the dilution ratio is the ratio of the concentration of a given dilution (the final concentration) to the concentration of the original sample (the initial concentration). In Figure 6-2, the concentration of solution **B** is 1/400th the concentration of the original sample, making the dilution ratio 1:400. Therefore, the dilution factor is 400, the reciprocal of the dilution ratio; this is the number by which we multiply the concentration of solution **B** to yield the concentration of the original sample.

Equation 6 allows for the fast calculation of a sample dilution. For example, if there are 10 tubes in the series and if the tube dilution is 1/4, then the sample dilution in tube #6 is $(1/4)^6$, or 1/4096. The usefulness of this equation, however, goes even further.

Suppose a technologist is going to test the susceptibility of a bacterial strain to various antibiotics, and she receives from the supervisor a suspension of the bacteria at a concentration of about 6.0×10^7 cells/mL. In order to inoculate agar plates with the bacteria, she needs a suspension of cells at a concentration between 50 and 100 per mL. Therefore, she must achieve a dilution of the original sample between 600,000-fold and 1,200,000-fold, a very large factor that calls for a serial dilution.

Using Equation 6, the technologist sets the value of D_{sample} at 1/600,000. After choosing a convenient tube dilution—say, 1:10—she calculates the number of tubes in the series necessary to bring the concentration of cells into the target range by substituting into Equation 6:

$$\frac{1}{600{,}000} = \left(\frac{1}{10}\right)^N$$

Algebraic manipulation of this equation gives

$$\frac{\log\left(\frac{1}{600{,}000}\right)}{\log\left(\frac{1}{10}\right)} = N$$

$$5.8 = N$$

Because 5.8 is close to 6, this result means that, if the technologist performs six dilutions in a series with a 1:10 tube dilution, the last tube should have a sample dilution in the target range of 1/600,000 to

1/1,200,000. She confirms this expectation by substituting into Equation 6 the values of 1/10 for D_{tube} and 6 for N, which do indeed give a D_{sample} of 1/1,000,000.

Serology also employs the technique of serial dilution in the semiquantification of antibody titers. An **antibody titer** represents the amount of antibody present in serum against a certain antigen and is defined as the reciprocal of the highest sample dilution ratio at which antibody is detectable. This technique is used to screen patients for exposure to a pathogen or to evaluate a vaccination.

In short, the procedure is to prepare a dilution series with a tube dilution usually of 1:2, giving sample dilutions of 1:2, 1:4, 1:8, 1:16, 1:32, 1:64, 1:128, and so forth. Then antigen is added at a fixed volume to each dilution and the presence or absence of a reaction is noted. If, for example, there is a reaction in every dilution from 1:2 up to and including 1:32, then the antibody titer is said to be "32," which is the reciprocal of the highest dilution ratio at which there is reaction. This means that there was enough antibody in the serum to react visibly with antigen when diluted 32-fold, but there was not enough to react when diluted 64-fold or more.

The titer goes up with the concentration of antibody in the serum because the dilution factor necessary to make the antibody undetectable increases. In other words, a titer of 128 indicates a larger concentration of antibody than does a titer of 16 because rendering the reaction undetectable required an 8-fold higher dilution.

☑ CHECKPOINT 6-2

1. When is serial dilution preferable to simple dilution?
2. Consider the serial dilution of a sample at 50,000 ng/dL. If the tube dilution is 1:10, what is the concentration in the fourth tube?

1. Serial dilution is preferred when the final volume required for a simple dilution would be inconveniently large.
2. $D_{sample} = (D_{tube})^N = (1/10)^4 = 1/10,000$. Thus, the concentration in tube #4 is 5 ng/dL.

Summary

1. Common reasons for making dilutions are (a) to bring back into range a test result that exceeded the upper limit of the analytical method, (b) to prepare standard solutions at various concentrations, (c) to prepare a suspension of cells at a concentration suitable for plating, and (d) to semiquantify antibody titers.
2. In a simple dilution, add together a volume of the liquid sample (e.g., serum, urine, peritoneal fluid) and a volume of liquid *diluent*.
3. The extent of dilution is quantified by the *dilution ratio:*

$$\text{dilution ratio} = \frac{V_{initial}}{V_{final}} = \frac{C_{final}}{C_{initial}}$$

4. Identify a dilution by its ratio. If the ratio is 1/4, the dilution is "1:4" (pronounced "1-to-4").
5. The *dilution factor* is the value by which one multiplies the concentration of a dilution to give the concentration of the original sample. It equals the reciprocal of the dilution ratio.
6. This equation expresses the relationship among the volumes and concentrations before and after dilution:

$$V_{final}C_{final} = V_{initial}C_{initial}$$

7. For dilutions with very large factors—for example, > 1000—it may be more practical to perform serial dilutions than simple dilutions.
8. A serial dilution is a progressive series of dilutions in which each dilution is less concentrated than the preceding one by a constant amount. The *tube dilution* is the dilution ratio from one tube to the next, whereas the *sample dilution* is the dilution ratio of a given tube relative to the original sample.
9. Calculate the tube dilution from this equation:

$$D_{tube} = \frac{V_{sample}}{V_{sample} + V_{diluent}}$$

10. When the tube dilution is constant, the sample dilution forms a geometric series; one calculates it from this equation:

$$D_{sample} = (D_{tube})^N$$

where N is the number of the tube in the sequence.

Practice and Contextual Problems

1. (LO 2) For each of the following dilutions, calculate the dilution factor between the original liquid and the final solution.

   (a) 20 mL of solution *Q* is diluted to 100 mL.

   (b) 500 μL of solution *X* is diluted to 2.0 mL.

   (c) 150 μL of serum is added to 300 μL of saline solution, and 20 μL of the resulting solution is added to 180 μL of saline solution.

   (d) 25 mL of liquid *W* is diluted with solution *Z* to 75 mL and then to 750 mL with saline solution.

   (e) 0.10 mL of plasma is diluted to 1.0 mL, and the resulting solution is brought to a final volume of 4.0 mL with diluent.

   (f) 50 μL of urine is added to 0.150 mL of water.

   (g) 300 μL of cerebrospinal fluid is added to 2.70 mL of diluent, and 0.50 mL of the resulting solution is added to 2.0 mL of saline solution.

   (h) 5 mL of liquid *K* is added to 5.0 L of water.

   (i) 10 μL of urine is added to 90 μL of diluent, and the resulting solution is brought to a final volume of 0.50 mL with water.

   (j) 5 μL of whole blood is pipetted into 1.0 mL of diluent.

   (k) 0.040 mL of serum is added to 260 μL of saline solution, and 150 μL of the resulting solution is added to 1.35 mL of saline solution.

   (l) 13 mL of solution *M* is brought to a final volume of 100 mL with solution *N*.

   (m) 0.55 mL of plasma is mixed with 0.45 mL of diluent.

   (n) 1.0 mL of saline solution is mixed with 0.50 mL of water.

2. (LO 2) Complete the following table.

	Volume of Serum (μL)	Volume of Diluent (mL)	Dilution Factor
a	20		10
b		0.18	7
c	45	0.090	
d		240	4
e	50		10
f	100	0.400	
g		380	20
h	150		3
i	65	0.455	

3. (LO 1, 2, 4) Nine serum samples (*a–i*) appear in the table below. Each was diluted serially, into tubes *A*, *B*, and *C*. For each sample, provide the missing information about the serial dilution.

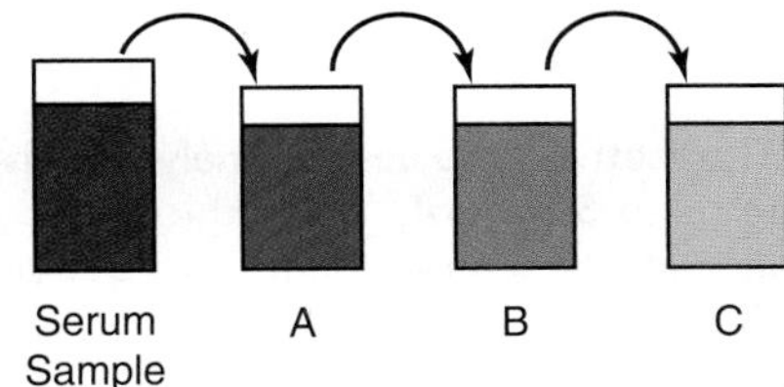

4. (LO 2, 4) Propose a procedure for carrying out each of the following dilutions.

   (a) In one step, dilute 10 μL of solution 1:50 such that the final volume is 0.50 mL.

   (b) In one step, dilute 20 μL of serum 1:6 such that the final volume is 120 μL.

	Tube *A*			Tube *B*			Tube *C*			
	Volume of Serum (mL)	Volume of Diluent (mL)	Tube Dilution	Volume From Tube *A* (mL)	Volume of Diluent (mL)	Tube Dilution	Volume From Tube *B* (mL)	Volume of Diluent (mL)	Tube Dilution	Sample Dilution
a	0.20	1.800		0.20	1.800		0.20	1.800		
b	0.50	4.50		0.10	0.90		0.05	0.100		
c	0.10	0.40		0.05	0.45		0.10	4.90		
d	0.10	4.90		0.10	4.90		0.10	0.30		
e	0.01		1:25	0.01		1:10	0.01		1:3	
f	0.02		1:50	0.02		1:40	0.02		1:3	
g	0.01	0.50		0.01	0.50		0.01	0.10		
h	0.40		1:10	0.02		1:30	0.02			1:9000
i	0.025		1:20	0.025		1:20	0.025			1:12,000

(c) In one step, dilute 15 μL of urine 1:30 such that the final volume is 450 μL.

(d) In a serial dilution of two equivalent steps, achieve a sample dilution of 1:100 starting with 50 μL of solution and ending with a final volume of 0.50 mL.

(e) In a serial dilution of three equivalent steps, achieve a sample dilution of 1:8000 starting with 10 μL of plasma and ending with a final volume of 0.20 mL.

(f) In a serial dilution of two equivalent steps, achieve a sample dilution of 1:25 starting with 1.0 mL of serum and ending with a final volume of 5.0 mL.

(g) In a serial dilution of five equivalent steps, achieve a sample dilution of 1:100,000 starting with 0.20 mL of solution and ending with a final volume of 2.0 mL.

5. (LO 1, 2, 3, 4) If the pipets available to you have variable volumes over the range 20–1000 μL, explain how to prepare the following dilutions of a patient serum that has a total volume of 1.5 mL. So as not to waste diluent, keep the final volume of the dilution no greater than 1.0 mL.

(a) 1:3 (b) 1:20

(c) 1:100 (d) 1:201

6. (LO 1, 2) The method you use for analyte *X* gives a reliable result from 5 to 50 ng/dL. After the raw first result for a particular patient sample comes out 59, you dilute the sample 1:5.

(a) If the raw second result (for the diluted sample) is 54 ng/dL, the concentration of *X* in the original sample is greater than what value?

(b) If the raw second result (for the diluted sample) is 6.2 ng/dL, what is the concentration in the original sample?

(c) If you dilute the 1:5 dilution by a factor of 2, and if the raw result for this further dilution is 52 ng/dL, the concentration of *X* in the original sample must be greater than what value?

(d) If you add 30 μL of the 1:5 dilution to 90 μL of diluent, and if the raw result for this further dilution is 46 ng/dL, what is the concentration in the original sample?

7. (LO 1, 2) A technologist mixes 100 μL of patient sample with 300 μL of diluent and then multiplies the result by 3 in an attempt to correct for the dilution. Explain whether the corrected concentration is accurate, too high, or too low. If inaccurate, by what percentage is it too high or too low?

8. (LO 1, 2) A technologist adds 40 μL of whole blood to 1.0 mL of diluent and then multiplies the result by 25 in an attempt to correct for the dilution. Explain whether the corrected concentration is accurate, too high, or too low. If inaccurate, by what percentage is it too high or too low?

9. (LO 1, 2, 4) A technologist is given a broth culture of bacteria believed to have about 100,000 viable cells per mL. In an attempt to determine this number more accurately, he decides first to carry out four serial dilutions, then to spread 0.10 mL from each dilution on an agar plate and let it incubate 24 hours, and finally to count the colonies.

He begins by adding 1.0 mL of the culture to tube **1**, which contains 9.0 mL of water; he mixes the resulting suspension well. From tube **1** he then transfers 1.0 mL to tube **2**, which also contains 9.0 mL of water. From tube **2**, in turn, he removes 1.0 mL and adds it to tube **3**, in which there is again 9.0 mL of water. From tube **3**, he transfers 1.0 mL into the 9.0 mL of water in tube **4**. Finally, from tube **4** he withdraws 0.10 mL, spreads it on an agar plate, and counts the bacterial colonies 24 hours later.

(a) If the original culture actually has bacteria at 92,300 cells/mL, what is their concentration in tube **3**?

(b) If tube **4** shows 190 cells/mL, what is their concentration in the original culture?

(c) If the original culture actually has bacteria at 5.2×10^5 cells/mL, which tube would give the technologist about 50 cells in 0.10 mL for spreading on an agar plate?

(d) Suppose the technologist mistakenly dispenses 10.0 mL of water, rather than 9.0 mL, into each of tubes **1–4**. What is the resulting sample dilution in tube **4**?

10. (LO 4) If the tube dilution is 1:3, how many tubes are required in a series to achieve a sample dilution of 1:243?

11. (LO 1, 2) A laboratory uses an automated analyzer for quantifying glucose in serum. The reportable range for the method is 20–600 mg/dL. The analyzer is programmed to dilute automatically any sample whose glucose result lies above that range and then to repeat the test on the diluted sample.

They receive a patient sample from the nephrology unit of the hospital. The analyzer reports the first (undiluted) result to be 1220 mg/dL. Because this lies beyond the method's reportable range, the analyzer automatically dilutes the sample 1:2 and repeats the test. Eight minutes later, the second (diluted) result comes out as 688 mg/dL.

A technologist takes the straight serum sample in hand and transfers 200 μL to another tube, to which he adds 800 μL of the proper diluent. After thoroughly mixing the manually diluted sample, he loads it on the analyzer for glucose quantification. Coming out eight minutes later, the result for the manually diluted sample is 275, which falls within the reportable range of 20–600.

(a) What is the corrected glucose concentration for this sample?

(b) The technologist notices something in the data that leads him to wonder whether the laboratory should extend the reportable range for this particular method beyond 600 mg/dL. Explain.

12. (LO 1, 2) For protein electrophoresis tomorrow, a technologist uses the technique of membrane dialysis to concentrate a urine sample from a patient who may have multiple myeloma. In this dialysis technique, she put the urine in contact with a semipermeable membrane, through which

the water, electrolytes, and small molecules pass from the urine. This gradually causes the volume of the urine to decrease and the protein concentration in the urine to rise. When the volume of the urine has decreased into the proper range, she transfers it to a fresh tube where it will remain until she uses it in the electrophoresis step tomorrow.

In this case, the protein concentration of the straight urine sample, that is, before membrane dialysis, is 86 mg/dL. The electrophoresis method she will use, however, requires the concentration to be 1.5–2.0 g/dL. Therefore, if the starting volume of the urine sample is 9.8 mL, what is the optimal range for the final volume?

13. (LO 1, 2) A laboratory uses a method for total serum protein that has a linearity range of 2.0–12.0 g/dL. After the serum for patient *Z* gives a result of > 12.0, a technologist dilutes 100 μL of the serum with 200 μL of the proper diluent and then repeats the test. The second result, uncorrected for dilution, is 3.0. After confirming the calculation, he immediately notifies his supervisor that something may be wrong with the instrument. What led him to raise this possibility?

14. (LO 1, 2) *N*-Telopeptide (NTx) is a product of bone resorption by osteoclasts, a process that normally occurs in balance with bone formation by osteoblasts. Released into the blood during resorption, NTx is specific to the degradation of type I collagen in bone. The quantification of NTx in urine is used in the diagnosis of osteoporosis, which can be caused by various diseases, hereditary conditions, and nutritional deficiencies.

    A technologist's laboratory uses company *Q*'s method for quantifying NTx in urine. When a sample's concentration is greater than 3000 nM BCE (bone collagen equivalents), he must dilute it and repeat the assay. The method calls for diluting a sample 1:5 with another urine sample of known BCE concentration that is between 200 and 500 nM.

    One of the urine samples (sample *A*) has a BCE concentration greater than 3000 nM. The following problem refers to this sample.

    He dilutes sample *A* 1:5 with another urine sample (sample *B*) having a BCE concentration of 331 nM. If the uncorrected concentration of sample *A* diluted with sample *B* is 1946 nM BCE, what is the BCE concentration in undiluted sample *A*?

15. (LO 1, 4) A commercial screening test for syphilis consists of the semiquantitative detection of a substance called "reagin" which is present in the serum of an individual infected with a treponemal pathogen. The technologist places sample at a different dilution on each of five circles that have been drawn on a white card and then adds reagent to each and, after a few minutes of shaking incubation, inspects for the presence of black clumps (a positive result) against the white background. Clumping is the result of agglutination caused by the presence of reagin in the specimen. Here is the layout of the card:

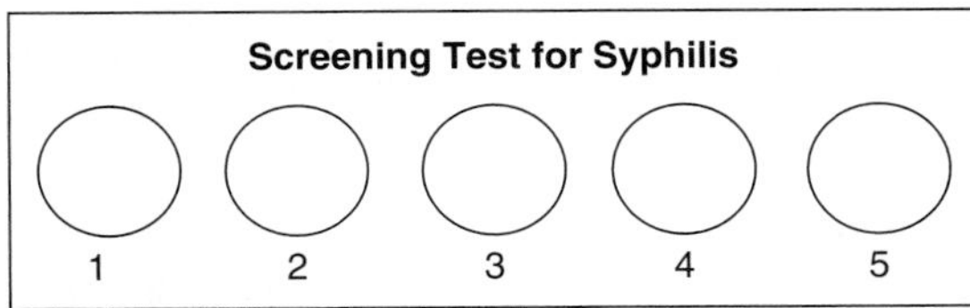

    Procedure: Pipet normal saline solution (50 μL) onto each of circles 2–5. Next, place 50 μL of straight sample on each of circles 1 and 2. Then pump the mixture on circle 2 in and out of the pipet tip about 10 times. Of the resulting solution, transfer 50 μL onto circle 3 and repeat the procedure for mixing and diluting through the fifth circle. From the fifth circle, remove and discard 50 μL, equalizing the volumes on all five circles. Then add reagent to each circle, mix well the solution within each circle, and incubate the card for 10 minutes.

    (a) Calculate the dilution ratio for each circle on the card.

    (b) If the antibody titer in the patient's serum is so high that even the most dilute circle gives a positive result, then carry the dilution further on a new card. First, dilute 100 μL of sample into 1.50 mL of normal saline solution in a test tube. Then, use a pipet to put 50 μL of diluent onto each of circles 2–5. Next, dispense 50 μL of the diluted sample onto each of circles 1 and 2. Then pump the mixture in circle 2 in and out of the pipet tip about 10 times. Of the resulting solution, transfer 50 μL onto circle 3 and repeat the procedure for mixing and diluting through the fifth circle. From the fifth circle, remove and discard 50 μL, equalizing the volumes on all five circles. Then add reagent to each circle, mix the solution within each circle well, and incubate the card for 10 minutes. Calculate the dilution ratio for each circle on the card.

    (c) Using only one card, outline an efficient serial dilution protocol that covers the range of 1:4 to 1:1024, with a constant dilution factor from circle to circle. After the serial dilution procedure and before addition of reagent, there should be no more than 75 μL of solution on each circle.

PEARSON **myhealthprofessionskit**™

Go to www.myhealthprofessionskit.com <http://www.myhealthprofessionskit.com/> to access the Companion Website created for this textbook. Simply select "Clinical Laboratory Science" from the choice of disciplines. Find this book and log in using your username and password to access additional practice problems, answers to the practice and contextual problems, additional information, and more.

7 Proportionality, Graphs, and Rates of Change

Learning Objectives

At the end of this chapter, the student should be able to do the following:

1. Recognize proportionality between two variables and calculate the proportionality constant
2. Plot data on a Cartesian graph
3. Relate the slope-intercept equation to its plot on a graph
4. Find the values of the slope and *y*-intercept from an equation or from a line on a graph
5. Use the slope as a rate of change, particularly as a reaction rate
6. Explain the purpose of standard curves
7. Interpolate properly
8. Relate a nonlinear equation to its plot on a graph

Chapter Outline

Key Terms

abscissa
absorbance
calibrator
Cartesian coordinate system
dependent variable
directly proportional
extrapolation
graph
independent variable
interpolation
linear
ordered pair
ordinate
proportionality
proportionality constant
slope
slope-intercept form
standard
standard curve
y-intercept

In practical terms, a **graph** is a visual summary of data. Its purpose is to simplify interpretation of the results by allowing us to see easily how one variable changes with another variable. In other words, a graph depicts the relationship between two or more variables. French philosopher and mathematician René Descartes (1596–1650) developed the graphing system we now use routinely, a system that unites algebra and geometry by representing numbers as points on a graph and equations as geometric shapes. In his honor, therefore, we call it the **Cartesian coordinate system**.

PROPORTIONALITY

Before considering graphs and the equations that describe them, we examine the phenomenon of **proportionality**, in which one variable changes in proportion to another. For example, consider the equation

$$y = 3x$$

The value of y is always three times the value of x. If x increases by a factor of 2, then y also increases by a factor of 2 (e.g., if x goes up from 5 to 10, then y goes up proportionally, from 15 to 30). Likewise, if x falls by a factor of 4, then y also falls by a factor of 4 (e.g., if x goes down from 12 to 3, then y goes down proportionally, from 36 to 9).

This relationship, of course, also holds true for negative values of x. If x increases from -6 to -2 (a factor of 3), then y increases from -18 to -6 (also a factor of 3).

Accordingly, the factor of 3 in the above equation is known as the **proportionality constant**. In this case, its effect is to set the value of y at three times the value of x. Furthermore, because y always moves in the same direction as x and always in proportion to it, we say that y is "**directly proportional**" to x, or that y "varies directly" with x.

In general, then, y is directly proportional to x when

$$y = kx$$

where k is a nonzero constant.

Now consider the consequence of putting a negative sign in front of the proportionality constant:

$$y = -3x$$

In this equation, the value of y is always the negative of three times the value of x. If x *increases* by a factor of 2, then y *decreases* by a factor of 2 (e.g., if x goes *up* from 5 to 10, then y goes *down* proportionally, from -15 to -30). Likewise, if x falls by a factor of 4, then y rises by a factor of 4 (e.g., if x goes down from -3 to -12, then y goes up proportionally, from 9 to 36).

As for the positive proportionality constant, this relationship holds true for negative values of x. If x increases from -6 to -2 (a factor of 3), then y decreases from 18 to 6 (also a factor of 3). Even though in this case y always moves in the opposite direction from x but in proportion to it, we again say that y is "directly proportional" to x, or that y "varies directly" with x because the two variables are still related by an equation of the form

$$y = kx$$

The term "inversely proportional" is often applied to the case in which k is negative in the above equation, but this is incorrect. Inverse proportionality involves the reciprocal of x:

$$y = \frac{k}{x}$$

where k is a nonzero constant.

STRAIGHT LINES

Let us first consider a simple example. Suppose we have the equation

$$y = 2x + 2$$

We regard x as the **independent variable** because it is the one we control; in other words, we choose values of x and then observe the resulting values of y. Therefore, we treat y as the **dependent variable** because its value is determined by the value we select for x; in other words, y depends on x. Table 7-1 ★ lists 10 chosen values of x and the corresponding values of y.

★ **TABLE 7-1** Corresponding Values of a Dependent and Independent Variable

x	y = 2x + 2
1	4
2	6
3	8
4	10
5	12
6	14
7	16
8	18
9	20
10	22

To see at a glance how y changes with x, we construct a graph of the data (Figure 7-1 ■), putting y on the vertical axis (the **ordinate**) and x on the horizontal axis (the **abscissa**). Each data point on the graph represents an **ordered pair** of corresponding (x,y) values from Table 7-1.

Notice that the data points are located such that we can draw a straight line through them. Because of this property, we call the data **linear**, and we say that the equation that generated these data points ($y = 2x + 2$) describes a straight line. Consequently, any ordered pair on that line satisfies the equation, an example being $x = 5.5$ and $y = 13$. Notice also that the line running through the data crosses the y-axis at $y = 2$ when $x = 0$ (Figure 7-1A). Thus, we say that the ***y*-intercept** of this line is "2," and we symbolize it as b.

Figure 7-1B depicts another property of our line. Notice that, for every change of 1 in x, the value of y changes by 2. For example, in going from $x = 5$ to $x = 6$, the graph goes from $y = 12$ to $y = 14$. Thus, the ratio of the change in y to the change in x is

$$\frac{\text{change in } y}{\text{change in } x} = \frac{14 - 12}{6 - 5} = \frac{2}{1} = 2$$

Likewise, in going from $x = 2$ to $x = 9$, the graph goes from $y = 6$ to $y = 20$. The ratio of the change in y to the change in x is still 2:

$$\frac{\text{change in } y}{\text{change in } x} = \frac{20 - 6}{9 - 2} = \frac{14}{7} = 2$$

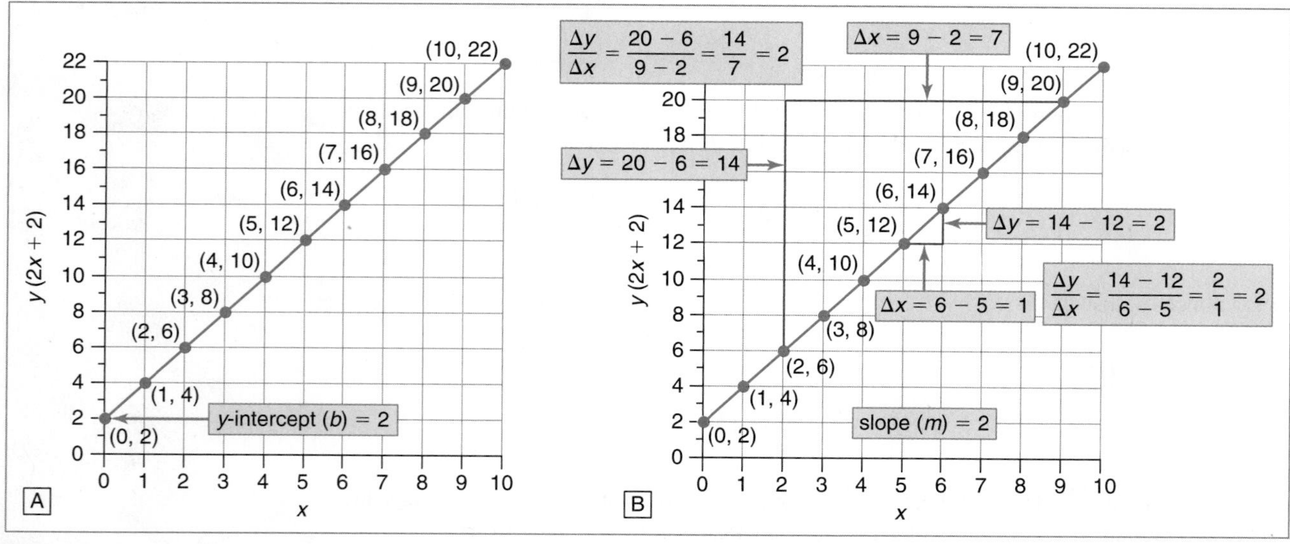

■ **FIGURE 7-1** A graph of the data in Table 7-1 (pink line), indicating the y-intercept (panel A) and the slope (panel B).

For a straight line, then, the ratio of the change in y (which we symbolize as Δy) to the change in x (which we symbolize as Δx) is the **slope** of the line. We represent the slope as m, the first letter in the French word *monter*, meaning "to rise."

$$\text{slope} = m = \frac{\Delta y}{\Delta x}$$

EQUATION 1

The slope is also sometimes called the "rise over the run" because it compares the vertical change (the rise) to the horizontal change (the run).

In our equation $y = 2x + 2$, y varies directly with x, and the slope is the proportionality constant. Whenever x increases, y increases proportionally. Therefore, as Table 7-1 and Figure 7-1 show, x and y in this equation are related by a straight line.

In general, the equation of any straight line is

$$y = mx + b$$

EQUATION 2

where m is the slope and b is the y-intercept. Equation 2 is the **slope-intercept form** of the equation of a straight line. See Appendix 7-1 on the website for the derivation of this equation.

APPENDIX 7-1
"Forms of the Equation of a Line"
www.myhealthprofessions.kit.com
PEARSON myhealthprofessionskit

Slope as the Rate of Change

In the laboratory, as in all of science and technology, *the slope is significant in that it represents the rate of change*. Consider, for example, the distance someone who is running has covered at various times after starting (Table 7-2 ★). Like the data in Table 7-1, these data give a straight line (Figure 7-2 ■).

★ TABLE 7-2 Hypothetical Data for a Person Running

Time (minutes)	Distance (miles)
0	0.00
9	0.72
16	1.28
25	2.00
31	2.48
38	3.04
49	3.92

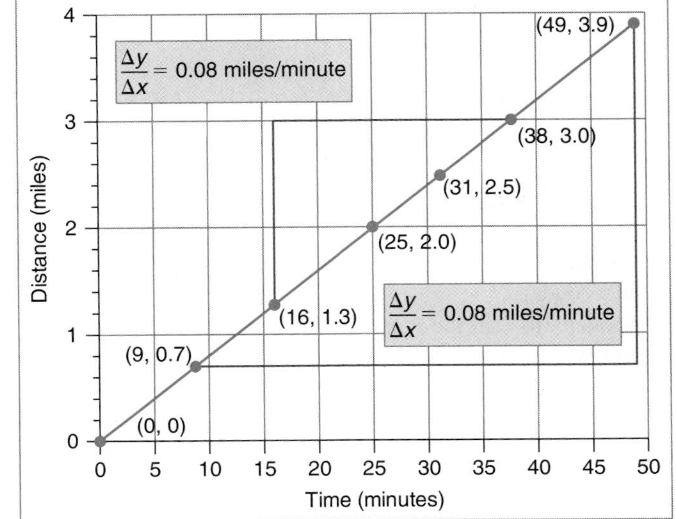

■ FIGURE 7-2 A graph of the data in Table 7-2 (pink line).

The slope of this line, $\Delta y/\Delta x$, is the runner's speed, which is simply the rate at which the distance (y) changes with time (x). Any two points on the line may be used in the calculation:

$$\text{slope} = m = \frac{\Delta y}{\Delta x} = \frac{3.9 \text{ miles} - 0.7 \text{ miles}}{49 \text{ minutes} - 9 \text{ minutes}} = \frac{3.2 \text{ miles}}{40 \text{ minutes}} = 0.08 \text{ miles/minute}$$

or

$$\text{slope} = m = \frac{\Delta y}{\Delta x} = \frac{3.0 \text{ miles} - 1.3 \text{ miles}}{38 \text{ minutes} - 16 \text{ minutes}} = \frac{1.7 \text{ miles}}{22 \text{ minutes}} = 0.08 \text{ miles/minute}$$

In the laboratory, a typical example of the slope as the rate of change occurs in assays that monitor the appearance of a reaction product as a function of time. Consider this chemical reaction:

$$A \rightarrow X$$

Suppose it is part of the assay for an analyte in serum. The instrument that runs this assay determines the amount of **X** (in "picomoles") present in the reaction vessel at the very moment all the components have been added together ("time zero") and then again at each of six time points thereafter. At the beginning of the reaction, there is no **X** present, whereas at 100 seconds, 20 picomoles have been generated.

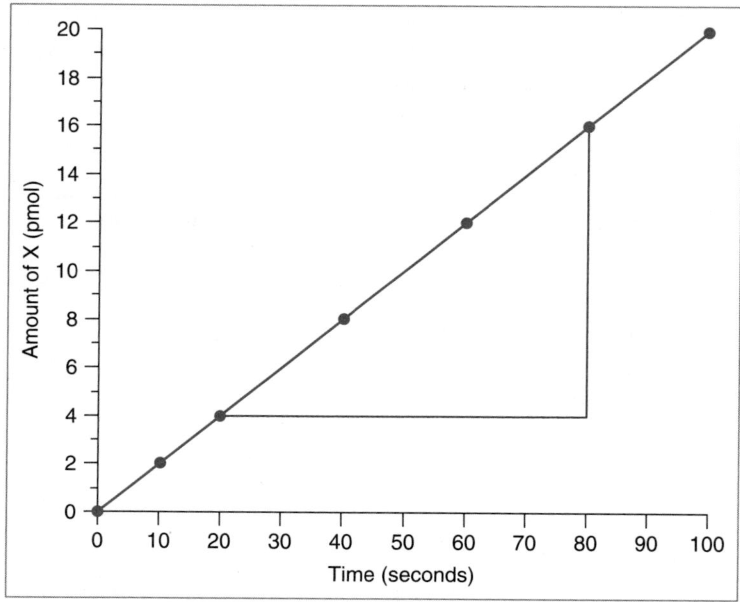

The slope of this line represents the rate at which the amount of **X** changes:

$$\text{slope} = m = \frac{\Delta y}{\Delta x} = \frac{16 \text{ pmol} - 4 \text{ pmol}}{80 \text{ seconds} - 20 \text{ seconds}} = \frac{12 \text{ pmol}}{60 \text{ seconds}} = 0.2 \text{ pmol/second}$$

What this value means is that the amount of **X** increases by 0.2 pmol every second for the duration of the assay (from 0 to 100 seconds).

Furthermore, it is possible to write the equation for this line because we know both the slope, which is 0.2, and the y-intercept, which is 0:

$$y = 0.2x + 0$$

or

$$y = 0.2x$$

The slope of 0.2 is the proportionality constant, and y varies directly with x. Remember, furthermore, that in the equation the "0.2" has units of "pmol/second" and the y-intercept has units of "pmol." Therefore, all the units in the equation are congruous:

$$\underset{y}{\underset{\uparrow}{\text{pmol}}} = \underset{m}{\underset{\uparrow}{\frac{\text{pmol}}{\text{second}}}} \times \underset{x}{\underset{\uparrow}{\text{seconds}}} + \underset{b}{\underset{\uparrow}{\text{pmol}}}$$

Suppose, however, that the assay monitors not the *appearance* of product but the *disappearance* of reactant. In this case, the instrument quantifies **A** rather than **X** at various times. For example, it shows that, at the beginning of the reaction, there are 100 picomoles of **A** in the reaction mixture, whereas, at 100 seconds, 80 picomoles remain.

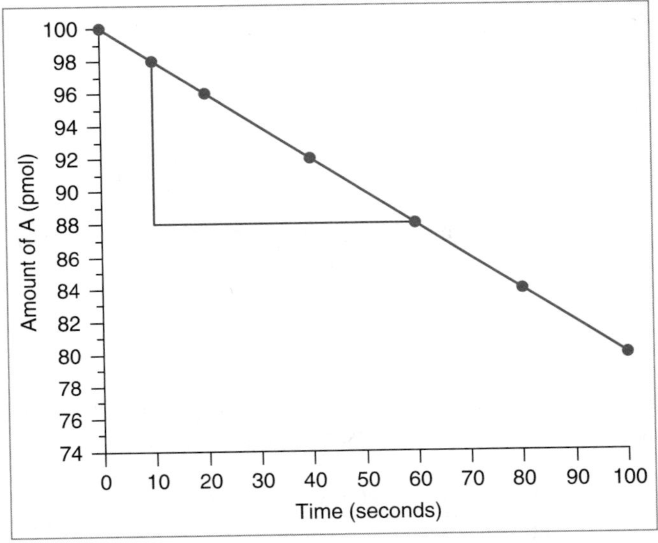

The slope of this line represents the rate at which the amount of **A** changes:

$$\text{slope} = m = \frac{\Delta y}{\Delta x} = \frac{88\text{ pmol} - 98\text{ pmol}}{60\text{ seconds} - 10\text{ seconds}} = \frac{-10\text{ pmol}}{50\text{ seconds}} = -0.2\text{ pmol/second}$$

What this value means is that the amount of **A** falls by 0.2 pmol every second for the duration of the assay (from 0 to 100 seconds).

As for the previous assay, it is possible to write the equation for this line because we know both the slope, which is -0.2, and the y-intercept, which is 100:

$$y = -0.2x + 100$$

The "-0.2" in the equation has units of "pmol/second," and the y-intercept has units of "pmol." Therefore, as in the assay with the positive slope, all the units in this equation are congruous:

$$\underset{y}{\underset{\uparrow}{\text{pmol}}} = \underset{m}{\underset{\uparrow}{\frac{\text{pmol}}{\text{second}}}} \times \underset{x}{\underset{\uparrow}{\text{seconds}}} + \underset{b}{\underset{\uparrow}{\text{pmol}}}$$

This example illustrates the fact that slopes can be negative (and that an axis of the graph does not have to start at a value of "0"). In this case, the two variables move in opposite directions but nevertheless proportionally.

Rather than the change in the amount of product or reactant, an assay might monitor the change in concentration. For example, consider the following graph of hypothetical data for the same reaction as above, **A** ⟶ **X**.

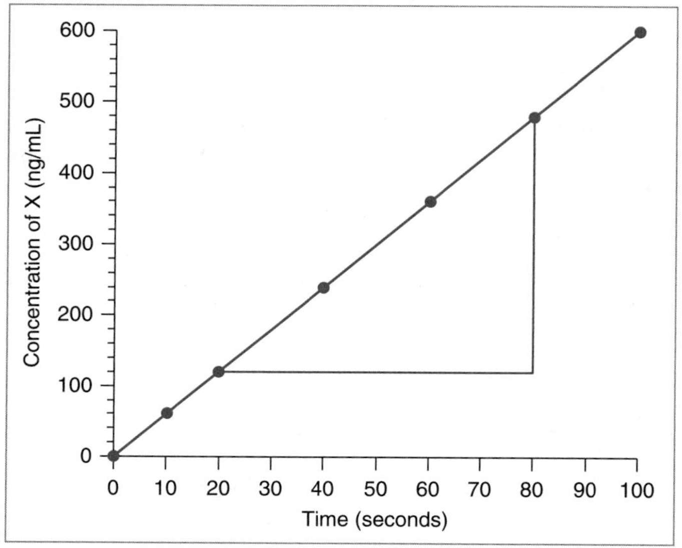

At the beginning of the reaction, there is no **X** in the reaction mixture, whereas at 100 seconds, **X** is present at 600 ng/mL. The slope of this line represents how fast the concentration of **X** changes:

$$\text{slope} = m = \frac{\Delta y}{\Delta x} = \frac{480\ \text{ng/mL} - 120\ \text{ng/mL}}{80\ \text{seconds} - 20\ \text{seconds}} = \frac{360\ \text{ng/mL}}{60\ \text{seconds}} = 6\ \text{ng/mL/second}$$

What this value means is that the concentration of **X** goes up by 6 ng/mL every second.

Because the slope is 6 and the y-intercept is 0, the equation of the line is

$$y = 6x + 0$$

or

$$y = 6x$$

The proportionality constant is "6 ng/mL/second," and y varies directly with x. All the units in this equation are congruous:

$$\underset{\substack{\uparrow \\ y}}{\text{ng/mL}} = \underset{\substack{\uparrow \\ m}}{\frac{\text{ng/mL}}{\text{second}}} \times \underset{\substack{\uparrow \\ x}}{\text{seconds}} + \underset{\substack{\uparrow \\ b}}{\text{ng/mL}}$$

☑ CHECKPOINT 7-1

1. Calculate the slope of the line in the following graph and write the equation.

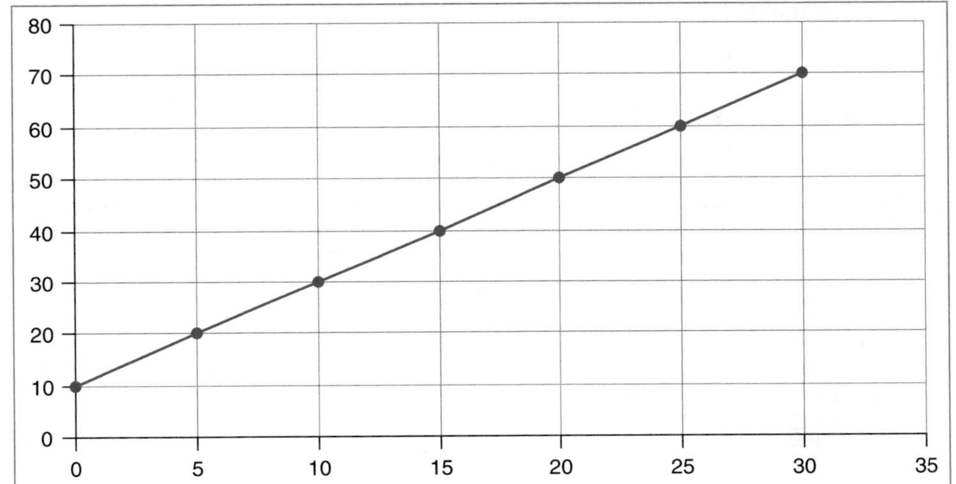

2. Calculate the slope of the line in the following graph and write the equation.

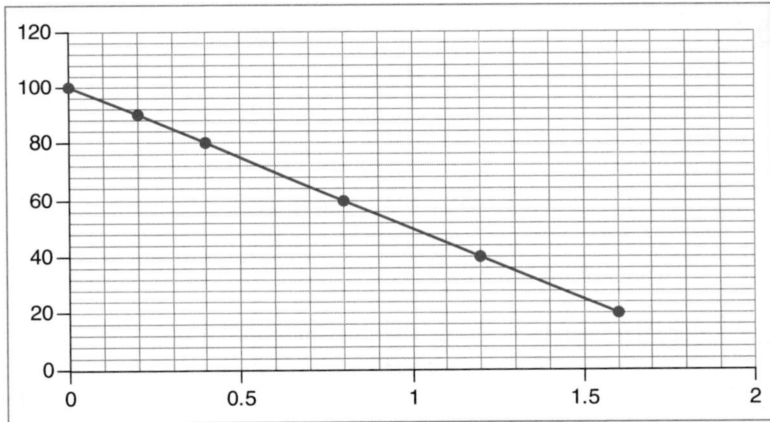

1. The slope is

$$\text{slope} = m = \frac{\Delta y}{\Delta x} = \frac{70 - 10}{30 - 0} = \frac{60}{30} = 2$$

and the equation is

$$y = 2x + 10$$

2. The slope is

$$\text{slope} = m = \frac{\Delta y}{\Delta x} = \frac{20 - 100}{1.6 - 0} = \frac{-80}{1.6} = -50$$

and the equation is

$$y = -50x + 100$$

STANDARD CURVES

As mentioned in connection with Figure 7-1, any point on this line satisfies the equation. Consequently, if we know the value of x, say, 50 seconds, we can quickly calculate the corresponding value of y to be 300 ng/mL:

$$y = 6x$$

$$y = 6(50 \text{ ng/mL})$$

$$y = 300 \text{ ng/mL}$$

The other way to find the y value that corresponds to an x value of 50 seconds is to draw a vertical line from the x value up to the data line and then to draw a horizontal line over to the y value:

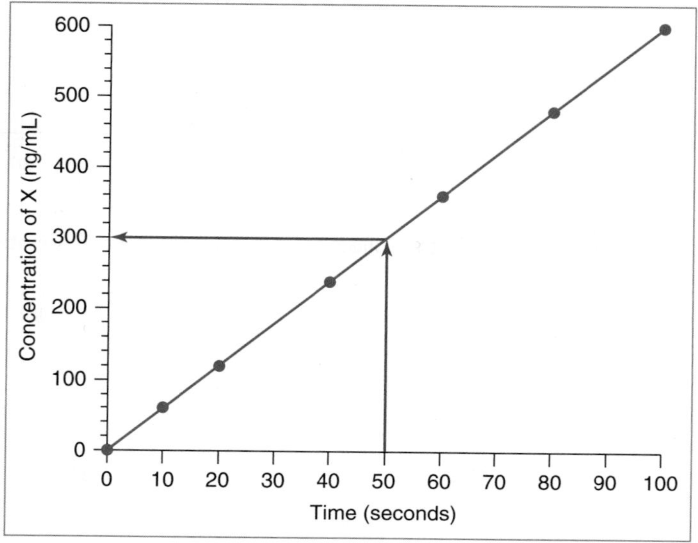

In the clinical laboratory, it is often necessary to determine the concentration of a substance from some property of the substance that can be directly measured. The most common ways to quantify a chemical substance exploit the interaction of matter and light. There are others, of course, but we will use light in order to demonstrate the purpose of standard curves.

Sometimes a chemical reaction emits light of a particular wavelength, a phenomenon called *chemiluminescence*. That light is measurable. Sometimes a chemical substance absorbs light in a process called *absorption*, discussed in a later chapter. The amount of absorbed light, called the **absorbance**, is also measurable. *Fluorescence* is the process of absorbing light of a certain wavelength and then emitting light at a lower wavelength. As in the other two cases, that light is measurable.

Thus, a chemical substance in a solution can be quantified by measuring the amount of light it absorbs or emits under well-defined conditions. The trick, however, lies in reasoning backward from the measurement of light to the amount of substance present. In other words, we must answer this question: from the amount of light we measure, how do we know how much substance is present?

Enter the standard curve. In the laboratory, we typically have several solutions of the substance we intend to quantify, each at a unique concentration. These solutions are called **standards** or **calibrators**, and the manufacturer has already determined their concentrations to high accuracy by some method other than the one we are using. What we do with these standards is to measure, say, their absorbances, and then to plot those values against concentration on a graph (Figure 7-3 ■). Often, but certainly not always, the data are linear. From this **standard curve** we discover the answer to the question posed in the previous paragraph because every point on a line satisfies the equation.

Suppose we have a solution of substance Q at an unknown concentration. If we measure the absorbance of this solution, we can then use the standard curve in Figure 7-3 to ascertain the concentration of substance Q from any value we might observe between 0 and 0.900. For example, if the absorbance

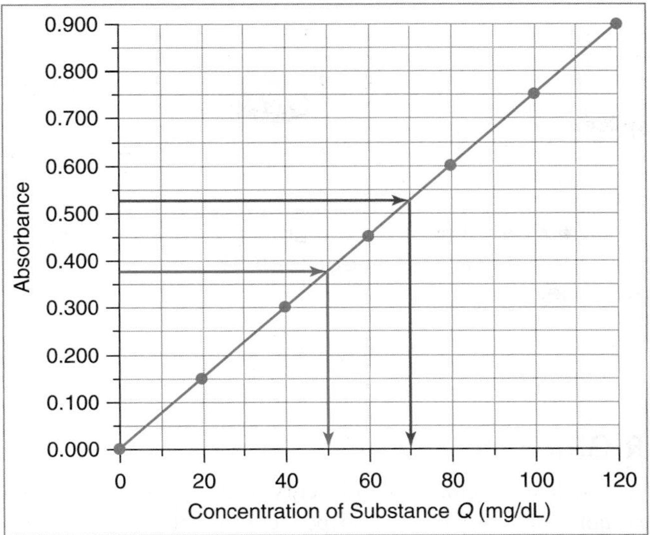

■ FIGURE 7-3 Hypothetical standard curve relating absorbance of a chemical substance to its concentration. Absorbance values of 0.375 (green line) and 0.525 (blue line) correspond, respectively, to concentrations of 50 mg/dL and 70 mg/dL.

of our solution is 0.525, then we know the concentration is 70 mg/dL; if the absorbance is 0.375, then the concentration is 50 mg/dL. This process of using a standard curve to predict the value of one variable from that of another is called **interpolation**.

Notice, however, that we have no information beyond a concentration of 120 mg/dL. We do not know whether the relationship between absorbance and concentration for substance *Q* remains linear. Therefore, if the absorbance of our solution falls above 0.900, say, 1.133, we cannot confidently predict the corresponding concentration from our standard curve. Doing so is known as **extrapolation**, and it is generally unacceptable.

We can reason to the equation for our standard curve in Figure 7-3. The *y*-intercept is 0 (or very close to 0) and the slope is

$$\text{slope} = m = \frac{\Delta y}{\Delta x} = \frac{0.750 - 0.150}{100 \text{ mg/dL} - 20 \text{ mg/dL}} = \frac{0.600}{80 \text{ ng/mL}} = \frac{0.0075}{\text{mg/dL}}$$

What this value means is that the absorbance increases by 0.0075 for every increase of 1 mg/dL in the concentration. This is a rate of change that does not involve the element of time. Realize, furthermore, that the units on the slope can be written in another way:

$$m = \frac{0.0075}{\text{mg/dL}} = 0.0075\left(\frac{\text{dL}}{\text{mg}}\right) = 0.0075 \text{ dL/mg}$$

Therefore, the equation for the standard curve in Figure 7-3 is

$$y = (0.0075 \text{ dL/mg})\, x + 0$$

or

$$y = (0.0075 \text{ dL/mg})\, x$$

We can confirm this equation by substituting our interpolated values for the *x* and *y* variables. We said that a *y* value of 0.525 corresponds to an *x* value of 70 mg/dL; these two values do indeed satisfy the equation:

$$0.525 = (0.0075 \text{ dL/mg})(70 \text{ mg/dL})$$

A later chapter in the book and online appendices discuss more-rigorous methods for finding equations—methods that do not rely on visual inspection of a plot. Such methods are especially important when the data do not fall neatly on a straight line.

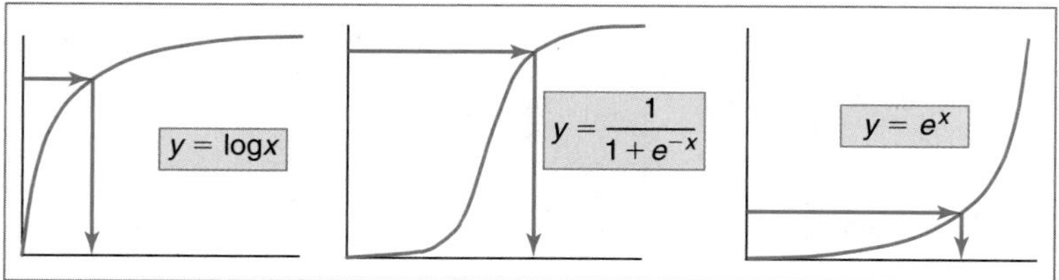

■ **FIGURE 7-4** Three examples of nonlinear graphs (pink curves) and their general equations, in which y is not proportional to x. Interpolation, however, is still possible (green lines).

NONLINEAR GRAPHS

In the clinical laboratory, data sometimes describe curves rather than lines. In nonlinear graphs, the dependent variable is not proportional to the independent variable, and their equations, accordingly, do not fit the model for a straight line, which is $y = mx + b$. Figure 7-4 ■ shows three examples. Even though finding their equations is often difficult (and sometimes impossible) without a computer, we can employ the same process of interpolation as we do on straight lines. Even so, it is generally easier to use straight lines as standard curves.

The strategy behind finding the equations for nonlinear data appears in a later chapter. At this juncture, suffice it to say that computers are very efficient at performing this task on our behalf.

☑ CHECKPOINT 7-2

Using the following standard curve, interpolate the concentrations corresponding to three specified absorbance values: 0.165, 0.621, and 0.997.

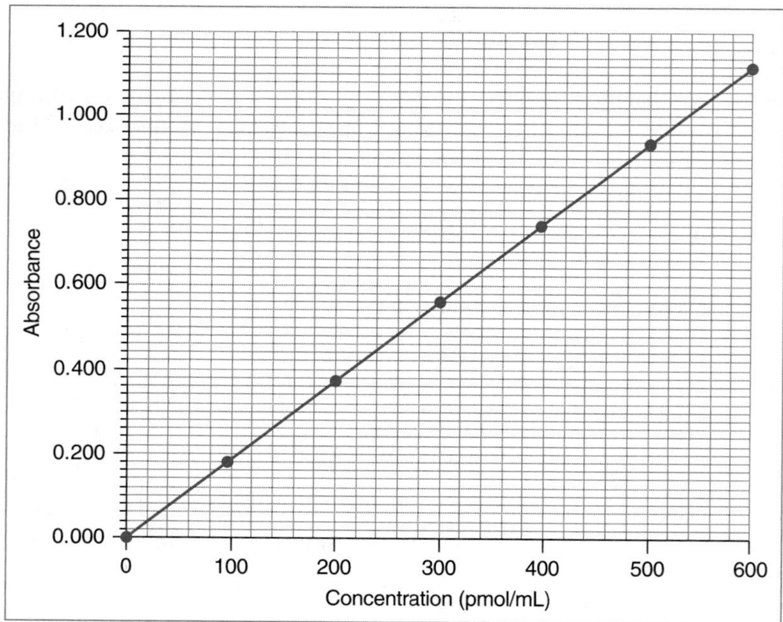

Absorbances of 0.165, 0.621, and 0.997 correspond to concentrations, respectively, of 90 pmol/mL, 340 pmol/mL, and 543 pmol/mL.

Summary

1. A *graph* is a visual summary of data. Its purpose is to simplify interpretation of the results by allowing us to see easily how one variable changes with another variable.
2. Two variables, x and y, are directly proportional when related by the equation:

$$y = kx$$

where k is the *proportionality constant.*

3. The *independent variable* is controlled; it determines the *dependent variable.*
4. Each data point on a graph represents an *ordered pair* of (x,y) values. The x value is usually plotted on the horizontal axis and the y value on the vertical axis.
5. Data are said to be *linear* when a straight line fits them.
6. The *slope-intercept form* of the equation of a straight line is

$$y = mx + b$$

where m is the *slope* and b is the y-intercept.

7. The slope of a line is

$$\text{slope} = m = \frac{\Delta y}{\Delta x}$$

8. The slope is significant in that it represents the rate of change.
9. A *standard curve* is usually a plot of a measurable property (e.g., absorbance) as a function of concentration. Its purpose is to allow the concentration to be determined by interpolation.
10. *Interpolation* is the process of predicting the value of one variable from the value of another by means of an equation or a graph.
11. Predicting the value of one variable from the value of another that lies outside the range of a standard curve is *extrapolation*, which is generally unacceptable.
12. In nonlinear graphs, the dependent variable is not proportional to the independent variable, and their equations, accordingly, do not fit the model for a straight line ($y = mx + b$).

Practice Problems

1. (LO 1) In which of the following cases is y directly proportional to x?

   (a) $y = 6 + x$ (b) $y = 18.3x - 9.6$

   (c) $y = 4x/(4 + x)$ (d) $y = 0.5 - (x/5)$

2. (LO 2) By means of graphing software or pen and paper, plot each of the following equations at $x = 1, 2, 3, 4$, and 5.

   (a) $y = 4x + 3$ (b) $y = 3x - 1$

   (c) $y = 0.62x + 2.6$ (d) $6x + 3y = 18$

   (e) $x = 0.25y + 4$ (f) $y = x$

   (g) $y = 5$ (h) $x = -10y$

   (i) $y = -2x + 15$

3. (LO 2, 3, 4) Plot each of the following data sets and write the equation for the line.

(a)

x	y
1	9
2	14
3	19
4	24
5	29

(b)

x	y
1	15
2	12
3	9
4	6
5	3

(c)

x	y
20	9
40	25
60	41
80	57
100	73

(d)

x	y
0. 066	209.9
0. 198	229.7
0. 396	259.4
0. 462	269.3
0. 660	299.0

4. (LO 4, 5) Each of the following lines represents the change in concentration in a chemical reaction. Calculate the reaction rate corresponding to each line.

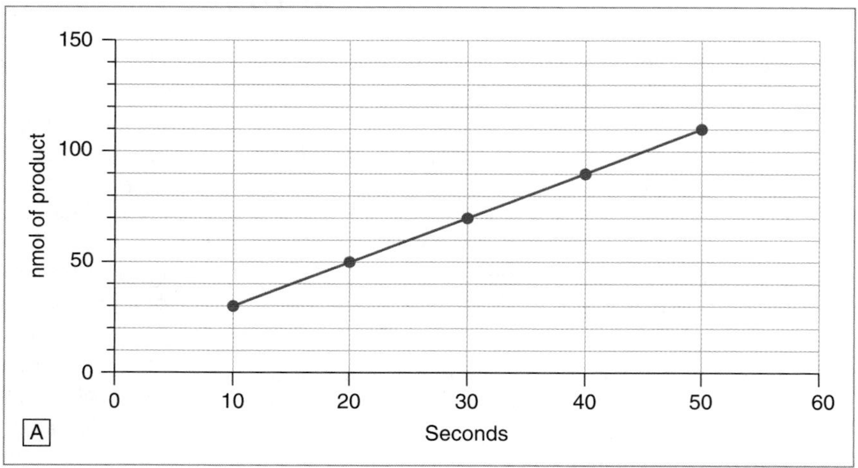

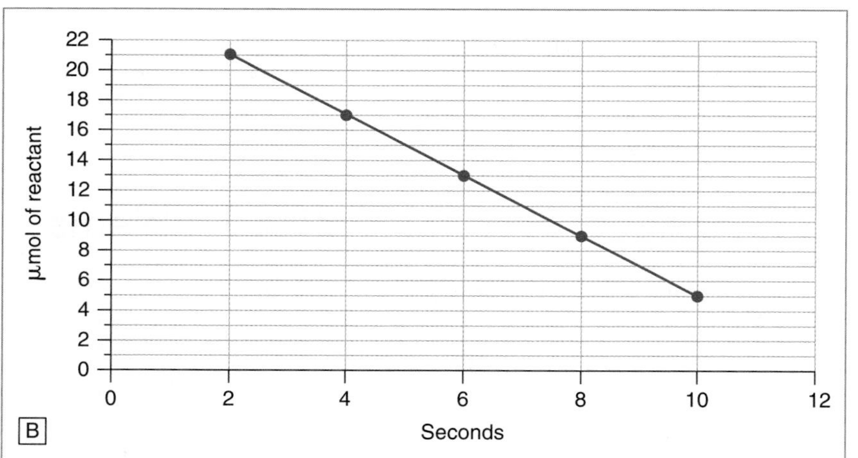

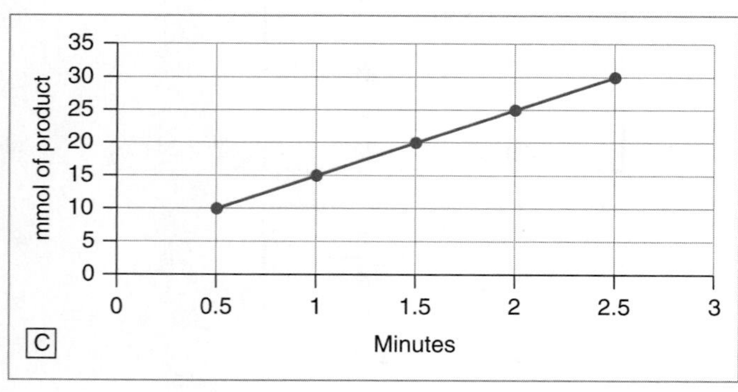

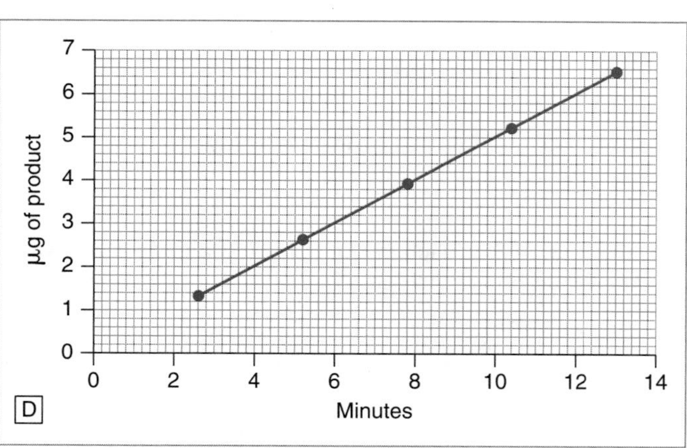

5. (LO 2, 7) From the following data, construct a standard curve. By inspection, interpolate the concentration of each solution below from the absorbance given.

Concentration (mmol/L)	Absorbance
0	0
3	0.151
6	0.299
9	0.448
12	0.602
15	0.750

(a) $A = 0.682$ (b) $A = 0.177$

(c) $A = 0.304$ (d) $A = 0.098$

6. (LO 2, 7) From the following data, construct a standard curve. By inspection, interpolate the concentration of each solution below from the luminescence given. (Luminescence is measured as the number of photons of light that strike the detector in a given second.)

Concentration (mmol/L)	Luminescence (counts/second)
0	0
5	7710
10	121,951
20	1,649,485
30	5,000,000
50	8,852,691
60	9,411,765
70	9,673,650
80	9,806,081
90	9,878,049
100	9,919,651

(a) 9,862,430 (b) 8,903,779

(c) 4,388,021 (d) 355,612

7. (LO 6, 7) Which of the interpolations in problem 6 is the most prone to error? Explain.

8. (LO 3, 4) Match the following 10 graphs with their equations. Assume that all the graphs have the same x-axis scales and the same y-axis scales.

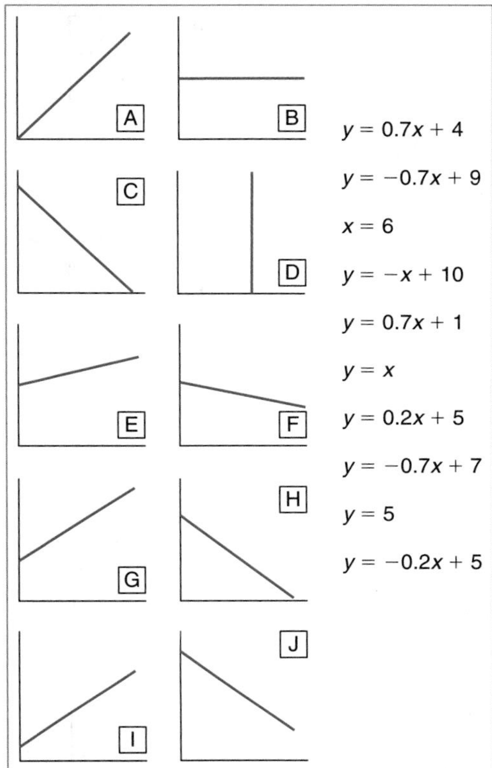

9. (LO 3, 4) Referring to the graph at the right, explain whether each of the following statements is true.

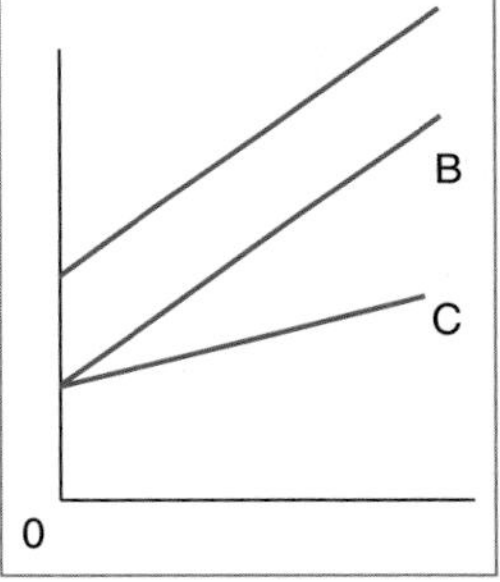

(a) If the equation for line **A** is $y = 2x + 5$, then the slope of line **C** must be less than 2.

(b) If the equation for line **C** is $y = x + 10$, then the y-intercept of line **B** is 10.

(c) If the equation for line **C** is $y = 2x + 6$, then the equation $y = 4x + 12$ is possible for line **A**.

(d) The equation $y = -3x + 8$ is possible for one of the three lines.

(e) The equation $y = 6x - 7$ is possible for one of the three lines.

10. (LO 8) Match the following nonlinear graphs with their equations.

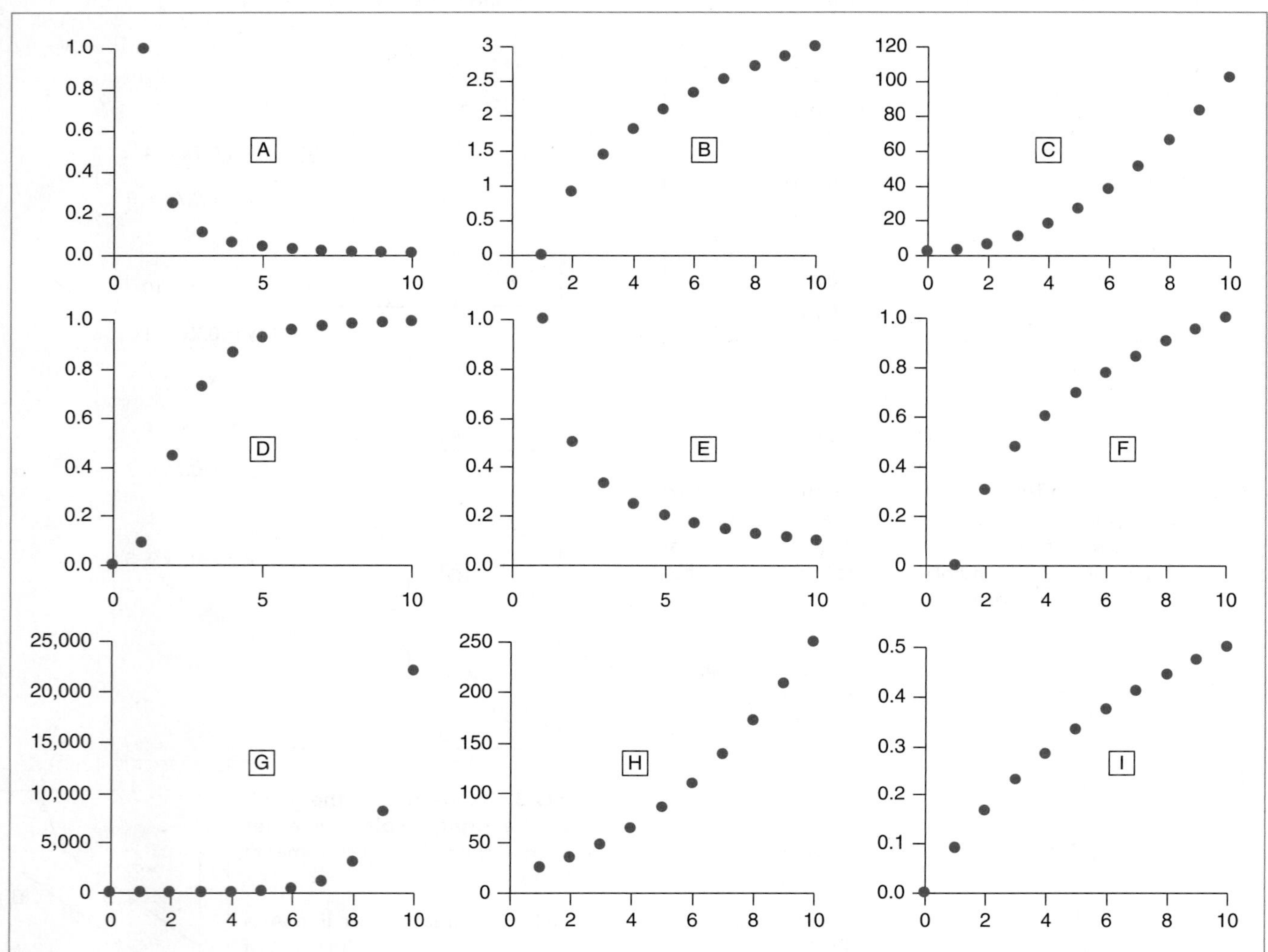

$y = \log x$

$y = 3 \log x$

$y = e^x$

$y = 2x^2 + 3x + 20$

$y = x^2 + 2$

$y = x / (x + 10)$

$y = x^3 / (x^3 + 10)$

$y = 1 / x$

$y = 1 / x^2$

Contextual Problems

1. (LO 6, 7) The following standard curve pertains to an assay for a hormone. The test employs chemiluminescence and reports "relative light units" (RLU) being emitted from the reaction mixture at the end. The technology is such that luminescence decreases as concentration of the hormone increases.

   (a) What is the concentration of a specimen whose luminescence is 700,000 RLU? 1,900,000 RLU? 200,000 RLU?

   (b) Notice that this graph is semilogarithmic (i.e., the *x*-axis is logarithmic). Plot the same data on arithmetic axes and compare the two graphs for usefulness as standard curves.

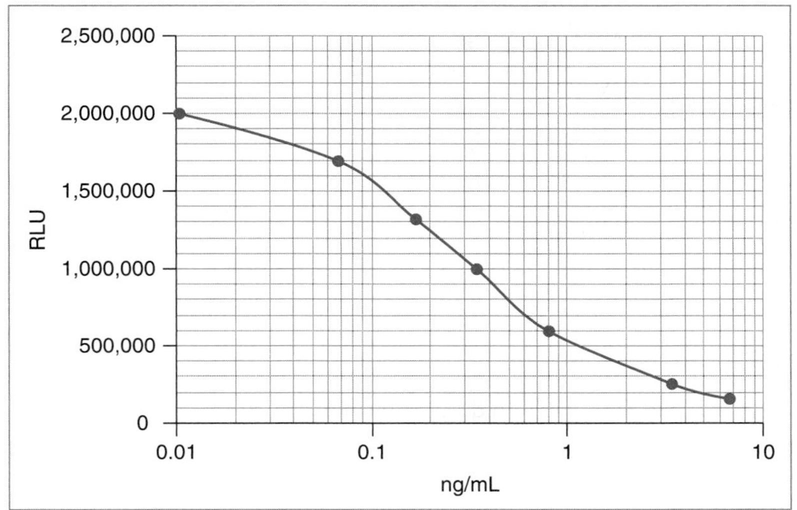

2. (LO 2, 3, 4) Your laboratory's assay for a particular analyte requires checking the standard curve weekly for shifting due to such factors as deterioration of the reagent. This process entails running two standards in the assay, drawing the line between them, and comparing that line to the existing standard curve. The standard curve is considered valid if the slope of the new line is within 10% of the previous slope and if the new *y*-intercept is within 10% of its previous value. (The measurement is in units of "counts per second.")

   (a) Plot the following data and calculate the slope and *y*-intercept of the standard curve.

Concentration (μmol/L)	Counts per second
5	42,972
20	47,142
40	52,702
80	63,822
120	74,942
160	86,062

   (b) The following results come from a two-standard check. Is the existing standard curve still valid?

Concentration (μmol/L)	Counts per second
20	50,117
120	80,046

   (c) Consider two hypothetical scenarios for the two-standard check.

   Scenario A: slope = 278, *y*-intercept = 35,193
   Scenario B: slope = 340, *y*-intercept = 41,582

   In which of these two scenarios is the new line closer to the existing standard curve at a concentration of 120 μmol/L and above? Explain.

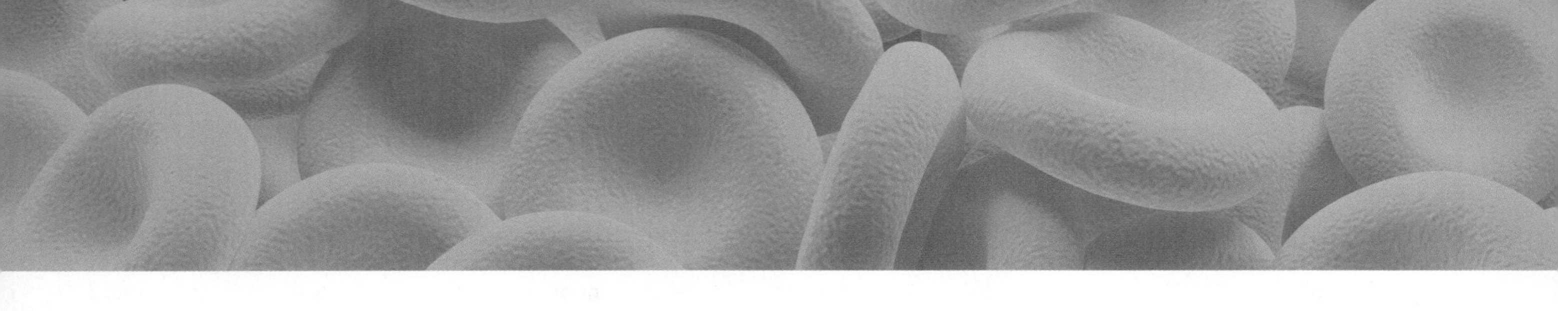

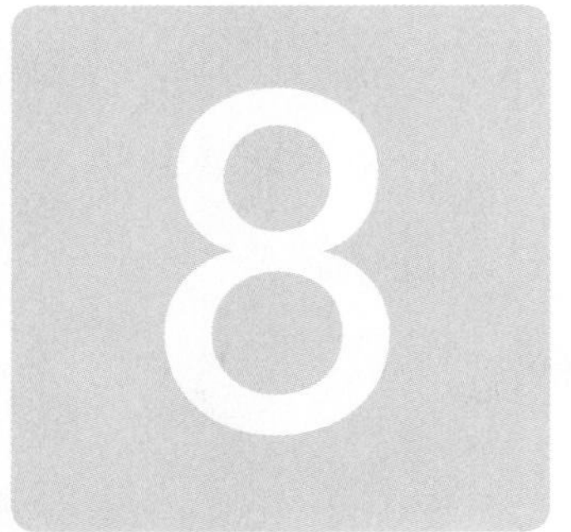

Statistics

Learning Objectives

At the end of this chapter, the student should be able to do the following:

1. Set forth the reasons that a laboratory professional should have a working understanding of statistics
2. Recognize the difference between accuracy and precision
3. Explain central tendency in data sets and the significance of typical values
4. Calculate, interpret, and properly use the three most common measures of center (mean, median, mode) and recognize the relationship between the mean and accuracy
5. For a normal distribution, explain (a) the equality of the mean, median, and mode, and (b) the 68-95-99.7 Rule
6. Explain the usefulness of the standard deviation as a measure of dispersion, carry out its calculation, and interpret it properly
7. Calculate and interpret the coefficient of variation and recognize its relationship to precision
8. Explain the usefulness of regression in the clinical laboratory
9. Generate linear regression equations (by means of a calculator or computer)
10. Explain the difference between linear and nonlinear regression
11. Interpolate properly from regression lines
12. Calculate the correlation coefficient (by means of a calculator or computer)
13. Interpret the correlation coefficient properly, recognizing its strengths and limitations
14. Explain the similarities and differences between regression and correlation
15. Explain the purpose of data weighting
16. Interpret the coefficient of determination properly
17. Use the basic techniques (visual inspection, root-mean-squared error, standard error of the slope, confidence intervals) for judging goodness-of-fit for regression lines
18. Explain the basic strategy behind nonlinear regression
19. State and interpret a null hypothesis
20. Select a significance test appropriate for the question to be answered

Chapter Outline

21. Interpret the probability represented by "*p* value"
22. Calculate values for the *F*, *t*, and χ^2 statistics
23. Use the values of *F*, *t*, and χ^2 to assess the statistical significance of differences
24. Explain the requirements and limitations of significance tests

Key Terms

accuracy
arithmetic mean
categorical
central tendency
coefficient of determination
coefficient of variation
confidence interval
contingency table
correlation
correlation coefficient
critical value
degrees of freedom
linear regression
mean
median
mode
nonlinear regression
normal distribution
null hypothesis
outlier
p value
precision
regression analysis
specimen pairing
standard deviation
statistically significant
t value
unimodal
variance

This chapter presents the statistics that are important in a medical laboratory. Below is a list of reasons that a clinical laboratory professional should develop a working understanding of statistics.

- To make rational decisions about whether laboratory instruments and reagents are functioning properly so that test results can be reported
- To manage the many other elements of quality control in the laboratory
- To understand the information in printed materials from manufacturers of test methods or laboratory instruments
- To compare a new method or instrument in the laboratory with the one already in use
- To follow the reasoning presented in research papers, scientific talks, and continuing-education courses

Implicit to all these reasons are two notions that are tightly connected to quality control in the laboratory: **accuracy**, which is the degree of correctness of a laboratory result, and **precision**, which is the degree of reproducibility in repeated measurements. In other words, accuracy refers to how close a laboratory value is to the true value, whereas precision refers to how tightly clustered several replicates are, whether or not they are close to the true value. One might say, then, that accuracy reveals the quality of a result, and precision reveals the quality of the measurement behind that result. The clinical laboratory seeks both accuracy and precision, in which case the measurements are all close to, and tightly grouped around, the true value.

THE CENTRAL TENDENCY

One of the paramount questions arising from every set of numerical data is this: if there is a typical value, what is it likely to be? The answer to this question lies in the **central tendency** of the data. There are three common measures of central tendency: (1) the **median**, which is the midpoint of the data; (2) the **mean**, which is the balance point of the data; and (3) the **mode**, which is the value that occurs most often in the data.

The Median

To find the median, arrange all the entries in the data set, including all repeats, in ascending or descending order and then locate the midpoint. If the number of entries in the data set is odd, the median is the middle entry. If the number is even, the median is the calculated value halfway between the two middle entries. Here are two examples:

Data	Median	Comment
2, 3, 4, 6, 8, 9, 10	6	Because the number of values is odd (7), the median is the middle value, or "6."
33.1, 33.8, 33.9, 41.5, 42.0, 42.4	37.7	Because the number of values is even (6), the median is the calculated value halfway between the two middle entries: 3.8 3.8 33.9 37.7 41.5

Note that when the number of entries is even, the median is calculable by adding the two middle entries and dividing the sum by 2 (this happens to be the mean of the two middle values, discussed next). For the second example above,

$$\frac{33.9 + 41.5}{2} = 37.7$$

The Mean

To find the mean, or the balance point, of the data, add all the values together and divide the sum by the number of those values:

EQUATION 1

$$\bar{x} = \frac{x_1 + x_2 + x_3 + \ldots + x_n}{n}$$

where $\bar{x}$ is the mean of the data and n is the number of entries in the data set. Consider, for example, this simple data set: 1, 2, 2, 4, 5, 6, 8. The mean is 4 (28 ÷ 7).

The mean is also the unique value that can replace every observed value in the data set without altering the total of those values. For example, replacing each member of the above data set with its mean, which is "4," gives the same total:

$$1 + 2 + 2 + 4 + 5 + 6 + 8 = 28 = 4 + 4 + 4 + 4 + 4 + 4 + 4$$

We can regard the mean as the "center of gravity" of the data. If we place the data points on a number line, like weights on a beam, then the mean is the fulcrum, or the balance point (Figure 8-1 ■).

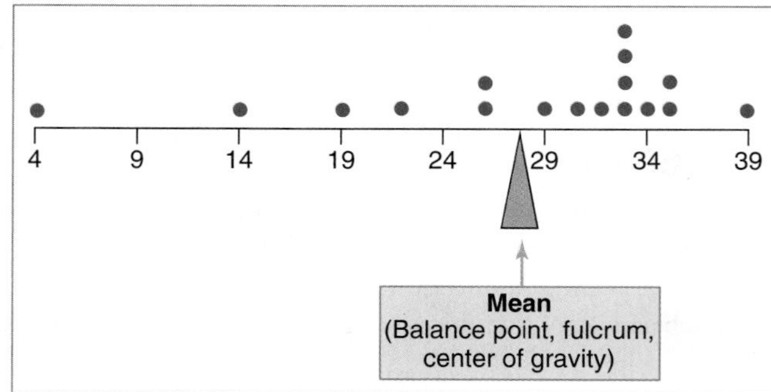

■ **FIGURE 8-1** The weights-on-a-beam analogy for the mean of a data set. The individual values: 4, 14, 19, 22, 26, 26, 29, 31, 32, 33, 33, 33, 33, 34, 35, 35, 39. The mean is 28.

The mean we discuss here is the **arithmetic mean** (pronounced "arith-MET-ic"), one of the three classical Pythagorean means; the other two are the *geometric* and *harmonic* means. The geometric mean, though encountered much less often than the arithmetic, does have functions in the clinical laboratory, one of which occurs in the calculation of the "International Normalized Ratio" (see Chapter 10). Appendix 8-7 on the website discusses the geometric mean in depth.

APPENDIX 8-7
"Arithmetic Means, Geometric Means, and Log-Normal Distributions"
www.myhealthprofessions.kit.com
PEARSON myhealthprofessionskit™

The Mode

The mode is the value that occurs most often. In Figure 8-1, that value is 33. Because it has only one mode, we call this data set **unimodal**, although it is possible for a data set to have more than one peak, in which case the set may be bimodal or even trimodal. Realize, however, that the mode may not be the center, or near the center, of the data; therefore, the mode is not necessarily a measure of central tendency.

How Outliers Affect the Central Tendency

An **outlier** is an extreme value, one that falls well above or below the other data. Consider the following three data sets.

	Data	Mean	Median	Mode
A	25, 27, 30, 30, 32, 35, 37	31	30	30
B	25, 27, 30, 30, 32, 35, 75	36	30	30
C	25, 27, 30, 30, 32, 35, 37, 75	36	31	30

Data sets **B** and **C** each have an outlier ("75," in pink). In set **B**, the outlier has replaced the final entry in set **A**; in set **C**, the outlier has merely been added to set **A**. As the table shows, the outlier markedly changes the mean, although it barely affects the median and does not disturb the mode at all. This illustrates a major difference among these three measures of central tendency. The median and mode resist the influence of outliers better than does the mean; in other words, the median and mode are generally more *robust*. This is so because an outlier goes directly into the calculation of the mean, whereas it may not change either the number of entries in the data set or the most frequent value.

☑ CHECKPOINT 8-1

1. Evaluate the mean, median, and mode for this data set: 1.9, 2.6, 2.3, 1.7, 2.0, 2.3, 1.8, 2.2, 2.3.
2. If the value of 2.6 in these data were replaced by 3.2, which of the measures of central tendency would change? Why?
3. If we added a data value of 1.8 to the original set of nine data, which of the measures would change? Why?

1. Mean = 2.1, median = 2.2, mode = 2.3
2. The mean would change because the new value of 3.2 goes directly into its calculation.
3. The mean would change because the additional value of 1.8 goes directly into its calculation. The median would change because the additional datum pushes the number of values up to 10, shifting the middle one.

DISPERSION

As explained earlier, the central tendency answers the question about what a typical value is for a data set. Now we face the corollary to that question: *how* typical is that typical value?

Summarizing a data set by reporting the mean (or median or mode) is often not enough. Although it locates the center of the data, the mean does not tell us how the data are dispersed around it; in other words, it does not tell us whether the data themselves are tightly clustered or widely spread. The following two data sets illustrate this point.

	Data	Mean
A	10, 11, 12, 13, 14, 15, 16	13
B	3, 5, 8, 13, 18, 21, 23	13

Despite having the same mean, the two data sets have different dispersions; the data are closer together in **A** than they are in **B**. Therefore, "13" is more typical of the data in **A** than it is of the data in **B**.

Standard Deviation

The most common measure of dispersion is the **standard deviation** (Equation 2). In a simple sense, what it represents is the average variation of the data around their mean. We can interpret the standard deviation as an indicator of the spread, as a typical distance between the data and the mean. A high value tells us that on average the data lie far from the mean, whereas a low value tells us they are clustered around it.

EQUATION 2

$$\text{standard deviation} = s = \sqrt{\frac{\sum_{i=1}^{n}(x_i - \bar{x})^2}{n - 1}}$$

where $\bar{x}$ is the mean of the data and n is the number of entries in the data set. The sigma (Σ) notation serves as shorthand for summation:

$$\sum_{i=1}^{n}(x_i - \bar{x})^2 = (x_1 - \bar{x})^2 + (x_2 - \bar{x})^2 + (x_3 - \bar{x})^2 + \ldots + (x_n - \bar{x})^2$$

The value under the sigma specifies the starting x, and the value above the sigma specifies the final x. In this case, then, we add the deviations together by starting with x_1 and finishing with x_n.

Data Set	n	x_1 (mg/dL)	x_n (mg/dL)	$\bar{x}$ (mg/dL)	$(x_1 - \bar{x})^2$ (mg^2/dL^2)	$\sum_{i=1}^{n}(x_i - \bar{x})^2$ (mg^2/dL^2)	Standard Deviation (s) (mg/dL)
A	7	10	16	13	9	28	2.2
B	7	3	23	13	100	378	7.9

For data set **A** above, $s = 2.2$. What this means is that, on average, the data values lie at a distance of 2.2 from their mean, which is 13. For data set **B**, $s = 7.9$; the larger standard deviation of **B** is consistent with the wider spread in the data.

Although calculators and spreadsheet software compute s for us, understanding Equation 2 goes a long way toward helping us avert misinterpretations of the standard deviation. The following sequence outlines the strategy within Equation 2, beginning with the numerator.

1. **Subtract the mean from each data value.** This measures the distance from that particular datum to the mean.
2. **Square each difference.** This eliminates any negative signs that may have arisen from the subtraction when the mean was greater than the data value. As the above table shows, however, this also squares the units, which consequently seem to make no sense; after all, what does a squared concentration mean? Step 5 solves this problem.
3. **Add together all the squared differences.** The numerator is the sum of all the squared deviations from the mean.
4. **Divide the numerator by $n - 1$.** This quantity, $n - 1$, is the number of **degrees of freedom**, which equals the number of independent values in the data set. Notice that it is one less than the number of members in the data set (n). As the size of the data set increases, the values of $n - 1$ and n become practically equal, and we may use either one in the denominator. For a more thorough explanation of degrees of freedom, consult Appendix 8-1 on the website. At the end of this step, what

APPENDIX 8-1
"Degrees of Freedom"
www.myhealthprofessions.kit.com
PEARSON myhealthprofessionskit

appears under the square-root sign is the average *squared* deviation from the mean, known as the **variance** (see the next section).

5. **Take the square root.** This solves the problem created in step 2 and restores the original units. Our measure of dispersion is now in the same units as the original data.

Variance

Although we rarely see the variance of a data set used to quantify dispersion, it appears in the *F* test, which this chapter addresses later, and in other contexts. Therefore, it is wise at this point to know that the variance is the square of the standard deviation:

$$\text{variance} = s^2 = \frac{\sum_{i=1}^{n}(x_i - \bar{x})^2}{n - 1}$$

Like the standard deviation, then, a high variance tells us that the data lie far from the mean, whereas a low variance tells us they are clustered around it.

Coefficient of Variation

The standard deviation can sometimes be misleading. For example, a standard deviation of 2 has quite a different impact when the mean is 5 than it has when the mean is 100. With a mean of 100, an s of 2 says that the average deviation is only 2% of the mean. With a mean of 5, however, the same value of s becomes a much larger 40% of the mean.

Therefore, in comparing two data sets with different means, it is necessary to have a measure of dispersion that relates the standard deviation directly to the mean. The **coefficient of variation** meets this need:

$$CV = \frac{s}{\bar{x}} \times 100\%$$

where CV = coefficient of variation, s = standard deviation, and $\bar{x}$ = mean.

In effect, the *CV* "standardizes" the standard deviation by expressing it as a percentage of the mean. As a dimensionless ratio, therefore, its value stays the same even when the units of measurement change. Suppose, for example, your assay results have a mean of 30 mg/dL with a standard deviation of 2 mg/dL. If you must report these values in units of g/L, the conversion would change the mean to 0.30 and the standard deviation to 0.02. The *CV*, however, would stay the same at 7%.

The coefficient of variation is the most common measure of *precision*, which tells us how tight the data are around their mean. This contrasts with *accuracy*, which tells us how close the mean is to the true or accepted value.

☑ CHECKPOINT 8-2

1. Why is it necessary to specify dispersion along with a measure of central tendency?
2. Calculate the standard deviation and coefficient of variation for this data set: 5.1, 9.6, 7.7, 6.3, 5.8, 6.6, 8.1, 7.4, 6.9, 6.2, 8.4, 6.5.

1. Dispersion gives information about how the data are distributed about the center.
2. SD = 1.2 (1.249), CV = 18% (17.7%) (mean = 7.05).

THE NORMAL DISTRIBUTION

Many variables in the physical, biological, and behavioral sciences adopt what is called a **normal distribution** (see Figure 8-2 ■). The word *normal* is used not because the distribution is proper or correct but (and this distinction is important) because it is considered typical or standard for a variable that depends on random processes.

In the clinical laboratory, the curve in Figure 8-2 might represent the serum cholesterol concentrations determined in 100 randomly selected patients. In that case, the independent variable (the *x*-axis)

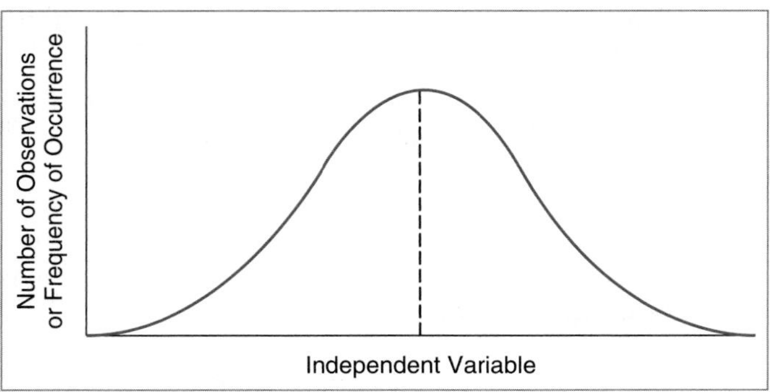

FIGURE 8-2 The normal distribution. The vertical dashed line indicates the mean, median, and mode of the independent variable.

would be the cholesterol concentration, and the dependent variable (the *y*-axis) would be the number of times each concentration was observed. In other disciplines—ecology, for example—the independent variable might represent the widths of maple leaves in southern Québec; in sociology, the mathematics test scores for all ninth-grade students in Chicago; in aeronautics, the ages of all passenger airplanes in the U.S. fleet.

Clearly, the lowest and the highest values of the independent variable occur least often, whereas values near the center occur most often. It is easy to see how this distribution acquired its nickname, "the bell curve."

The curve in Figure 8-2 is defined by the mean and standard deviation. Theoretically, given only those two numbers, one could draw the entire curve. It would be the same as if one knew the value of every data point. Although many variables in the sciences adopt this distribution, some variables do not, and there is a tendency among some researchers to invoke the normal distribution even before there is enough evidence to support it.

The normal distribution has several important properties, two of which we discuss now.

- *The mean, median, and mode are equal.* In other words, the balance point, the middle value, and the most common value are all the same (Figure 8-2, dashed line). This is so because the curve is symmetrical. In fact, the curve can be wider, narrower, taller, or shorter, and its peak may shift in one direction or the other, but the normal distribution is always symmetrical.
- *The normal distribution follows the 68-95-99.7 Rule.* In a normal distribution of data (Figure 8-3), 68% of the values fall between the mean plus one standard deviation ($\bar{x} + s$) and the mean minus one standard deviation ($\bar{x} - s$). Moreover, 95% of the data are between ($\bar{x} + 2s$) and ($\bar{x} - 2s$), and 99.7% are between ($\bar{x} + 3s$) and ($\bar{x} - 3s$).

In the clinical laboratory, the standard deviation guides the acceptance and rejection of quality control runs and determines whether patient specimens are tested. Suppose, for example, that your laboratory runs a test for ferritin in serum. Before running any patient specimens, you must ensure that your analytical method is functioning properly. You run your ferritin control solution and compare the result

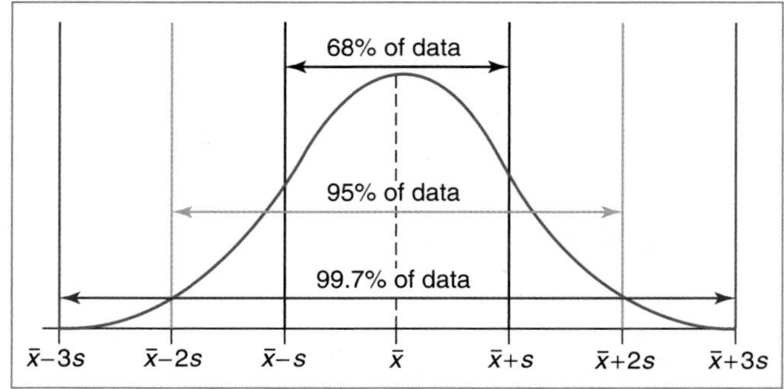

FIGURE 8-3 The 68-95-99.7 Rule for a normal distribution. The mean is $\bar{x}$ and the standard deviation is s.

(147 ng/mL) with the mean (151 mg/dL) for the 60 other ferritin control results that have been recorded for the previous 6 weeks. If the standard deviation of those control results is 3 ng/mL, then 68% of the data fall between 148 and 154 ng/mL, or between $\bar{x} - 1s$ and $\bar{x} + 1s$ (i.e., between 151 − 3 and 151 + 3). Moreover, 95% of the data would fall between 145 and 157 ng/mL, or between $\bar{x} - 2s$ and $\bar{x} + 2s$ (i.e., between 151 − 6 and 151 + 6).

Your result of 147 ng/mL falls between one and two standard deviations below the mean. At this point, the question is whether your result is close enough to the mean to conclude that the analytical method is functioning properly, and, therefore, whether to proceed with patient specimens. Laboratories have policies governing this decision based on the deviation of a given result from the mean. If your laboratory's established limit for the ferritin assay is $\pm 2s$, then your result of 147 ng/mL passes the standard-deviation test, and you proceed to run patient samples. However, if the limit is $\pm 1s$, then your result fails, and you do not run patient samples until the malfunction is rectified.

☑ CHECKPOINT 8-3

1. What is true about the mean, median, and mode in a normal distribution and what property of the normal distribution curve accounts for this?
2. What dimension of a normal distribution curve does the standard deviation measure?
3. How many of the data lie within two standard deviations of the mean?

1. They are all equal because of the property of symmetry.
2. Width
3. 95%

REGRESSION

In the clinical laboratory, it is often necessary to construct a standard curve, to compare two methods for quantifying the same analyte, to examine interference by some substance in an assay for another, or to ascertain for some other reason the relationship between two variables. In such a case, we use **regression analysis** to discover the mathematical equation that relates the independent and dependent variables. Moreover, when that equation describes a straight line, **correlation** specifies the strength and direction of the relationship.

Linear Regression

Linear regression by the least-squares method is a technique that fits a straight line to a set of data points consisting of values for a dependent variable, y, and corresponding values for an independent variable, x. For a detailed explanation of linear regression, consult Appendix 8-2 on the website.

APPENDIX 8-2
"The Reasoning Behind Linear Regression"
www.myhealthprofessions.kit.com
PEARSON myhealthprofessionskit

In fitting a straight line, regression establishes the mathematical relationship between the two variables and thereby makes it possible to calculate a value for one variable from a value for the other. An important use of regression lines lies in determining the unknown concentration of a substance from some response variable, such as absorbance, fluorescence, or radioactivity. In such a case, the line functions as a standard curve.

For example, one might measure the absorbance of the substance at each of several concentrations, plot the concentration against the absorbance, and then fit a line to the data points (Figure 8-4 ■). If a solution of the same substance at an unknown concentration has an absorbance of, say, 0.295, the regression line shows the corresponding concentration to be 5.6 mg/L. This process of using a standard curve to predict the value of one variable from that of another is interpolation.

Another important use of regression lines is in the comparison of two methods or instruments for the same analyte. The results from one method are plotted against the results from the other, and the agreement between the two methods is evaluated (Figure 8-5 ■).

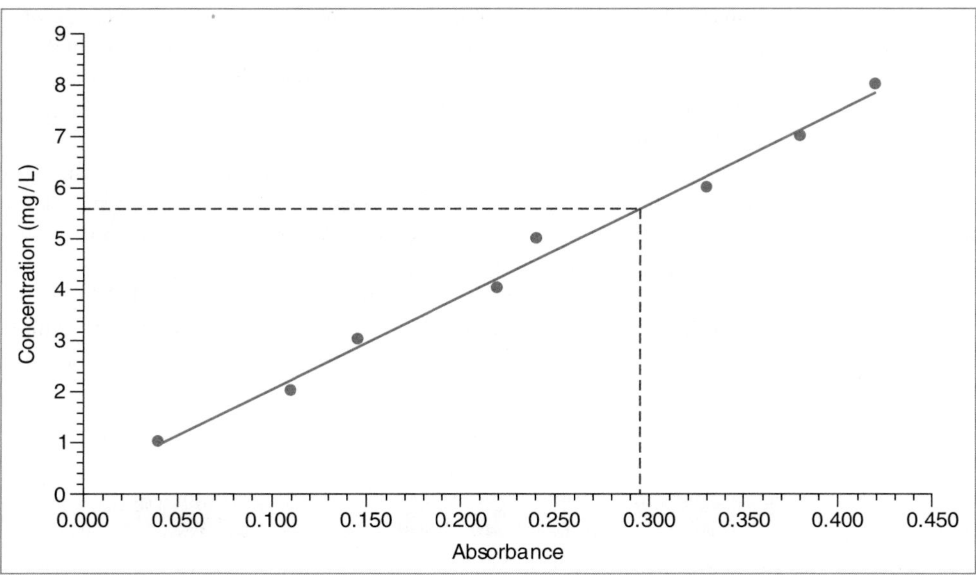

FIGURE 8-4 Regression line functioning as a standard curve. The data points (pink) are plotted, and then the regression line that fits the data best is drawn through the points. The broken line shows interpolation of a concentration of 5.6 mg/L at $A = 0.295$.

In simplest terms, the goal in drawing the best-fit line is to find the one closest to the data points. Though one can accomplish this fairly well by using his or her eye, there are established mathematical techniques that deliver uniformity, accuracy, and precision in the results. Because a straight line is defined by the equation $y = mx + b$, linear regression finds the slope (m) and y-intercept (b) of the

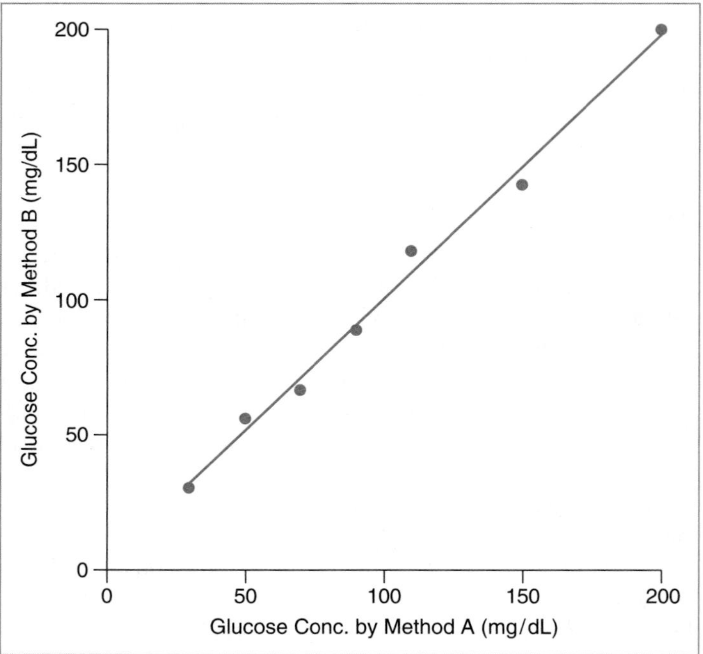

FIGURE 8-5 Regression line in comparison of two methods for the same analyte. The data points (pink) are plotted, and then the regression line that fits the data best is drawn through the points.

theoretical line such that the distance between the actual points and the line is as small as it can be. Equations 3 and 4 show how to calculate the slope and y-intercept:

$$\text{slope} = m = \frac{\sum_{i=1}^{n} x_i y_i - n\bar{x}\bar{y}}{\sum_{i=1}^{n} x_i^2 - n\bar{x}^2}$$

EQUATION 3

$$y\text{-intercept} = b = \frac{\bar{y}\sum_{i=1}^{n} x_i^2 - \bar{x}\sum_{i=1}^{n} x_i y_i}{\sum_{i=1}^{n} x_i^2 - n\bar{x}^2}$$

EQUATION 4

where x_i is the ith value of x, y_i is the ith value of y, $\bar{x}$ is the mean of the x values, $\bar{y}$ is the mean of the y values, and n is the number of data pairs. Fortunately, spreadsheet software can compute these values in the blink of an eye. For calculating the y-intercept, moreover, we can use an easier formula once we know the value of the slope. Because the regression line goes through the center of the data, which is the point $(\bar{x}, \bar{y})$, the formula for the y-intercept is simply a rearrangement of $y = mx + b$, with the values for x and y being their respective means:

$$y\text{-intercept} = b = \bar{y} - m\bar{x}$$

Caveats

There are two risks of which one should be aware in using regression lines. The first is the direction of interpolation. Equations 3 and 4 calculate the best-fit line in such a way that the *dependent* variable may be interpolated from the *independent* variable, as in Figure 8-4. The reverse, however, can be risky. Nevertheless, interpolating the independent variable from the dependent variable is commonly done on standard curves when all the data points are so close to the line that the two directions of interpolation give practically the same result. For more detail on the direction of interpolation, consult Appendix 8-3 on the website.

APPENDIX 8-3
"Classical and Inverse Calibrations"
www.myhealthprofessions.kit.com
PEARSON myhealthprofessionskit

The second caveat lies in the difference between interpolation and extrapolation. Interpolation makes a prediction *within* the range of values of the independent variable that were used to generate the standard curve. In Figure 8-4, this range is 0.040–0.4200. Extrapolation, however, makes predictions *outside* that range. Accordingly, extrapolation is unacceptable because the relationship between the two variables may not be linear outside the range of x values used to find the best-fit line.

Nonlinear Regression

When a linear model fails to fit the data, one of two courses of action might offer a solution:

1. linear transformation of the data, although sometimes no transformation succeeds and at other times the procedure is prohibitively difficult, and
2. **nonlinear regression**, a technique that fits a curve rather than a straight line to the data points.

Before high-speed computers were easily accessible, fitting nonlinear data to a curve was so difficult that standard practice was to linearize the data, rendering them much easier to analyze. Among the more-common linear transformations were Scatchard plots of binding data and Lineweaver-Burk plots of enzyme kinetics data. Although they are still used, methods like these have become almost obsolete, given the ease with which computers can fit nonlinear regression models to experimental data.

The weakness of linear transformations lies in their tendency to distort uncertainty in the data. Even so, linear transformations are very useful for *displaying* data because visual interpretation of such plots is often easy and quick and because straight lines can expose features of the data that curves obscure.

As explained above, linear regression finds values for the slope and y-intercept of the straight line that fits the data best. Unlike linear regression, however, nonlinear regression is iterative; it starts with an estimate of each variable in the equation of the curve and then adjusts those values repeatedly until the curve is as close as possible to the data points. Spreadsheet software has built-in nonlinear regression algorithms that carry out the procedure, draw the curve, and display the equation.

There are sophisticated programs that fit curves to data with no guidance from the user. Such programs fit the data to perhaps thousands of reasonable equations and then, at the end, present those equations with the best fits. But computers cannot go further because they do not understand the scientific context of the data. Thus, even though one curve might fit the data somewhat better than another, the other curve might be a more suitable choice because it makes assumptions that are in line with the underlying science.

Most spreadsheet software, however, asks the user to tell the algorithm where to begin, by selecting the curve (and its basic equation) most likely to fit the points. Here are five examples of the various curves sometimes encountered in the laboratory:

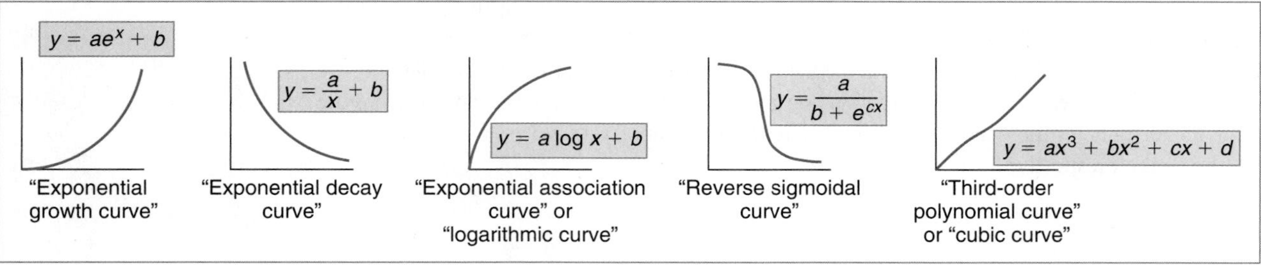

The quantities *a*, *b*, *c*, and *d* are constants whose values the algorithm adjusts in order to fit the data points to the curve as closely as it can. Here is an example of the above reverse sigmoidal curve for which spreadsheet software has found values for the constants *a*, *b*, and *c*:

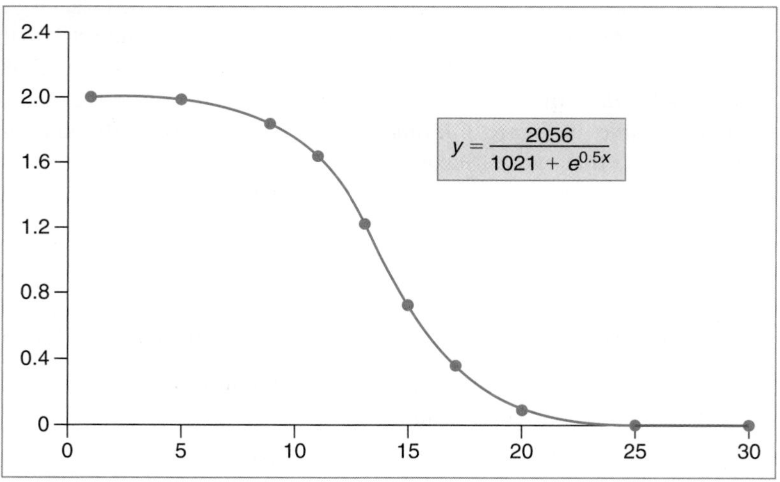

Data Weighting

In the above explanations of regression, it was assumed that every point on the line (or curve) has the same weight, or reliability, as every other point. This assumption is acceptable if the uncertainty at any point is the same as it is at any other point (i.e., if the uncertainty is *uniform*).

Often, however, the uncertainty is not uniform across the data points. Consequently, the points with greater uncertainty in their values influence the regression calculations more than do the points with less uncertainty. The resulting regression line, therefore, may be wrong.

An effective way to circumvent this problem is to *weight* the data equally. To do so, a weighting factor is incorporated into the least-squares calculations—a factor that has the effect of equalizing the uncertainty across all the data points. Even though the computers that control laboratory instruments usually weight data automatically when necessary, there are some techniques and instruments that require the user to choose the data-weighting factor. For more detail on data weighting, see Appendix 8-4 on the website.

APPENDIX 8-4
"Data Weighting"
www.myhealthprofessions.kit.com
PEARSON myhealthprofessionskit

☑ CHECKPOINT 8-4

1. What is interpolation?
2. Using the equations of linear regression, calculate the slope and y-intercept of the best-fit line through the following data.

x	y
10	61.5
20	93.2
30	115.7
40	148.3
50	183.6
60	212.9

1. The practice of predicting the value of one variable from that of another.
2. Slope = 29.8; y-intercept = 3.03.

JUDGING GOODNESS-OF-FIT

Finding the best-fit straight line through a set of data points does not necessarily mean that the line is useable. There are various tools the scientist can employ to test the suitability of the line as a model for the data, that is, to test its goodness-of-fit. After all, a line can be drawn through any set of points, no matter how reasonable or ridiculous the result.

Visual Inspection

Consider, for example, the three attempts at line-fitting in Figure 8-6 ■. The fit is reasonable only for the data points in Figure 8-6A, giving a line that is reliable throughout the range of x values. By contrast, the data points in Figures 8-6B and 8-6C clearly describe curves for which the regression lines drawn through them are nearly useless for interpolation. Either of those lines would predict from an x value a y value that, in almost every case, is too far from the actual y value. Therefore, the first test for goodness-of-fit should always be visual inspection: look at a plot of the data and ascertain whether the points trace out a straight line. If the data points do not look linear, the regression line fails the first test, and you should consider a nonlinear model instead.

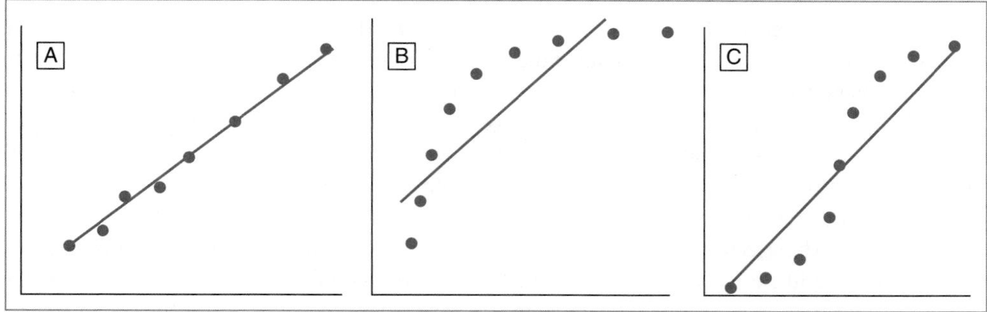

■ FIGURE 8-6 Proper and improper line-fitting to data points. Panel *A:* Reasonable fit because data look linear. Panel *B:* Unreasonable fit because data look curved. Panel *C:* Unreasonable fit because data look sigmoidal.

Root-Mean-Squared Error

Another test for goodness-of-fit is the root-mean-squared error (RMSE), which is known also as the *standard error of the estimate* or the *residual standard deviation:*

EQUATION 5

$$\text{RMSE} = \sqrt{\frac{\sum_{i=1}^{n}(y_i - \hat{y}_i)^2}{n - 2}}$$

where y_i is the actual value of y at x, and $\hat{y}_i$ is the predicted value of y at x. As the standard deviation of a data set is the average deviation from the mean, the RMSE represents the average deviation of the y values from the line. When the regression model fits the data well, the points lie close to the line, and the RMSE is small. Although there is no fixed criterion for accepting or rejecting the RMSE, we use it in conjunction with other statistics to evaluate a given regression line.

Standard Error of the Slope

The third test for goodness-of-fit is the *standard error of the slope* (S_m):

EQUATION 6

$$S_m = \frac{RMSE}{\sqrt{\sum_{i=1}^{n}(x_i - \bar{x})^2}}$$

APPENDIX 8-5
"Example: How the Range of *x* Values Affects Uncertainty in a Regression Line"
www.myhealthprofessions.kit.com

PEARSON myhealthprofessionskit™

Equation 6 says that, as the range of variable x widens, the denominator increases, and the RMSE has a smaller influence on the error in the slope. What this means is that one can draw a line more confidently through data points that are spaced farther apart because it is easier to see the trend. For an example, see Appendix 8-5 on the website.

Confidence Intervals

The fourth test for goodness-of-fit is the confidence interval. A **confidence interval** is a range that contains the true value of some parameter a large proportion of the time. For example, the 95% confidence interval for the slope of a regression line encloses the true slope 95 times out of 100. A confidence interval can be computed with any limit, such as 90% or 99%, although the 95% limit is most common.

Understand what "95%" means and what it does not mean. What it means is that, because of the way in which confidence intervals are computed, if data are independently gathered 100 times from the same population and a 95% confidence interval is calculated each time, then 95 of those intervals will contain the true slope. It does *not* mean that any one of the 100 confidence intervals has a 95% probability of containing the true slope.

A confidence interval for the slope is calculated from this formula:

EQUATION 7

$$CI = m \pm \underbrace{t \times S_m}_{\text{margin of error}}$$

where CI is the confidence interval, m is the calculated slope, t is the t-score, and S_m is the standard error of the slope. The product of t and S_m is called the *margin of error*. Thus, what Equation 7 says is that the confidence interval is the slope of the line plus and minus the margin of error.

By this point in the process, both m and S_m have already been computed, leaving only t to be determined. Again, if the slope is calculated for each of 100 samplings, and if a 95% confidence interval is computed each time, then 95 of those intervals will contain the true slope. The ***t* value** is, in this case, the number of standard errors at which a calculated slope lies from the mean of all 100 calculated slopes.

The t value to be selected is gleaned from a table that was established long ago and is now available in many printed and electronic resources; a small section of that table appears in Table 8-1 ★. The selection of a t value depends on the following two factors. (This chapter discusses the t value again in the sections on Student's t test and the paired t test.)

- **The number of degrees of freedom**(discussed above in the section on the standard deviation and in more detail in Appendix 8-1 on the website): for the slope of a line, this is $n - 2$ (where n is the

★ **TABLE 8-1** *t* Values for Confidence Intervals

Degrees of Freedom	*p* 0.10	0.05	0.01
1	6.31	12.71	63.70
2	2.92	4.30	9.92
3	2.35	3.18	5.84
4	2.13	2.78	4.60
5	2.01	2.57	4.03
6	1.94	2.45	3.71
7	1.89	2.36	3.50
8	1.86	2.31	3.36
9	1.83	2.26	3.25
10	1.81	2.23	3.17
20	1.72	2.09	2.85
30	1.70	2.04	2.75
120	1.66	1.98	2.62
∞	1.64	1.96	2.58

number of data points) because the slope and intercept have already been calculated. As mentioned above, the number of degrees of freedom in the standard deviation of a data set is $n - 1$.

- **The probability (p) that the true slope lies outside the confidence interval:** for a 95% confidence interval, p is 0.05, meaning that the true slope has no more than a 5% probability of falling outside the confidence interval. (See "Significance Testing" for more detail on p values.)

Consider the following example. Suppose that for a regression line the calculated slope is −23.6, the standard error is 0.93, and the number of data points is 10. To find the appropriate t value, locate the row for 8 ($n - 2$) degrees of freedom and go across to the column for $p = 0.05$. The t value is 2.31. Substituting these numbers into Equation 7 gives

$$CI = -23.6 \pm (2.31 \times 0.93) = -23.6 \pm 2.15$$

Thus, the 95% confidence interval for the slope extends from −25.8 up to −21.5.

Calculating the 95% confidence interval for the y-intercept is similar. First, the *standard error of the intercept* (S_b) is computed:

$$S_b = RMSE \times \sqrt{\frac{\sum_{i=1}^{n} x_i^2}{n\sum_{i=1}^{n}(x_i - \bar{x})^2}}$$

EQUATION 8

Then, we substitute the value of S_b into an equation analogous to Equation 7:

$$CI = b \pm \underbrace{t \times S_b}_{\text{margin of error}}$$

EQUATION 9

Calculation of the 95% confidence interval proceeds as it does for the slope, with a t value corresponding to $p = 0.05$ at $n - 2$ degrees of freedom.

Figure 8-7A ■ shows that, for any regression line, the confidence interval (whether at the 95% level or some other) resulting from the combined uncertainties in the slope and intercept is concave. The upper and lower boundaries of the confidence interval are themselves curves, not because they include possible regression curves along with straight lines but because they enclose all possible regression lines from the combined uncertainties (Figure 8-7B ■).

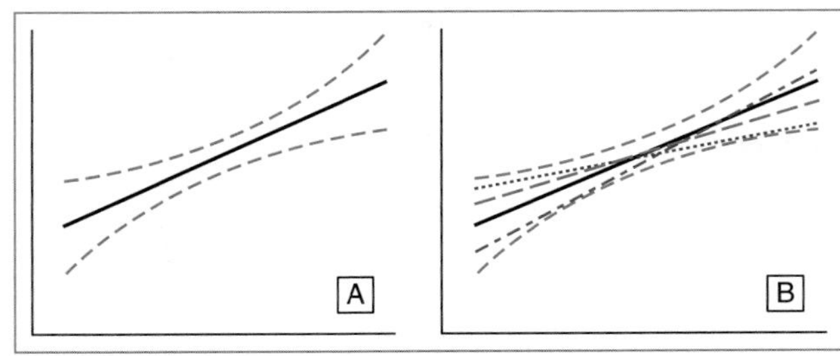

■ FIGURE 8-7 Panel *A:* A typical confidence interval (pink dashed) around a regression line (solid black). Panel *B:* Concavity of the confidence interval. The calculated regression line (solid black) is shown with three other possible regression lines within the confidence interval (pink dashed).

☑ **CHECKPOINT 8-5**

1. What is the significance of the RMSE?
2. In calculating the 90% confidence interval for the slope, with 32 data points, what is the *t* value?

1. The RMSE represents the average deviation of the *y* values from the regression line.
2. For a 90% confidence interval, the *p* value is 0.10. For 32 data points, there are 30 degrees of freedom in the slope. Thus, the *t* value is 1.70.

CORRELATION

Correlation gauges the strength of association between measured variables by evaluating their joint behavior. In other words, it shows the strength of their tendency to change together. The **correlation coefficient**, which is represented as r (Equation 10), ranges from -1 to 1, with a negative value meaning that one variable decreases as the other increases and a positive value meaning that the two variables move in the same direction. When $r = 1$, the correlation is positive and perfect, with all the data points lying on a line that has a positive slope, meaning that x and y rise together (Figure 8-8A ■). When $r = -1$, the correlation is negative and perfect, with all the data points lying on a line that has a negative slope, meaning that y falls as x rises (Figure 8-8B). When $r = 0$, there is no linear relationship between the variables (Figure 8-8C).

EQUATION 10

$$r_{xy} = \frac{\sum_{i=1}^{n}(x_i - \bar{x})(y_i - \bar{y})}{\left(\left[\sum_{i=1}^{n}(x_i - \bar{x})^2\right]\left[\sum_{i=1}^{n}(y_i - \bar{y})^2\right]\right)^{1/2}}$$

APPENDIX 8-6
"The Reasoning Behind the Coefficients of Correlation and Determination"
www.myhealthprofessions.kit.com

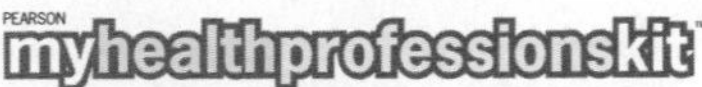

Equation 10 allows calculation of r directly from the original data. Because the calculation is tedious, we allow calculators and computers to carry it out at lightning speed. Appendix 8-6 on the website lays out the reasoning behind Equation 10 in detail.

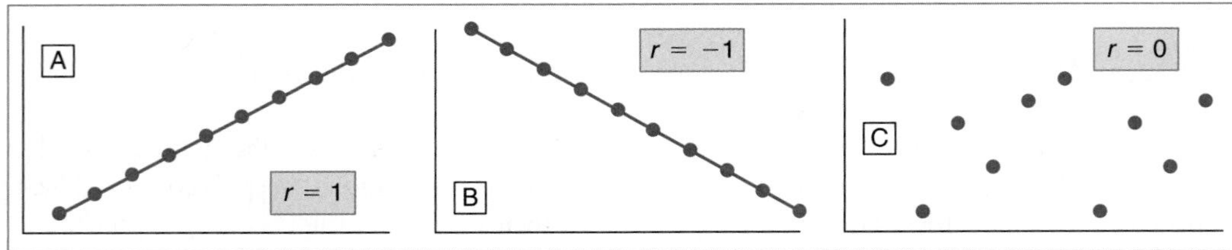

■ FIGURE 8-8 Panel *A:* Perfect positive correlation. Panel *B:* Perfect negative correlation. Panel *C:* No linear correlation.

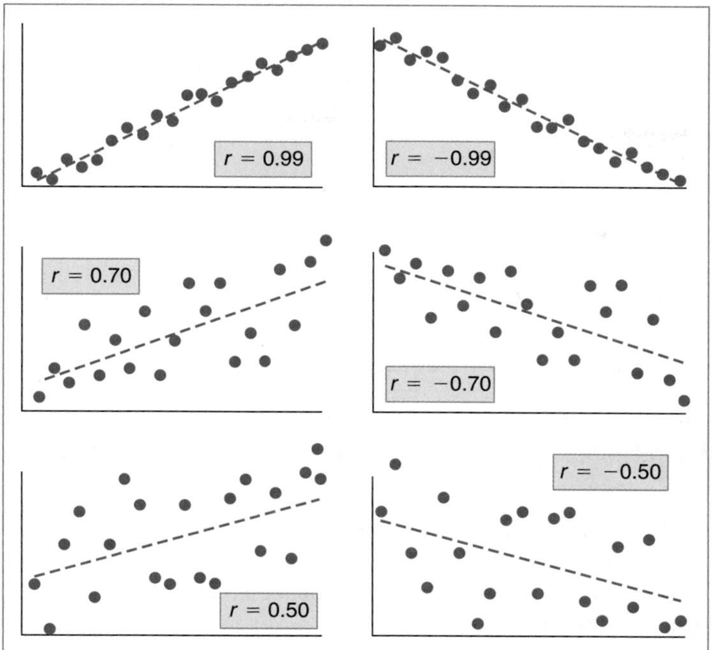

■ **FIGURE 8-9** Increase in scatter as *r* approaches 0 from either −1 or +1.

How do values other than −1, 0, and +1 look on a plot and what do they mean? Figure 8-9 ■ shows examples. As *r* moves closer to zero, either from −1 or from +1, the data fit a linear model less well; as a result, predicting the value of one variable from a value of the other becomes less reliable.

Caveats

The correlation coefficient is sometimes used improperly, especially when applied to standard curves. Strictly speaking, the use of *r* is appropriate when the data represent random samples drawn from a larger population. In other words, it is suitable when each variable has been measured, as, for example, in a comparison of the results from one method with those from another method for randomly chosen patient samples (Figure 8-5). The correlation coefficient is generally not appropriate when one variable is measured and the other is selected *a priori*, as in the case of a standard curve (Figure 8-4).

Nevertheless, the correlation coefficient is often reported for standard curves, perhaps for several reasons: (1) it is expected, (2) computers can calculate it fast, (3) it is easy to communicate as a single number, and (4) it can help give a coarse evaluation of the linearity along with other statistics. However, to judge the goodness-of-fit of a regression line for standard curves, the measures discussed in the previous section (e.g., RMSE, confidence intervals) are better. Table 8-2 ★ summarizes the differences between regression and correlation.

There is one final caveat. *Always look at the plot of the data* before interpreting the value of *r* because the coefficient is useful only to the extent that it reveals how tightly the two variables are coupled to each

★ **TABLE 8-2 A Brief Comparison of Regression and Correlation**

Regression	Correlation
Finds the best-fit line, whether or not the data are linear.	Does not find a line through the data. Shows how tightly two variables are coupled to each other (i.e., how strong their tendency is to change together).
Values for independent variable are selected. Values for dependent variable are measured.	Values for both x and y are measured. Does not distinguish between independent and dependent variables.
Appropriate for standard curves.	Appropriate for method comparisons.
Values of slope and intercept depend on units.	Value of coefficient does not depend on units.

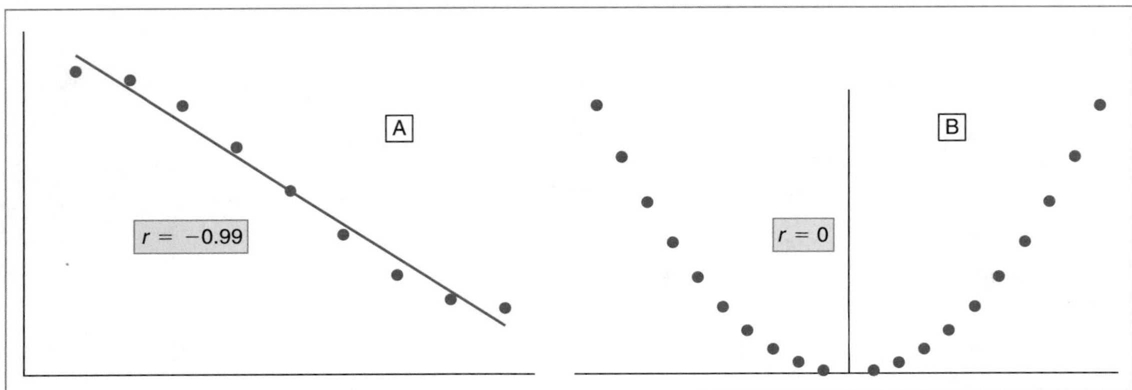

■ FIGURE 8-10 Examples of misleading *r* values. Panel *A:* Strong negative correlation but nonlinear relationship (reverse-sigmoidal or backward "S"). Panel *B:* No linear correlation but definite relationship (parabola, $y = x^2$).

other. Strong correlation, whether positive or negative, does not guarantee linearity; even curved data can give an *r* value close to +1 or −1 (Figure 8-10A ■). Furthermore, a value of *r* close to zero does not preclude a relationship between the variables; definite nonlinear relationships can show weak correlation or none at all (Figure 8-10B).

☑ CHECKPOINT 8-6

1. What does correlation show about two variables?
2. What is the range of values for the correlation coefficient?
3. If *y* decreases as *x* increases, how does the value of *r* relate to zero?
4. Calculate the correlation coefficient for the following data.

x	y
4.4	64.5
19.6	91.2
35.3	110.7
41.2	155.3
66.1	189.6
69.8	222.9

5. What is true about the variables when the correlation coefficient is most meaningful?
6. What is the most important step to take before interpreting the correlation coefficient for a set of data? Why?

1. It shows how strongly they tend to change together.
2. −1 to +1
3. $r < 0$
4. $r = 0.977$
5. Each variable has been measured.
6. Visual inspection. Nonlinear data can have *r* values close to +1 or −1, and data with clear relationships can have *r* values close to zero.

APPENDIX 8-6
"The Reasoning Behind the Coefficients of Correlation and Determination"
www.myhealthprofessions.kit.com
PEARSON myhealthprofessionskit™

COEFFICIENT OF DETERMINATION

The square of the correlation coefficient (r^2, albeit often symbolized as R^2) has a special interpretation. Appendix 8-6 on the website explains this in detail.

Known as the **coefficient of determination**, r^2 is the proportion of the total variation in y that is explained by the variation in x.

$$r^2 = \frac{\text{variation in } y \text{ explained by variation in } x}{\text{total variation in } y}$$

What does this mean? Obviously, y changes as x changes; that is to say, as x moves away from its own average, y moves away from its own average. If r^2 is 1.0, then the variation in x explains 100% of the variation in y, and all the data points lie on the regression line. But if r^2 is, say, 0.86, then the variation in x explains only 86% of the variation in y, and the data points do not all fall exactly on the regression line. The other 14% of the variation in y is accounted for by factors known or unknown; in other words, factors other than the change in x push the actual y values off the regression line.

This leads to another interpretation of r^2. If there were no correlation whatsoever, then predicting the value of y from a value of x would be no better than just citing the mean of the y values. If the correlation were perfect, however, then three conclusions would follow: (1) r^2 would equal 1, (2) the variation in x would explain all the variation in y, and (3) using the line to predict the value of y from a value of x would have 100% less error than just citing the mean of the y values. *Therefore,* r^2 *can be regarded as the proportional reduction in error that comes from using the regression line to predict* y *over using the mean.* An r^2 of 0.81 means not only that the variation in x accounts for 81% of the variation in y, but also that the error in predicting y from the regression line is 81% smaller than it would be in predicting y from the mean.

☑ CHECKPOINT 8-7

Consider the data in Checkpoint #6, item 4. How much of the variation in y is due to factors other than the variation in x?

The value of r^2 is 0.955. This means that the variation in x accounts for 95.5% of the variation in y; thus, 4.5% is due to other factors.

SIGNIFICANCE TESTING

Clinical laboratory work sometimes entails deciding whether an observed result from a study or an experiment is due to chance alone; that is, sometimes one has to decide whether an *apparent* difference, such as that between two laboratory methods or between a control group and a test group, is a *true* difference. Significance testing is a systematic approach that, when used properly, can become part of the evidence that helps us make these decisions. Beware, however, that even though significance testing has been, is being, and will continue to be, conducted by most researchers and laboratory professionals, it is sometimes misapplied and overemphasized.

Let us discuss the basics of significance testing, especially as it is used in the real world, before addressing the dangers. We begin by considering the following examples of questions that significance testing might help settle.

- Your laboratory is comparing a new cell counter to the one currently in use. For 20 randomly chosen patients, the new instrument gave a mean RBC count of 4.13×10^6 per μL, whereas for the same 20 patients the current instrument gave 4.28×10^6 per μL. Is the difference between the RBC counts due to chance or does the new instrument return counts that are truly higher?
- Volunteers taking drug **X** after 3 months had a mean serum cholesterol concentration of 180 mg/dL, whereas other volunteers taking a placebo had a mean concentration of 184 mg/dL. Is the difference between the two cholesterol concentrations due to chance or to the drug?
- Your laboratory is comparing a manual method for quantifying estriol in serum with an automated method. For 10 repeated measurements on a standard estriol solution, the manual method gave a mean concentration ($\pm$ SD) of 9.9 $\pm$ 1.1 ng/mL, whereas the automated method gave 11.4 $\pm$ 1.4 ng/mL. Is the difference between the two standard deviations a statistical anomaly or is the manual method truly more precise?

There are three steps to each significance test presented in this chapter:

1. Define the **null hypothesis** (H_0), which states that there is no difference between the results being compared.
2. Summarize the data, execute any preliminary calculations, and then compute the test statistic.
3. Assuming the null hypothesis to be true, use the test statistic from step 2 to determine the probability (p) of observing the results that were actually obtained.

The *F* Test

There are times when a clinical laboratory must compare the precisions of two different instruments, techniques, or methods. One widely used tool for performing such a comparison is the *F* test, named in honor of Sir Ronald Fisher, who invented the method in the 1920s.

The strategy is straightforward. If method *A* is more precise than method *B*, then *A*'s variance (the square of the standard deviation) is lower than *B*'s variance.

Step 1. We state the null hypothesis (H_0), that there is no difference between the two variances:

$$H_0\text{: } s_1^2 = s_2^2$$

Step 2. We calculate our test statistic, the *F* value. To do so, we take the ratio of the larger s^2 to the smaller s^2:

EQUATION 11

$$F = \frac{\text{larger } s^2}{\text{smaller } s^2}$$

If the two methods have the same precision, then their variances are equal and the value of *F* is 1. Notice that, whenever the two variances are unequal, the value of *F* is greater than 1 because we have taken the ratio of the larger to the smaller. Thus, as one of the methods becomes more precise than the other, their variances diverge, and the value of *F* rises above 1. But how much greater than 1 must the ratio be for us to conclude that the two variances are truly different and, therefore, that one of the methods is more precise than the other?

Step 3. To answer this question, we select a *p* value and compare the calculated value of *F* with a predetermined value of *F*, which is called the **critical value**. The ***p* value** represents the probability of our having observed this difference between the two variances if the two methods were equally precise.[1] If greater than the critical value, our calculated *F* value is high enough for us to reject the null hypothesis and to conclude that one method is probably more precise than the other—at the level of certainty we chose in the *p* value. If less than or equal to the critical value, our calculated *F* value is not high enough for us to reject the null hypothesis (H_0); therefore, we treat the two variances as statistically equal. Take, for example, the following hypothetical data.

Method	Number of Samples	Mean	Variance
A	6	22.9	3.66
B	8	25.1	6.13

The calculated value of *F* is

$$F = \frac{6.13}{3.66} = 1.675$$

In the table below, we find the critical value of *F* that applies to our data. The numerator has 7 degrees of freedom ($n - 1$) and the denominator has 5. The corresponding box in the table contains two numbers, 4.8759 and 10.455, the latter being italicized. They are the critical values at two levels of certainty, and those levels of certainty are reflected in the *p* value.

[1] For Equations 7 and 9, the *p* value answers this question: what would be the probability of obtaining, in a random sample, the slope (or intercept) actually found if there were no linear relationship between *x* and *y*?

Critical Values for the *F* Statistic

Roman type: $p = 0.05$; italic type: $p = 0.01$

		Degrees of Freedom in Numerator						
		1	2	3	4	5	7	10
Degrees of Freedom in Denominator	1	61.45 *4052.2*	199.50 *4999.5*	215.71 *5403.4*	224.58 *5624.6*	230.16 *5763.6*	236.77 *5928.4*	241.88 *6055.8*
	2	18.513 *98.503*	19.000 *99.000*	19.164 *99.166*	19.247 *99.249*	19.296 *99.299*	19.353 *99.356*	19.396 *99.399*
	3	10.128 *34.116*	9.5522 *30.817*	9.2766 *29.457*	9.1172 *28.710*	9.0135 *28.237*	8.8867 *27.672*	8.7855 *27.229*
	4	7.7086 *21.198*	6.9443 *18.000*	6.5915 *16.694*	6.3882 *15.977*	6.2560 *15.522*	6.0942 *14.976*	5.9644 *14.546*
	5	6.6078 *16.258*	5.7862 *13.274*	5.4095 *12.060*	5.1922 *11.392*	5.0504 *10.967*	4.8759 *10.455*	4.7351 *10.051*
	7	5.5914 *12.246*	4.7375 *9.5467*	4.3469 *8.4513*	4.1202 *7.8466*	3.9715 *7.4605*	3.7871 *6.9929*	3.6366 *6.6201*
	10	4.9645 *10.044*	4.1028 *7.5594*	3.7082 *6.5523*	3.4780 *5.9944*	3.3259 *5.6363*	3.1354 *5.2001*	2.9782 *4.8492*

If the null hypothesis is true and the two variances are the same, then p is the probability that a calculated F value above the critical value would have occurred. An F value above the critical value can still appear *even if the two methods are equally precise*, although it is unlikely. In the case of our data, therefore, we can say that, if our two variances are statistically the same, then there is only a 5% probability of observing an F value of at least 4.8759. What this means is that, if our two methods have the same precision and if we run the comparison experiment 100 times, each time calculating an F value, then only five of the 100 F values we calculate would be at least 4.8759.

If our calculated F value is higher than 4.8759, then the likelihood is small that it came about without a difference in precision. If that likelihood is small enough, we *do* reject the null hypothesis and conclude that the ratio reflects a true difference between the two variances. We say that the difference is **statistically significant**. But we must always specify the level of certainty that determined the critical value; in this case, it is $p = 0.05$.

The italicized number, 10.455, is the critical value when p is 1%. It is logical that achieving this greater level of certainty requires the calculated F value to be even higher than for $p = 5\%$. For us to be even more certain about the conclusion, the difference between the two variances must be greater.

For a p of 0.05, our calculated F value, 1.675, is less than the critical value, 4.8759, preventing us from rejecting the null hypothesis. Therefore, we say that the difference observed between the two methods is *statistically nonsignificant* and that we cannot conclude, from this information alone, that methods *A* and *B* have different precisions.

Student's *t* Test

This statistical test is a good example of necessity being the mother of invention. William S. Gosset, who published under the pseudonym "Student," developed this tool in the early 1900s to help him solve problems in his work as a statistician for a brewery. We use Student's *t* test to compare the means of two groups when one variable is *categorical* (non-numerical) and the other is numerical. An example of this is a comparison of turnaround times for the same test in two different laboratories; in this case, the categorical variable is the laboratory and the numerical variable is turnaround time.

Step 1. State the null hypothesis, which is that there exists no real difference between the two means (i.e., no difference between the turnaround times).

$$H_0: \bar{x}_1 = \bar{x}_2$$

Step 2. Calculate the *t* value, which compares the difference that was actually observed between the means with the difference that would have been expected for randomly selected specimens. The equation is already programmed into calculators and spreadsheet software.

EQUATION 12

$$t = \frac{\bar{x}_1 - \bar{x}_2}{\sqrt{\left(\dfrac{\sum_{i=1}^{n_1}(x_i - \bar{x}_1)^2 + \sum_{j=1}^{n_2}(x_j - \bar{x}_2)^2}{n_1 + n_2 - 2}\right)\left(\dfrac{1}{n_1} + \dfrac{1}{n_2}\right)}}$$

where *i* refers to the *i*th value in data set #1 and *j* to the *j*th in data set #2.

This formula assumes that the variances of the two groups are equal. To decide whether a given data set meets this criterion, employ the *F* test. Compare the calculated *F* value with the critical value. If the *F* value is less than the critical value, consider the variances equal. If the *F* value exceeds the critical value, consider the two variances to be different and use the *t* test for unequal variances (also known as the "Welch test"):

EQUATION 13

$$t = \frac{\bar{x}_1 - \bar{x}_2}{\sqrt{\dfrac{s_1^2}{n_1} + \dfrac{s_2^2}{n_2}}}$$

where

$$s_1^2 = \frac{\sum_{i=1}^{n_1}(x_i - \bar{x}_1)^2}{n_1 - 1}$$

and

$$s_2^2 = \frac{\sum_{j=1}^{n_2}(x_j - \bar{x}_2)^2}{n_2 - 1}$$

As the difference between the two means increases, so does the probability that they are significantly different (Figure 8-11A ■). Furthermore, a smaller variability raises the likelihood that the difference is significant (Figure 8-11B), whereas a larger variability can nearly overwhelm a difference between the means and erase our confidence that the apparent difference is real (Figure 8-11C). So, when the difference between two means is real, the observed difference between the means is greater than the expected difference. This, in turn, makes the numerator larger than the denominator and pushes the ratio up, which is the *t* value.

Step 3. Choose a *p* level and compare your calculated *t* value with the critical value. If the calculated *t* value is more extreme than the critical value, then the difference between the means is statistically significant. If not, then the difference is statistically nonsignificant.

If Student's *t* test (Equation 12) was used, then the number of degrees of freedom is the total number of data entries minus 2:

$$d.f. = n_1 + n_2 - 2$$

However, if the unequal-variances *t* test (Equation 13) was used, then the number of degrees of freedom is rather complex to compute. This is another reason to let a computer carry out the *t* test.

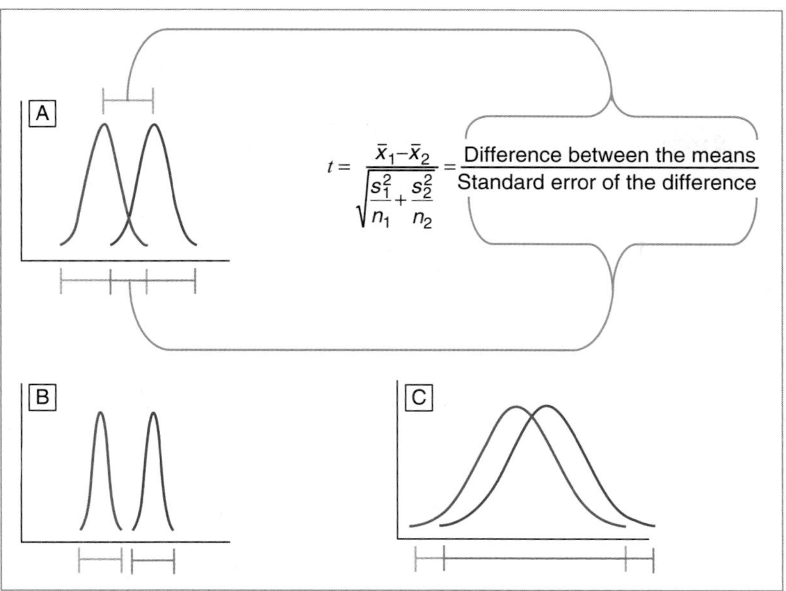

FIGURE 8-11 Graphical representation of the t value in Equation 13. (**A**) Numerator is the difference between the two means. Denominator contains the sum of the variabilities of the two groups. (**B**) Smaller variability *increases* likelihood that observed difference between means is real. (**C**) Larger variability *decreases* likelihood that observed difference between means is real.

$$d.f. = \frac{\left(\frac{s_1^2}{n_1} + \frac{s_2^2}{n_2}\right)^2}{\left\{\frac{\left(\frac{s_1^2}{n_1}\right)^2}{n_1 - 1} + \frac{\left(\frac{s_2^2}{n_2}\right)^2}{n_2 - 1}\right\}}$$

Round the result down to the nearest integer before consulting a *t* table.

Let us consider the example mentioned above: a comparison of the turnaround times for the same test performed in two different laboratories.

	Turnaround Time (min)	
	Laboratory Q	Laboratory *R*
	106	100
	107	102
	108	103
	111	97
	103	94
	101	93
	98	
SAMPLE MEAN	105	98

For our data in the table above, the *t* statistic is <u>**2.781**</u> by Equation 12 (built into a spreadsheet), and there are 11 degrees of freedom (7 + 6 − 2). The corresponding critical values in the *t* table are 3.106 at $p = 0.01$ and 2.201 at $p = 0.05$. Therefore, the difference between the means in our data is statistically significant at $p = 0.05$ but statistically nonsignificant at $p = 0.01$.

Critical Values for the t Value (two-tailed)

		Value of p		
		0.10	0.05	0.01
Degrees of Freedom	1	6.314	12.706	63.657
	2	2.920	4.303	9.925
	3	2.353	3.182	5.841
	4	2.132	2.776	4.604
	5	2.015	2.571	4.032
	6	1.943	2.447	3.707
	7	1.895	2.365	3.499
	8	1.860	2.306	3.355
	9	1.833	2.262	3.250
	10	1.812	2.228	3.169
	11	1.796	2.201	3.106
	15	1.753	2.131	2.947
	25	1.708	2.060	2.787
	50	1.676	2.009	2.678
	100	1.660	1.984	2.626

We interpret significance at $p = 0.05$ this way: the difference we observed between the two mean turnaround times would have occurred five out of every hundred times we ran the experiment, *even if, on average, the two laboratories returned results in the same amount of time.* Significance did not, however, extend to a p of 0.01; thus, we cannot conclude that the difference would have occurred only *one* out of every hundred times.

Technically, the t test presented here is *two-tailed* because it tests for a difference without assuming which mean is greater than the other. Although the table summarizing the critical values for the two-tailed t value lists only positive numbers, *each value represents both the positive and negative cutoffs for statistical significance.* Therefore, the null hypothesis is rejected whenever t is more extreme than either cutoff, that is, whenever t is greater than the positive critical value or more negative than (less than) the negative critical value.

The Paired *t* Test

One of the most important tasks facing the clinical laboratory is the comparison of two instruments or methods for a given analyte. In such a comparison, each of the specimens is tested on one instrument and then on the other. This **specimen pairing** creates a one-to-one correspondence between the two instruments for every individual specimen.

Step 1. State the null hypothesis, which is that there exists no real difference between the two means (i.e., no difference between the two instruments).

$$H_0 : \bar{x}_1 = \bar{x}_2$$

Step 2. Carry out the necessary preliminary calculations and then compute the t statistic

EQUATION 14

$$t = \frac{\overline{D}}{\sqrt{\frac{s^2}{n}}}$$

where $\overline{D}$ is the mean of the differences, s^2 is the variance of the differences, and n is the number of differences.

Step 3. Compare the calculated t value with the critical value.

For example, suppose we are comparing two instruments for quantifying substance M in whole blood, and we want to know whether their results differ statistically:

	Concentration of Substance M (ng/mL)			
Specimen	**Instrument A**	**Instrument B**	$A - B$	$B - A$
1	4.60	4.82	−0.22	0.22
2	4.53	4.62	−0.09	0.09
3	4.47	4.70	−0.23	0.23
4	4.55	4.61	−0.06	0.06
5	4.72	4.79	−0.07	0.07
6	4.51	4.78	−0.27	0.27
7	4.63	4.70	−0.07	0.07
8	4.61	4.66	−0.05	0.05
9	4.49	4.69	−0.20	0.20
10	4.66	4.73	−0.07	0.07
		MEAN	−0.133	0.133
		VARIANCE	0.007357	0.007357
		t-STATISTIC (paired, Eq. 14)	−4.904	4.904

The number of degrees of freedom for this test is $n - 1$. Equation 14 returns a t value of -4.904 or 4.904, depending on whether B is subtracted from A or A from B. At 9 degrees of freedom and a p value of 0.01, the value of -4.904 is more negative than the critical value of -3.250. Therefore, we reject the null hypothesis that there is no difference between the results from instruments A and B and conclude that the observed difference between the two means is statistically significant. In other words, the results coming from instrument A probably differ truly from those coming from instrument B.

The Chi-Square Test

The chi-square (χ^2) test is used on qualitative or categorical data, which, as stated above for Student's t test, are non-numerical in nature. For example, suppose there is concern that a new drug, Q, may interfere in the method our laboratory uses to detect the presence of antibodies against hepatitis C in serum. To answer this question, we gather relevant data on 97 patients and summarize them in a **contingency table** (Table 8-3 ★), which in general is a tabular summary of categorical data.

★ **TABLE 8-3** Effect of Drug Q on Qualitative Test for Antibodies Against Hepatitis C in Serum

		Response Variable (presence of antibodies against hepatitis C)			
		Positive	**Equivocal**	**Negative**	**Total**
Explanatory Variable	Taking Drug Q	8 (9.68)	3 (4.85)	36 (32.5)	47
	Not Taking Drug Q	12 (10.3)	7 (5.15)	31 (34.5)	50
	TOTAL	20	10	67	97

Note: Each orange cell of the table shows the *observed* number of specimens and, in parentheses, the *expected* number of specimens (calculated in step 2).

Step 1. State the null hypothesis.

H_0: The observed counts do not differ from the expected counts.

Step 2. Compute the expected frequency in each cell on the assumption that the null hypothesis is true, and then calculate the χ^2 statistic. If there is no relationship between the drug and the hepatitis test result, then it is immaterial whether a given specimen came from a patient taking the drug or from a patient not taking the drug: all 20 "positive" specimens would have tested "positive" regardless of the patients from whom they were drawn. There could just as easily have been 10 specimens from the group taking the drug and 10 from the group not taking the drug. Thus, if the null hypothesis is true, the expected frequency of "positive" results is 0.206:

$$\text{expected frequency of "positive" results} = \frac{\text{number of observed "positive" results}}{\text{number of specimens tested}}$$

$$0.206 \text{ positives per specimen} = \frac{20 \text{ positives}}{97 \text{ specimens}} = 20.6\%$$

This means that, if the drug has no effect on our hepatitis assay, then about 21% (rounded up from 20.6%) of all results should be "positive," whether or not the patients are taking the drug.

Therefore, if the null hypothesis is true, we expect the number of patients who test "positive" while taking the drug to be about 10:

$$\begin{matrix}\text{expected number of} \\ \text{patients who test} \\ \text{"positive" while on} \\ \text{drug Q}\end{matrix} = \begin{matrix}\text{expected frequency of} \\ \text{"positive" results}\end{matrix} \times \begin{matrix}\text{number of patients} \\ \text{taking drug Q}\end{matrix}$$

$$9.68 \text{ expected positives} = \begin{matrix}0.206 \text{ positives} \\ \text{per specimen}\end{matrix} \times 47 \text{ specimens}$$

Likewise, the expected number of patients who test "positive" while not taking the drug is also about 10 ($0.206 \times 50 = 10.3$). The other expected numbers in the table are calculated similarly.

Next, calculate the χ^2 statistic.

EQUATION 15

$$\chi^2 = \sum \frac{(\text{observed result} - \text{expected result})^2}{\text{expected result}}$$

What this equation tells us is that, when the drug does *not* affect the hepatitis test, that is, when there is no relationship between the explanatory and response variables, (a) every observed result is the same as its expected result, (b) each difference in the numerator is zero, (c) χ^2 is zero, and (d) we do not reject H_0. However, if the drug *does* affect the hepatitis test, then the differences between observed and expected results widen, and the value of χ^2 increases until it exceeds the critical value, at which point we do reject H_0.

By Equation 15, the value of χ^2 for our hypothetical data in Table 8-3 is

$$\chi^2 = 2.674$$

Step 3. For any contingency table, the number of degrees of freedom is

$$d.f. = (\text{number of rows} - 1)(\text{number of columns} - 1)$$

There are many explanations of this formula in printed and electronic resources. As for Table 8-3, then, the number of degrees of freedom is

$$d.f. = (2 - 1)(3 - 1) = 2$$

To determine whether our observed results differ significantly from the expected results, we compare our value of χ^2 with the critical value in the following table. For a p value of 0.05, which is the customary threshold for significance, and with 2 degrees of freedom, the critical value of χ^2 is 5.991. Because our value of 2.674 is less than the critical value, we do not reject the null hypothesis, which says that there is no relationship between the drug and our test results. Instead, we let the null hypothesis stand.

Critical Values for the χ^2 Statistic

		Value of *p*		
		0.10	0.05	0.01
Degrees of Freedom	1	2.706	3.841	6.635
	2	4.605	5.991	9.210
	3	6.251	7.815	11.345
	4	7.779	9.488	13.277
	5	9.236	11.070	15.086
	6	10.645	12.592	16.812
	7	12.017	14.067	18.475
	8	13.362	15.507	20.090
	9	14.684	16.919	21.666
	10	15.987	18.307	23.209
	25	34.382	37.652	44.314
	50	63.167	67.505	76.154
	100	118.498	124.342	135.807

When the χ^2 statistic exceeds the critical value, we know only that somewhere in the table a count is significantly higher than expected. Visual inspection is then necessary to identify it.

The χ^2 test has several implicit unique requirements; if any of them is not met, the test is invalid.

- Each subject may contribute data to only one cell in the contingency table. For example, consider an experiment, summarized in the table below, in which each of 100 patients is tested for antibodies against hepatitis C at 10 and 15 weeks after suspected exposure.

		Antibodies Against Hepatitis C		
		Positive	Negative	TOTAL
Time After Exposure	10 weeks	35	65	100
	15 weeks	71	29	100
	TOTAL	106	94	200

  This χ^2 test is invalid because each patient is present in more than one cell. The total number of counts in the table is 200 even though there are only 100 patients. The χ^2 test cannot be used for correlated data (e.g., before/after treatment, paired samples).
- Each number in the contingency table must be a raw count (not a percentage).
- The sample size must be adequate. There is no universally accepted minimum, but many researchers insist on at least 20.
- The cell size must be adequate. A common minimum is five samples in every cell in a 2 × 2 table. In larger tables, 80% of the cells should each have at least five samples.
- The total number of observed counts must equal the total number of expected counts.

Caveats

1. **Significance thresholds are arbitrary.** The bifurcation of results into those that are significant or nonsignificant is artificial. Therefore, the value of *p* should be interpreted in view of all the other evidence and *should never be regarded as the final arbiter*. Even when *p* is 0.05 and the actual results have only a 5% probability of being observed when the null hypothesis is true, they will still come

up one in 20 times (5 in 100 times). So, if H_0 is indeed true and we choose to reject it whenever $p = 0.05$, then we would be wrong about every 20th time we ran the experiment. Clearly, a lower p value such as 0.005 or 0.001 is much more convincing. Rejecting the null hypothesis is a gamble: when $p = 0.05$, one is betting that he or she has not stumbled upon that one time in 20 that represents mere coincidence.

2. **The *p* value is ambiguous.** As the value of n goes up (as sample size increases), the value of p goes down. Conversely, as n goes down, p goes up. This means that almost any difference between two groups will become statistically significant if the sample size increases far enough. Therefore, a significant result might be due to a real effect or it might be due to an increase in the power of the test simply because n is very large.
3. **Statistical significance is not clinical significance.** The fact that the difference between two results is statistically significant does not make the difference clinically meaningful. For example, consider two laboratory instruments used for quantifying a protein in plasma. Comparison studies reveal that instrument #1 returns a concentration of 881 ng/dL, whereas instrument #2 gives 894 ng/dL, with $p < 0.005$. The difference can be considered statistically significant, but it is only 13 ng/dL, or 1.5% of the mean (887.5 ng/dL). The question of whether such a small difference would have any clinical significance must be taken into account when the laboratory is selecting one instrument over the other, especially if cost, space, or some other factor is a consideration.
4. **Nonrejection of the null hypothesis does not mean it is true.** Remember, H_0 states that there is no difference between the results. Strictly speaking, we can never accept the null hypothesis or prove it true; we can only fail to reject it. Although the distinction may seem petty, it reminds us of the need to keep significance testing in perspective. Even if the difference between two results proves to be statistically nonsignificant, it is risky to conclude that there is *no* difference between them.

Summary

1. There are two paramount questions arising from a set of numerical data.
   - What is a typical value, that is, what is the *central tendency* or middle of the data set?
   - How typical is a typical value or how far from the center do the data lie?
2. *Accuracy* is the degree of correctness of a laboratory result, whereas *precision* is the degree of reproducibility in repeated measurements. Accuracy refers to how close a laboratory value is to the true value, whereas precision refers to how tightly clustered several replicates are, whether or not they are close to the true value.
3. The three most-common measures of central tendency are the *mean*, *median*, and *mode*. The mean is more sensitive to extreme values (*outliers*) than is the median or mode.
4. The mean, usually represented as $\bar{x}$, can be considered the data set's center of gravity. It is calculated by adding all the data values together and dividing the sum by the total number of values in the data set:

$$\bar{x} = \frac{x_1 + x_2 + x_3 + \ldots + x_n}{n}$$

   where n = number of values in the data set. The mean is also the unique value with which every observed value in the data set can be replaced without altering the total of those values.
5. The median is the midpoint of the data set. To locate the midpoint, all the entries in the data set, including all repeats, are arranged in ascending or descending order. If the number of entries in the data set is odd, the median is the middle entry. If the number is even, the median is the calculated value halfway between the two middle entries.
6. The mode is the value that occurs in the data set most often. Sometimes a data set has more than one mode. Because the mode may not be near the center of the data, it is not necessarily a measure of central tendency.
7. A *normal distribution* is symmetrical. Therefore, its mean, median, and mode are all equal. The *standard deviation*, which has the same units as the x-axis variable, is a measure of the average distance between the data points and the mean. In a normal distribution, 68% of the values lie within a distance of one standard deviation from the mean in both directions; 95% lie within two standard deviations and 99.7% within three.
8. The standard deviation is the most commonly used measure of dispersion. It is defined as the square root of the *variance:*

$$\text{variance} = s^2 = \frac{\sum_{i=1}^{n}(x_i - \overline{x})^2}{n - 1}$$

$$\text{standard deviation} = s = \sqrt{\frac{\sum_{i=1}^{n}(x_i - \overline{x})^2}{n - 1}}$$

where n is the number of values in the data set.

9. The *coefficient of variation* relates the standard deviation directly to the mean.

$$CV = \frac{s}{\overline{x}} \times 100\%$$

It standardizes the standard deviation and offers a measure of precision.

10. *Linear regression* is a technique that fits a straight line to a set of data points. One variable is independent (x) and the other is dependent (y). In the clinical laboratory, straight lines are used most often to generate standard curves and to compare methods.
11. Regression proceeds by finding a pair of values for the slope and y-intercept that define a line as close as possible to the data points. There are standard equations for calculating the slope and y-intercept, and they are integrated into computer algorithms.
12. Technically, a regression line is valid only for interpolating the dependent variable from the independent variable. However, interpolating in the opposite direction may be acceptable if the regression line is close to the data points.
13. Extrapolation is risky because the relationship between the variables is unknown outside the data range.
14. *Correlation* is a measure of how tightly the variables are coupled to each other (how strong their tendency is to change together). The *correlation coefficient* (r) ranges in value from -1 to $+1$. When $r = +1$, the correlation is perfect, the two variables move in the same direction, and all the data points lie on the line. When $r = -1$, the correlation is again perfect, and all the points lie on the line, but the two variables move in opposite directions. When $r = 0$, there is no linear relationship between the variables. Because r can be misleading, one should always look at the plot before drawing any conclusions.
15. Technically, the correlation coefficient should be calculated only when both variables are measured. It is inappropriate when one variable is measured and the other is controlled, as for standard curves, although it can nevertheless give a coarse estimate of goodness-of-fit for a regression line.
16. The *coefficient of determination* (r^2) is the proportion of the total variation in y explained by the variation in x. It is also the proportional reduction in error that comes from using the regression line to predict y over merely citing the mean of the y values.
17. The basic tools for judging how well a regression line fits the data are (a) visual inspection, which serves to verify the linearity of the points, (b) the root-mean-squared error, which represents the average deviation of the y-values from the line, (c) the standard error of the slope or intercept, which functions as the standard deviation and which depends on the sample size, and (d) the *confidence interval* of the slope or intercept, which is a range that contains the true value a large proportion of the time.
18. Generally, linear transformations of nonlinear data are more useful for displaying data than they are for analyzing data because computers can execute nonlinear regression quickly.
19. *Nonlinear regression* employs the same strategy as linear regression, except that it adjusts values iteratively until the curve is as close as possible to the data points.
20. Data weighting equalizes the influence of all data points on the calculation of a regression line or curve.
21. Significance testing helps determine whether an apparent difference between data sets is a true difference.
22. There are three steps to each significance test presented in this chapter:
    (1) Define the *null hypothesis*, which states that there is no difference between the results in question.
    (2) Summarize the data, execute any preliminary calculations, and then compute the test statistic.
    (3) Assuming the null hypothesis to be true, use the test statistic from step 2 to determine the probability (p) of observing, by coincidence alone, results more extreme than those that were actually observed.
23. A *p value* of 0.05 is the cutoff used most often, though certainly not always, especially in biological sciences.
24. The F test compares the precisions of two different instruments, techniques, or methods.
25. The F statistic is calculated with this formula:

$$F = \frac{\text{larger } s^2}{\text{smaller } s^2}$$

26. The calculated F value is compared with the critical value at a selected p and number of degrees of freedom. If F exceeds the critical value, the difference is *statistically significant*.
27. A t test compares the means of two data sets when one variable is *categorical* (non-numerical) and the other is numerical.
28. Student's t test assumes equality in the variances of the two data sets, using the following formula to calculate the t value. The number of degrees of freedom is $n_1 + n_2 - 2$.

$$t = \frac{\overline{x}_1 - \overline{x}_2}{\sqrt{\left(\frac{\sum_{i=1}^{n_1}(x_i - \overline{x}_1)^2 + \sum_{j=1}^{n_2}(x_j - \overline{x}_2)^2}{n_1 + n_2 - 2}\right)\left(\frac{1}{n_1} + \frac{1}{n_2}\right)}}$$

29. If the variances of the two data sets are *not* equal, use this formula to calculate the *t value:*

$$t = \frac{\bar{x}_1 - \bar{x}_2}{\sqrt{\frac{s_1^2}{n_1} + \frac{s_2^2}{n_2}}}$$

30. In the unequal-variances *t* test, use this formula to calculate the number of degrees of freedom:

$$d.f. = \frac{\left(\frac{s_1^2}{n_1} + \frac{s_2^2}{n_2}\right)^2}{\left\{\frac{\left(\frac{s_1^2}{n_1}\right)^2}{n_1 - 1} + \frac{\left(\frac{s_2^2}{n_2}\right)^2}{n_2 - 1}\right\}}$$

31. The calculated *t* value is compared with the critical value at a selected *p* and number of degrees of freedom. If *t* is more extreme than the critical value, the difference is statistically significant.

32. In the table of critical values for the two-tailed *t* value, each value represents both the positive and negative cutoffs for statistical significance. The null hypothesis is rejected whenever *t* is greater than the positive critical value or more negative than (less than) the negative critical value.

33. The paired *t* test is used to compare results for the same specimens under two different conditions. In the clinical laboratory, this is usually a comparison on two different instruments. Such *specimen pairing* creates a one-to-one correspondence between the two instruments for every individual specimen.

34. The formula for the paired *t* value is this:

$$t = \frac{\bar{D}}{\sqrt{\frac{s^2}{n}}}$$

where $\bar{D}$ is the mean of the differences, s^2 is the variance of the differences, and *n* is the number of differences.

35. The χ^2 test is used on qualitative or categorical data. It compares the observed results with the expected results.

36. In a χ^2 test, we summarize the data in a *contingency table* and then calculate the expected frequencies.

37. We use this formula to calculate the χ^2 statistic:

$$\chi^2 = \sum \frac{(\text{observed result} - \text{expected result})^2}{\text{expected result}}$$

38. In a χ^2 test, the number of degrees of freedom is

$d.f.$ = (number of rows − 1)(number of columns − 1)

39. The calculated χ^2 value is compared with the critical value at a selected *p* and number of degrees of freedom. If χ^2 is greater than the critical value, the difference between the observed results and expected results is statistically significant.

40. Though very helpful in decision-making, significance tests do not substitute for sound scientific judgment. There are at least four important caveats pertaining to significance testing:

(1) Significance thresholds are arbitrary.
(2) The *p* value is ambiguous.
(3) Statistical significance is not practical significance.
(4) Nonrejection of the null hypothesis does not mean it is true.

Practice Problems

1. (LO 3, 4) Consider the following three data sets. For each set, calculate the mean and median. What do these results say about resistance to outliers?

   (1) 100, 120, 140, 160, 180, 200

   (2) 100, 120, 140, 160, 180, 2000

   (3) 10, 120, 140, 160, 180, 200

2. (LO 4) Determine the mean, median, and mode for each of the following data sets.

(1) 2.3	2.6	1.9	3.5	2.6	2.0
2.8	2.5	2.6	2.2	2.4	
(2) 101	119	106	108	107	113
103	107	109	106	106	
(3) 44.8	44.1	44.6	33.9	45.1	44.0
44.8	44.0	44.1	44.8	43.9	

3. (LO 4, 6) Calculate the mean and standard deviation ($n - 1$) for each of the following sets of numbers.

   (a) 6, 6, 9, 4, 6, 4, 3, 2, 5, 7, 8, 6

   (b) 88.3, 85.6, 90.2, 99.1, 89.7, 94.0, 89.4, 96.1, 93.5, 95.7

   (c) 0.033, 0.046, 0.022, 0.039, 0.031, 0.028, 0.026, 0.040, 0.030, 0.037

   (d) 9.91×10^5, 9.86×10^5, 1.01×10^6, 9.80×10^5, 9.97×10^5, 1.12×10^6, 9.77×10^5, 9.84×10^5, 9.82×10^5

   (e) 1022, 4375, 2998, 893, 2245, 1836, 3661, 2718, 970, 2056

4. (LO 3, 4) Using the weights-on-a-beam analogy, determine whether each of the following sets of numbers is balanced on its *median*, and if not, whether the set tips to the left or the right.

   (a) 1, 2, 3, 4, 5, 6, 7, 8, 9

   (b) 1, 5, 5, 6, 7, 8, 9, 9, 9

(c) 100, 105, 105, 105, 108, 108, 108, 125, 160

(d) 0.45, 0.61, 0.64, 0.67, 0.81, 0.84

(e) 2.3×10^4, 6.6×10^4, 9.2×10^4, 1.5×10^5, 1.9×10^5, 3.4×10^5

5. (LO 6) Consider the following five data summaries. In the third column appears one of the data values from the data set. Calculate the number of standard deviations at which the single data value lies from the mean.

Data Set	Mean ± SD	One of the Data Values
A	554 ± 26	580
B	0.033 ± 0.005	0.039
C	13.6 ± 1.5	12.1
D	647 ± 31	699
E	8.22 ± 0.57	9.79
F	0.336 ± 0.045	0.240

6. (LO 5, 6) If a normal distribution has a mean of 50 and a standard deviation of 10, what percentage of the data values fall between 30 and 70?

7. (LO 1, 2, 7) There are three 200-µL mechanical pipets in your laboratory that you and your colleagues use routinely to prepare reagents and calibrators. In the regular quality assurance procedure, you test these pipets for accuracy and precision. You dispense deionized water 20 times from each pipet and summarize the results. Pipet *A* gives 202.4 ± 2.2 µL (mean ± SD), pipet *B* gives 197.2 ± 3.0 µL, and pipet *C* gives 192.4 ± 1.6 µL. Which pipet is the most accurate? Which is the most precise?

8. (LO 9) For each of the following sets of data, write the least-squares linear regression equation in the form $y = mx + b$ and calculate the correlation coefficient.

(a)

x	1	2	3	4	5	6	7	8	9	10
y	8	7	12	14	15	17	18	22	23	26

(b)

x	0.1	0.3	0.5	0.7	0.9	1.1	1.3	1.5	1.7	1.9
y	44	37	35	29	31	25	22	15	10	7

(c)

x	9.8	19.6	31.2	42.8	49.1	60.5	69.6	83.2	91.3	96.7
y	0.2	0.4	0.8	0.9	1.4	1.7	2.2	2.4	2.5	2.9

(d)

x	0.06	0.11	0.14	0.23	0.26	0.30	0.36	0.42	0.47	0.51
y	810	2608	1746	3122	4565	3901	5539	6782	6413	7990

(e)

x	102	209	288	389	517	620	731	798	866	1010
y	91	180	277	364	476	589	690	765	843	969

(f)

x	10.0	10.2	10.4	10.6	10.8	11.0	11.2	11.4	11.6	11.8
y	69	49	59	40	31	37	17	15	14	3

9. (LO 11) For the data sets in problem 8 above, predict the values of *x* from the following values of *y*.

(a) 22.6 (b) 34.1 (c) 1.6 (d) 7119 (e) 333 (f) 50.2

10. (LO 8, 9, 11, 12) The following data represent a comparison of two methods, *P* and *Q*, for quantifying potassium in serum. Twelve randomly selected patient samples were tested by each method. Each datum is a concentration in units of mmol/L.

	Patient											
	1	2	3	4	5	6	7	8	9	10	11	12
P	2.2	2.4	2.9	3.4	3.9	4.3	4.7	4.8	5.0	5.1	6.3	6.9
Q	2.4	2.5	3.1	3.6	4.1	4.2	4.7	4.7	4.9	5.0	6.2	7.0

(a) Treating *P* as the independent variable, calculate the slope, *y*-intercept, and r^2 of the regression line. Predict the results for method *Q* when the results for method *P* are 5.5 and 2.5.

(b) Treating *Q* as the independent variable, calculate the slope, *y*-intercept, and r^2 of the regression line. Predict the results for method *P* when the results for method *Q* are 5.5 and 2.5.

(c) At which value of the independent variable (5.5 or 2.5) do the two regression lines agree more closely? Explain.

11. (LO 8, 9, 11, 12) The following data are intended for construction of a standard curve for analyte *Z*. The concentration is in units of mg/dL.

conc.	2.0	4.0	6.0	8.0	10.0	12.0	14.0	16.0	18.0	20.0
abs.	0.060	0.121	0.173	0.218	0.266	0.338	0.368	0.444	0.516	0.583

(a) Treating concentration as the independent variable, calculate the slope, *y*-intercept, and r^2 of the regression line. Predict the concentration when the absorbance is 0.300 and 0.547.

(b) Treating absorbance as the independent variable, calculate the slope, *y*-intercept, and r^2 of the regression line. Predict the concentration when the absorbance is 0.300 and 0.547.

(c) Might either regression line be suitable for predicting concentration from absorbance? Explain.

12. (LO 8, 13, 15) Your laboratory is comparing serum and plasma results in the assays for analytes *A* and *B*. The data fit straight lines, and the statistics are tabulated below. Which assay shows stronger agreement between the results for serum and plasma? Explain.

Analyte	Regression Equation	r	n
A	$y = 1.012x + 0.882$	0.961	38
B	$y = 2.647x + 0.014$	0.999	44

13. (LO 8, 17) Substance V is suspected of interfering in the assay for analyte M. An experiment is conducted in which the measured concentration of M (μg/dL) is plotted as a function of the known concentration of V (μg/dL). The data fit a straight line, the regression equation is $y = -8.23x + 66.52$, and $n = 32$.

   (a) If the standard error of the slope is 0.041, what is the 99% confidence interval for the slope?

   (b) What does this confidence interval for the slope say about the interference of V in the assay for M?

   (c) If the standard error of the intercept is 2.92, what is the 90% confidence interval for the y-intercept?

14. (LO 8, 9, 11, 17) Your laboratory's assay for a certain endocrine marker involves constructing a standard curve at six known concentrations (pg/mL). The response variable is absorbance. Shown below are the data from one run of this assay.

Concentration (pg/mL)	Absorbance
10	0.040
30	0.092
100	0.303
250	0.697
500	1.334
1000	2.480

   (a) Plot the data directly.

   (b) Plot the logarithm of absorbance against the logarithm of the concentration.

   (c) How is the log-log plot superior to the direct plot? Calculate the regression equation for the log-log plot. What concentrations correspond to absorbances of 0.844 and 0.107?

15. (LO 8, 9, 11, 12, 17) Consider the following data, which a technologist gathered to construct a standard curve for a heavy metal in serum.

Concentration (μg/dL)	Absorbance
1.0	0.06
2.0	0.08
3.0	0.130
4.0	0.220
5.0	0.330
6.0	0.440
7.0	0.530
8.0	0.580
9.0	0.600

   (a) Calculate the least-squares linear regression equation and the correlation coefficient.

   (b) What concentrations does the regression line predict for absorbances of 0.130, 0.330, and 0.530?

   (c) Plot absorbance against concentration.

   (d) Comment on the suitability of the line for use as a standard curve.

16. (LO 8, 9) The time required for a population of bacteria to double (d) can be calculated from this equation:

$$c_i \times 2^{t/d} = c_t$$

where c_i is the initial cell number, t is the elapsed time, d is the time required for one doubling, and c_t is the cell number at time t. Rearranging this equation to make t the independent variable gives

$$\log c_t - \log c_i = \frac{\log 2}{d} t$$

$$\log c_t - \log c_i = \frac{0.301}{d} t$$

$$\log c_t = \frac{0.301}{d} t + \log c_i$$

By means of linear regression, use the following data for bacterial cell growth to determine the doubling time.

Elapsed Time (min)	Cell Number
0	19
11	32
26	66
43	122
55	257
72	435
88	822
131	3343
154	6934

17. (LO 13) Match the scatterplots below with their correlation coefficients.

0.997, 0.914, 0.071, −0.980, −0.541

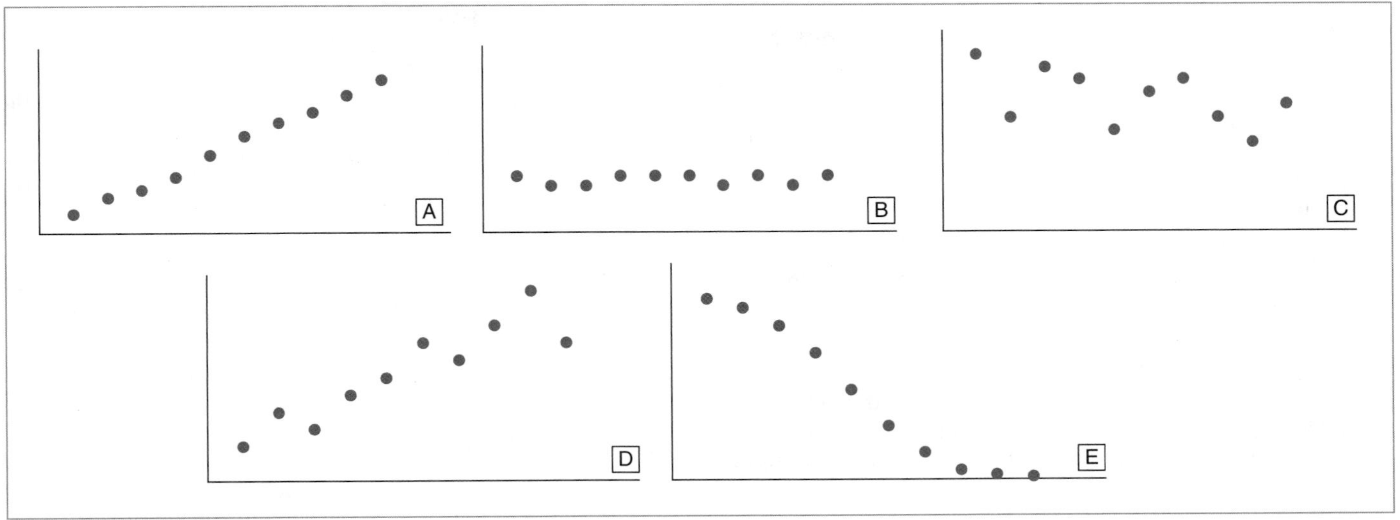

18. (LO 23) Each row in the following table represents a Student's *t* test. For each test, determine whether the difference between the means is statistically significant at $p = 0.05$.

	t value	n_1	n_2	$\bar{x}_1$	$\bar{x}_2$
(a)	1.933	5	5	63.1	64.9
(b)	2.307	13	14	0.18	0.22
(c)	1.615	4	4	2.04	3.12
(d)	2.009	10	7	167	148
(e)	4.184	26	24	0.0278	0.0189

19. (LO 23) For a set of data, there are six specimens in one group and seven in the other. Student's *t* test returns a *t* value of 2.445. Is there a significant difference between the means of the two groups at $p = 0.05$? At $p = 0.01$?

20. (LO 20, 22, 23, 24) Is Student's *t* test appropriate for comparing the means of the following two groups of data? Explain.

Group	N	Variance
1	21	13.34
2	21	14.78

21. (LO 22, 23) Five instrument comparisons appear in the table below. In each comparison, different samples were run on two instruments. Calculate the *F* value for each comparison and determine whether precision differs significantly between the two instruments ($p = 0.05$). All distributions are normal.

	Instrument #1		Instrument #2			Is Difference Significant?
	Variance	n	Variance	n	F	(yes / no)
(a)	0.0446	21	0.0793	21		
(b)	8.094	8	10.772	11		
(c)	46.812	11	23.004	11		
(d)	0.3755	61	0.4217	61		
(e)	16.17	21	15.112	21		

22. (LO 19, 22, 23) Consider the following contingency table. State the null hypothesis and then calculate the χ^2 statistic. Decide whether we may reject the null hypothesis.

		Response Variable			TOTAL
		X	Y	Z	
Explanatory Variable	A	12	26	83	
	B	18	34	91	
	C	15	45	76	
	TOTAL				

23. (LO 19, 22, 23) For each of the following contingency tables, state the null hypothesis and then calculate the χ^2 statistic. Decide whether the null hypothesis may be rejected.

(a)

442	108	627
299	451	820

(b)

34	67	90
29	72	94
38	69	86

(c)

101	423	669	87
625	710	472	95

24. (LO 23) Each row in the following table represents a *t* test for equal variances. For each test, determine whether the difference between the means is statistically significant at $p = 0.01$.

	t value	n_1	n_2	$\overline{x}_1$	$\overline{x}_2$
(a)	1.934	48	54	0.846	0.912
(b)	2.735	5	4	2.78	3.26
(c)	4.077	6	7	89	70
(d)	3.406	5	6	13.3	16.2
(e)	1.028	24	28	522	559

25. (LO 21) Suppose Student's *t* test shows the difference between two means to be statistically significant at $p = 0.05$. Decide whether each of the following statements is necessarily true.

    (a) The difference that was observed between the means will appear one in 20 times even if there is no real difference between the two groups.

    (b) If the null hypothesis is true, the results have a 5% probability of being as extreme as they were in this experiment.

    (c) The difference observed between the means is greater than would be observed if *p* were 0.01.

26. (LO 21) In a study of a new antihypertensive agent, one group of patients is given the drug and another group is given a placebo. A paired *t* test is carried out on the two groups, revealing a statistically significant difference between the means at $p = 0.01$. Is the following statement true?

    "If the drug has no effect, then the probability is 1% that random sampling by itself would have produced an effect as large as that seen in this experiment."

27. (LO 21, 23) Consider these results of a *t* test: $t = 2.046$, $d.f. = 10$. Is the following conclusion true?

    "The difference was statistically significant ($p < 0.10$)."

28. (LO 21, 23) Consider these results of a *t* test: $t = 2.880$, $d.f. = 7$. Is the following conclusion true?

    "There was a statistically significant difference between the means ($p < 0.05$)."

Contextual Problems

1. (LO 1, 6) Your LIS (laboratory information system) has gone down for several hours. Because calculations must be performed manually in the interim, you yourself have to ascertain whether the result for your control solution is within two standard deviations of the mean, the limit that your manager has set to permit the release of patient results. Over the past month, 16 values (in "ng/dL") for the control solution have been obtained in the test you are running, including yours from today, which is 40.4:

    55.1, 56.4, 61.5, 43.7, 52.0, 55.2, 59.0, 70.1, 53.2, 50.9, 53.3, 48.6, 49.7, 66.0, 52.2, 40.4

    Can you begin running patient samples and releasing results?

2. (LO 1, 6) Your laboratory's control solution for the cardiac marker troponin-T is prepared by adding 2.00 mL of deionized water directly to a manufacturer-supplied bottle containing the preweighed dehydrated material. You and your colleagues have been using this lot of control solution for the last 30 days, having gathered 90 data values; the concentration is 2.94 ± 0.03 ng/mL (mean $\pm$ SD). Your laboratory policy allows for running patient samples and releasing results if the control value falls within 2*s* of the mean.

    (a) Suppose someone prepares a bottle of fresh control solution today, but mistakenly adds only 1.90 mL of water, rather than 2.00. Is this pipetting error negligible? Explain.

    (b) Suppose that a single drop of water from the pipet has a volume of 0.05 mL. If the technologist dispenses 2.00 mL of water into the bottle of dehydrated material but inadvertently allows one extra drop of water to fall in, will the test result for the control solution be affected appreciably? Explain.

3. (LO 1, 2, 3, 5) Your laboratory uses a manual method for quantifying analyte *Z* in plasma. It requires pipetting 50.0 μL of sample into 2.0 mL of reagent. For this purpose, there are two 50-μL pipets available on the bench top: one calibrated correctly to deliver 50.0 ± 1.0 μL (mean $\pm$ SD) and the other accidentally miscalibrated such that it actually delivers 55.0 ± 1.0 μL. Each technologist randomly chooses a pipet whenever he or she runs the assay. A correctly calibrated pipet gives a mean result for analyte *Z* of 100 ng per dL of plasma.

    (a) Over the course of several weeks, you and your colleagues run the assay on a control solution, generating 80 results. One day, your supervisor plots the results as a distribution curve and becomes alarmed. How does the curve look? Explain.

    (b) If each pipet were more precise, how would the distribution curve change?

    (c) If the technologists had used the correctly calibrated pipet more often than the miscalibrated one, how would the distribution curve have differed?

4. (LO 1, 5) If the leukocyte count is 6240 ± 480 cells/μL (mean $\pm$ standard deviation) for the population of city *X*, how many patients in a random sample of 100 would have a count below 5760 cells/μL? (Assume the distribution to be normal.)

5. (LO 1, 6, 7) Your laboratory manager is considering buying one of three competing analyzers. In an effort to evaluate their reproducibilities, you run a different patient sample on each analyzer for the concentration of total bilirubin. From the following data, identify the analyzer with the greatest precision.

Analyzer	Mean (mg/dL)	Standard Deviation (mg/dL)
A	5.4	0.22
B	1.3	0.10
C	12.3	1.1

6. (LO 1, 6, 7) The following tables present data for an analytical method, manufactured by company *W*, for quantifying lead (Pb) in whole blood. The first table shows values obtained for the same standard solution taken on 4 consecutive days ("day-to-day performance"), whereas the second table shows data for nine replicates of the solution taken in the same run on the same day ("within-run performance").

   Which of the data sets shows greater precision? Offer a reasonable explanation.

Day-to-Day Performance

Date	May 1	May 2	May 3	May 4	May 5	May 6	May 7	May 8	May 9
Value (μg/dL)	20	17	19	21	19	22	21	21	18

Within-Run Performance

Replicate	1	2	3	4	5	6	7	8	9
Value (μg/dL)	22	21	22	21	23	21	22	23	21

7. (LO 19, 21, 22) In an assay comparison, you quantified cholesterol in a quality-control solution in quadruplicate on 4 consecutive days by each of two methods. From the following data, use an appropriate significance test to decide whether the two methods have different precisions at $p = 0.05$. (Visual inspection of the data reveals a normal distribution.)

	Method 1	Method 2
Cholesterol Concentration (mg/dL), Mean ± SD	224 ± 4.7	227 ± 5.7

8. (LO 19, 21, 22, 24) To solve this problem, use statistical software, as is widely available in spreadsheets. Your laboratory is establishing a reference range for substance *X* in the serum of adults. In so doing, it is necessary to check for a difference in the average concentration between men and women. From the data in the table to the right use an appropriate significance test to decide whether the concentration of *X* differs between the sexes. Have the software calculate a *p* value. (Visual inspection of the data reveals a normal distribution.)

Concentration of X (pg/mL)	
Men	**Women**
5.53	6.02
5.68	6.22
5.21	5.79
6.28	5.98
5.75	6.09
5.48	5.81
6.10	5.97
5.59	5.74
5.44	5.66
5.72	6.11
5.59	6.20

9. (LO 19, 20, 21, 22) A diagnostics company hires your laboratory and one other to analyze 10 whole-blood specimens for hemoglobin. Each specimen is divided into two aliquots, and each laboratory analyzes one. The company wants to know, at the 99% confidence level, whether there is a significant difference between the two instruments used at the laboratories.

Specimen	Concentration of Hemoglobin (g/dL)	
	Laboratory 1	Laboratory 2
1	14.1	14.6
2	16.8	16.9
3	14.9	15.8
4	15.5	15.9
5	13.9	14.4
6	16.7	17.0
7	17.0	17.6
8	15.6	16.2
9	16.1	16.3
10	17.6	18.0

10. (LO 19, 21, 22) A laboratory manager wants to assess the skill of a job applicant to perform a manual differential (i.e., to differentiate and count white blood cells on a glass slide under a microscope). To carry out this assessment, the manager will compare the new technologist's results with those of two seasoned technologists for the same specimen. The data appear below. Using an appropriate test, determine whether the differences seen among the technologists are statistically significant at $p = 0.05$.

Technologist	Neutrophils	Lymphocytes	Monocytes
#1 (new)	64	30	6
#2	60	33	7
#3	59	34	7

11. (LO 19, 21, 22) Your laboratory is comparing its recently purchased instrument with the current one for determining urine osmolality. At a p value of 0.05, ascertain whether results from the two instruments differ significantly.

Specimen	Urine Osmolality (mOsm/kg)	
	Current Instrument	New Instrument
1	446	450
2	307	299
3	661	648
4	537	555
5	498	494
6	410	431
7	372	401
8	526	540
9	462	450
10	602	619

12. (LO 19, 21, 22) Statistics software will be very helpful in solving this problem. Your laboratory is investigating the possible interference of caffeine in the assay for drug *G* in serum. Therefore, you run 16 specimens from randomly chosen patients who drink coffee regularly and 16 from randomly chosen patients who abstain. All the patients are taking drug *G* at the same prescribed dose. The caffeine concentration in each of the 16 serum specimens from the coffee drinkers is in the range 0.5–0.9 mg/dL. The serum specimens from the abstainers have no detectable caffeine. Is there a significant difference between the means of the two data sets?

Concentration of Drug *G* (ng/mL)	
Coffee Drinkers	Abstainers
14.5	9.4
16.9	12.6
15.7	8.3
16.3	10.9
16.5	11.6
14.9	8.7
15.2	10.5
16.0	13.2
17.1	14.3
15.8	10.1
16.6	15.4
14.9	9.7
17.6	12.8
13.4	16.2
16.1	10.4
17.0	11.3

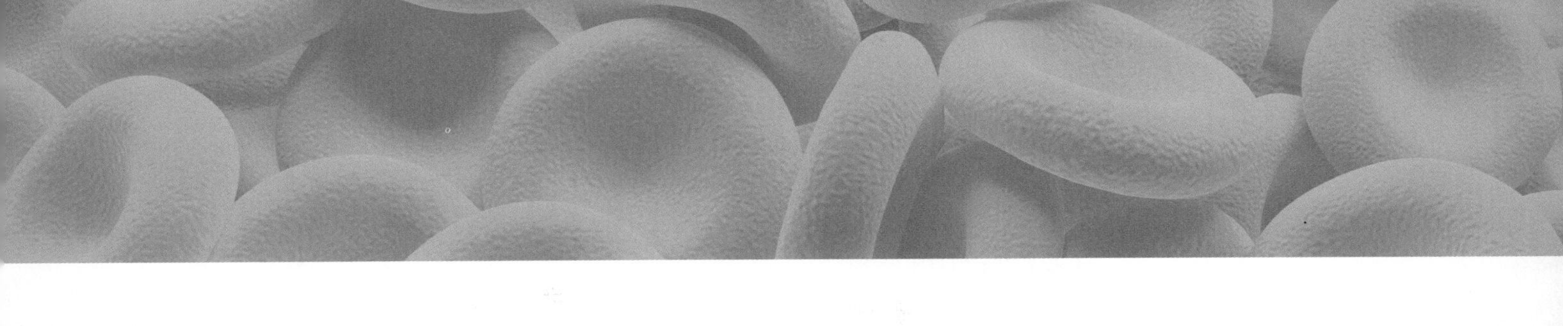

9 Chemistry

Learning Objectives

At the end of this chapter, the student should be able to do the following:

1. Explain and use the relationship between transmittance and absorbance
2. Explain the proportionality between absorbance and molar absorptivity, concentration, and path length
3. Use Beer's law properly
4. Explain when to use a standard curve, the molar absorptivity method, or the single-standard method to quantify a chromophore
5. Explain the strengths and weaknesses of end-point, two-point, and kinetic assay modes
6. Explain the significance of initial rate, K_M, and V_{max}
7. Relate the Michaelis-Menten equation to its plot and to its underlying model of enzyme catalysis
8. Explain the strengths and weaknesses of Lineweaver-Burk plots
9. Estimate K_M and V_{max} from a Michaelis-Menten plot and from a Lineweaver-Burk plot
10. Define the phenomenon of *p*H buffering
11. Use K_a and pK_a to compare the strengths of acids
12. Using the Henderson-Hasselbalch equation, calculate the concentrations of an acid and its conjugate base necessary to prepare a buffer at a given *p*H
13. Use the Henderson-Hasselbalch equation to calculate any one of these quantities from the other three: *p*H, pK_a, concentration of acid, concentration of conjugate base
14. Properly apply the Henderson-Hasselbalch equation to the CO_2-bicarbonate buffering system in the blood
15. Differentiate among respiratory and metabolic acidosis and alkalosis by *p*H, PCO_2, and bicarbonate concentration
16. Calculate the anion gap, with and without potassium
17. Calculate the osmolarity of a solution from the molarity
18. Calculate the osmolarity and osmolality of plasma, given the concentrations of sodium, glucose, and BUN
19. Calculate the osmolality gap

Chapter Outline

20. Calculate the concentration of LDL cholesterol by means of the Friedewald equation
21. Calculate the creatinine clearance rate, given the required information

Key Terms

absorbance
acid dissociation constant
acidosis
alkalosis
anion gap
Beer-Lambert law
buffered
chromophore
conjugate acid
conjugate base
creatinine clearance
double-reciprocal plot
end-point assay
enzyme
enzyme kinetics
Friedewald equation
glomerular filtration rate
HDL
Henderson-Hasselbalch equation
hypertonic
hypotonic
initial rate
K_a
K_M
kinetic assay
lag phase
LDL
linear phase
Lineweaver-Burk plot
lipoprotein
maximal velocity (V_{max})
metabolic acidosis/alkalosis
Michaelis-Menten equation
molar absorptivity
molar absorptivity method
molar extinction coefficient
osmolality
osmolality gap
osmolarity
osmole
osmosis
osmotic pressure
partial pressure
pK_a
respiratory acidosis/alkalosis
single-standard method
substrate
substrate-depletion phase
transmittance
two-point assay
VLDL

ANALYTICAL SPECTROSCOPY

Among the most important techniques in the clinical laboratory is analytical spectroscopy. It is based on the phenomenon that many chemical substances absorb light of a particular wavelength. A beam of light of known intensity (I_0) is directed into a solution, and the intensity (I) of the light emerging from the solution is then measured.

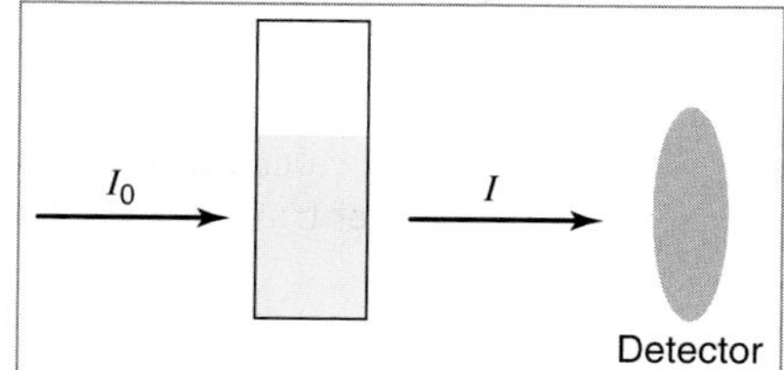

The fraction of light transmitted (I/I_0) is called the **transmittance** (T):

$$T = \frac{I}{I_0}$$

Being a fraction, T ranges in value from 0 to 1. The light that did not pass through the sample was absorbed. For example, if $T = 0.80$, then 80% of the light passing through the sample was transmitted and 20% was absorbed. Although transmittance goes down as concentration goes up, the relationship is not linear (Figure 9-1A ■).

Therefore, a plot of T against concentration is more difficult to use as a standard curve than is a straight line. But the logarithm of T as a function of concentration is a straight line and, as a result, is more useful for this purpose (Figure 9-1B). Accordingly, **absorbance** (A) is defined as the logarithm (base 10) of the transmittance:

$$A \equiv -\log\frac{I}{I_0} = -\log T$$

Thus, if $T = 0.648$, then 64.8% of the light passing through the sample is transmitted and 35.2% is absorbed. The absorbance, then, or A, is

$$A = -\log T = -\log 0.648 = 0.188$$

Absorbance depends, logically, on the following three factors.

- *The concentration of the absorbing chemical substance (the* ***chromophore****).* At higher concentrations, there is more of the chromophore present to absorb the light.
- *The length of the path the light takes passing through the solution.* In a longer container, the light stays in contact with the chromophore for a longer period of time and, accordingly, has more opportunity to be absorbed.
- *The inherent ability of the chromophore to absorb the light.* This ability is quantified in the **molar absorptivity** or the **molar extinction coefficient**. For every chromophore, it is unique and constant under a given set of conditions (solvent, wavelength, temperature).

The **Beer-Lambert law** (also called "Beer's law") is the mathematical relationship among absorbance and the three factors listed above:

EQUATION 1

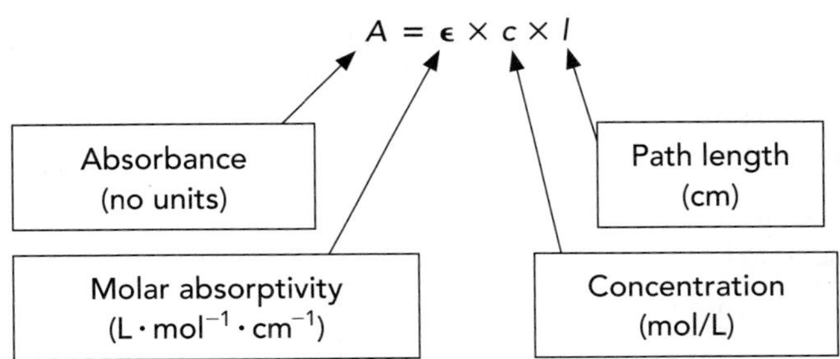

Equation 1 is linear. As Figure 9-1B shows, absorbance is directly proportional to concentration (as it is to path length), with ϵ functioning as the proportionality constant.

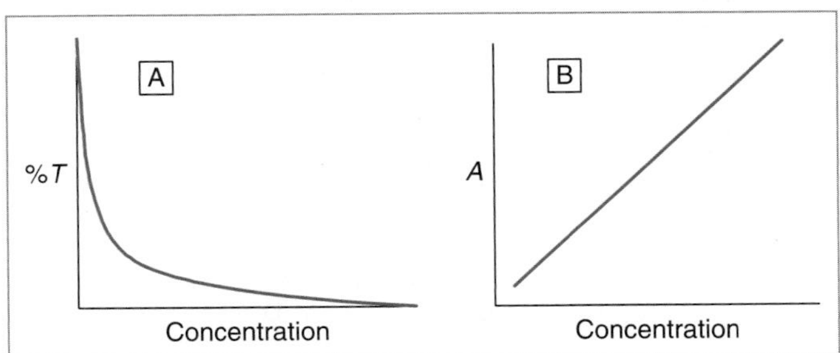

■ FIGURE 9-1 Panel *A*: The relationship between transmittance and concentration is nonlinear; %T is not proportional to concentration. Panel *B*: Absorbance *is* directly proportional to concentration.

If A has been measured, and if the molar absorptivity and path length are known, then the concentration of a chromophore can be calculated by solving Equation 1 for c:

$$c = \frac{A}{\epsilon \times l}$$

Suppose, for example, that we have a solution of all-*trans*-retinol (vitamin A) in isopropyl alcohol and we want to ascertain its concentration. In a reference book, we find that retinol in isopropyl alcohol has a molar absorptivity of 52,300 $L \cdot mol^{-1} \cdot cm^{-1}$. If we measure the absorbance of our solution to be 0.628, and if the path length is 1 cm, then the concentration is

$$c = \frac{0.628}{(52{,}300\ L \cdot mol^{-1} \cdot cm^{-1})(1\ cm)}$$

$$= 0.000012\ mol/L$$

$$= 1.2 \times 10^{-5}\ mol/L$$

$$= 12\ \mu mol/L$$

Beer's law is especially useful when the analyte is too unstable to generate a standard curve of absorbance versus concentration. In such a case, we calculate the concentration directly from its absorbance in the solution. This is the **molar absorptivity method**.

An alternative to the molar absorptivity method is the **single-standard method**, in which the absorbance of only one standard solution is measured and a line is drawn through it as the standard curve. This method is useful only if we know the standard curve to be linear.

Even though absorbance is directly proportional to concentration, the relationship does not remain linear as concentration continues going up (Figure 9-2 ■). For any chromophore, the concentration range in which absorbance is linear must be determined experimentally, and any absorbance reading above that range should not be trusted when used in Beer's law.

Sometimes a chemical substance does not obey Beer's law at any concentration, giving instead a curve across the entire range. The reasons for this behavior we leave to a chemistry textbook.

Therefore, generating a standard curve from several data points has at least two major advantages over the single-standard method.

- It can reveal nonlinearity that might be present so that (1) the sample may be diluted into the linear range or (2) the data may be fit to a curve by means of nonlinear regression.
- It averages out random errors over all the standards.

However, the additional time and cost represent one disadvantage of the standard-curve method over the single-standard method.

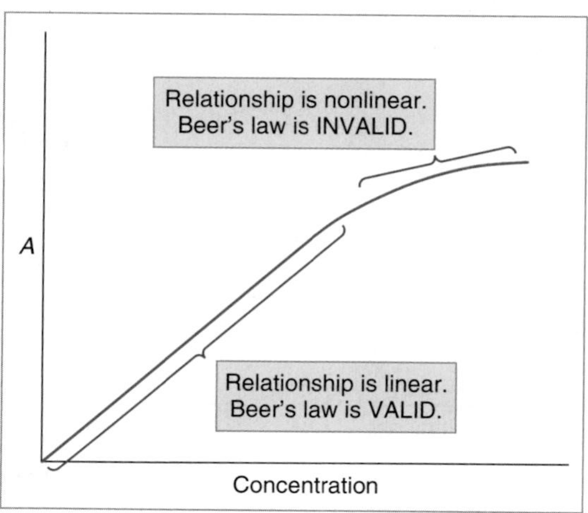

■ **FIGURE 9-2** Relationship between absorbance (A) and concentration eventually becomes nonlinear.

☑ CHECKPOINT 9-1

1. Calculate the concentration of a solution whose absorbance is 0.388, when the path length is 1 cm and the molar absorptivity is 2500 $L \cdot mol^{-1} \cdot cm^{-1}$.
2. Calculate the concentration of a solution whose absorbance is 0.917, when the path length is 1 cm and the molar absorptivity is 22,100 $L \cdot mol^{-1} \cdot cm^{-1}$.
3. If the concentration of a solution whose absorbance is 0.600 is diluted 1:2, what is the final absorbance?
4. Calculate the absorbance of a solution whose transmittance is 0.22.

1. We use the equation

$$c = \frac{A}{\epsilon \times l}$$

$$c = \frac{0.388}{(2500\ L \cdot mol^{-1} \cdot cm^{-1})(1\ cm)} = 1.55 \times 10^{-4}\ mol/L$$

2. The procedure is the same as for problem 1. The answer is 4.14×10^{-5} mol/L.
3. Because absorbance is directly proportional to concentration, the two variables change by the same factor. A dilution of 1:2 brings the concentration down to one-half of its original value. Therefore, the absorbance also goes down one-half, to 0.300.
4. The absorbance is

$$A = -\log T = -\log 0.22 = 0.658$$

ENZYME KINETICS

Because few reactions would otherwise proceed fast enough to sustain life, nearly every chemical reaction that occurs in a living thing is catalyzed. And almost all known biological catalysts, called **enzymes**, are proteins. In fact, until the discovery of catalytic ribonucleic acid in the 1980s, all enzymes were thought to be proteins.

The significance of enzymes in the clinical laboratory is two-fold. First, the activity of an enzyme in a patient specimen can give clues to a diagnosis. Examples are the enzyme alanine aminotransferase in liver damage, glucose-6-phosphate dehydrogenase in hemolytic anemia, alkaline phosphatase in bone disease, amylase in pancreatitis, and aetylcholinesterase in insecticide poisoning.

Second, selected enzymes are intentionally incorporated into assays as reagents. For example, the enzyme alkaline phosphatase is used in some assays to generate a fluorescent product whose quantity is directly proportional to the concentration of the analyte in the specimen.

Enzymes are strikingly efficient as catalysts. They can increase the reaction rate as much as 10^{20}-fold and are often many orders of magnitude more efficient than synthetic catalysts. The quantitative study of enzyme catalysis, or **enzyme kinetics**, which has been developed over decades, enables us to understand not only how enzymes accomplish their extraordinary feats but also how we can measure their activity and exploit them in the clinical laboratory.

Reaction Rates

The rate is a measure of how fast a reaction is going. (Rates are sometimes incorrectly described as "fast" or "slow," even though it is the reactions that are fast or slow; rates themselves are "high" or "low.") Consider the simple reaction **A** $\rightarrow$ **Z**. In practical terms, the rate of a reaction is determined by rapidly mixing the reactants in a tube or other vessel and then determining the concentration either of a reactant (called a "**substrate**" if the reaction is enzyme-catalyzed) or of a product after a certain amount of time has passed (Figure 9-3 ■).

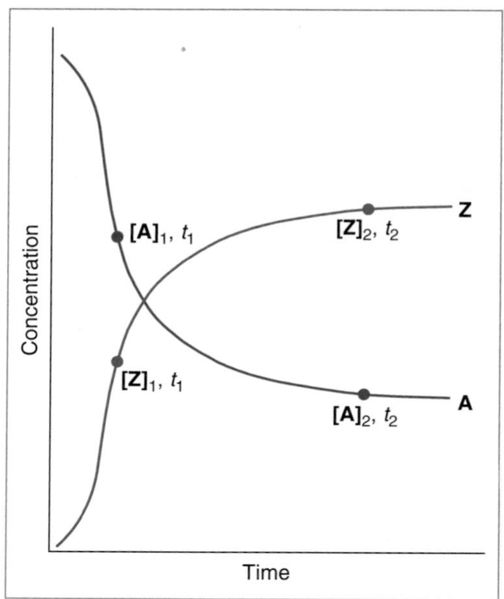

FIGURE 9-3 The change in concentration of the reactant **A** (blue curve) and the product **Z** (pink curve), as a function of time, for the reaction **A** → **Z.**

The reaction rate is the change in concentration of **A** or **Z** divided by the corresponding change in time:

$$\frac{[Z]_2 - [Z]_1}{t_2 - t_1} = \frac{\Delta[Z]}{\Delta t}$$

or

$$\frac{[A]_2 - [A]_1}{t_2 - t_1} = \frac{\Delta[A]}{\Delta t}$$

Appendix 9-1
"Elementary Chemical Kinetics"
www.myhealthprofessions.kit.com
PEARSON myhealthprofessionskit

The units, of course, are those of concentration per time, examples being "μmol/L/second," "mg/dL/minute," and "mEq/mL/minute." Realize, however, that the reaction rate is not necessarily constant; rather, it is only an average over the time interval specified. Appendix 9-1 on the website discusses chemical kinetics in more detail.

Assay Modes

In the clinical laboratory, chemical reactions are used to quantify many analytes, and a good number of those reactions employ enzymes as reagents. In an **end-point assay** (Figure 9-4A ■), we measure absorbance at a fixed time point, which may be several minutes or several hours after the reaction begins. We then calculate the concentration either from a standard curve, from a single standard, or from the molar absorptivity. From that concentration, then, we compute a reaction rate. A **two-point assay** (Figure 9-4B), by contrast, measures the absorbance at each of two time points; we then calculate the reaction rate between them. A **kinetic assay** (Figure 9-4C) takes absorbance readings at several time points, from all of which we then compute the rate.

Of these three, the kinetic assay is most reliable because it can confirm linearity between absorbance and time, in which case the reaction rate would be constant and one could conclude that (a) all reaction conditions are the same from one measured absorbance to the next and that (b) the assay depends only on the analyte's concentration. The two-point and end-point assays are less reliable because they assume linearity.

Reaction Phases

An enzyme-catalyzed reaction typically has three phases (Figure 9-5 ■). During the **lag phase**, which is the earliest and which may last for 1 or 2 minutes, various processes may be under way, such as

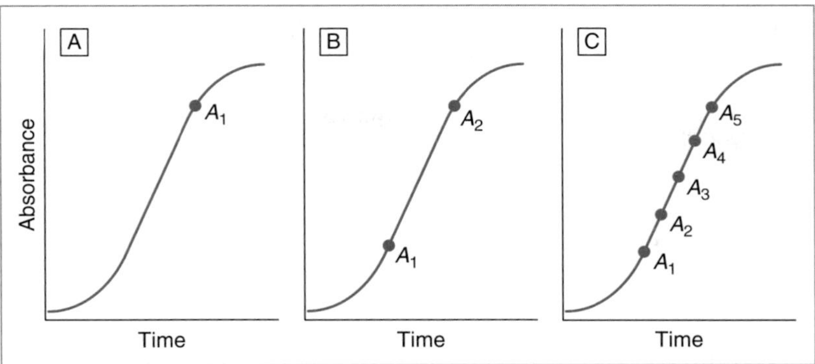

■ **FIGURE 9-4** Assay modes. (**A**) End-point assay. Absorbance is measured at only one time point after the reaction starts. (**B**) Two-point assay. Absorbance is measured at each of two time points. (**C**) Kinetic assay. Several absorbance readings are taken.

temperature stabilization and enzyme activation by cofactors or coenzymes. The reaction rate increases during this phase until it reaches a constant value, at which point the **linear phase** begins. Throughout this phase, the concentration of product is directly proportional to time, which means that the relationship between concentration and time is linear. As more time passes, the reaction enters the **substrate-depletion phase**, in which the substrate supply has diminished so much that product formation slows down, eventually becoming a plateau where its rate approaches zero.

The Michaelis-Menten Equation

As explained earlier and in Figure 9-5, the rate is constant only in the linear phase. In this phase, the rate is called the **initial rate**. Figure 9-6 ■ shows the change in concentration of **Z** as a function of time at three starting substrate concentrations. Not surprisingly, the initial rate increases with the substrate

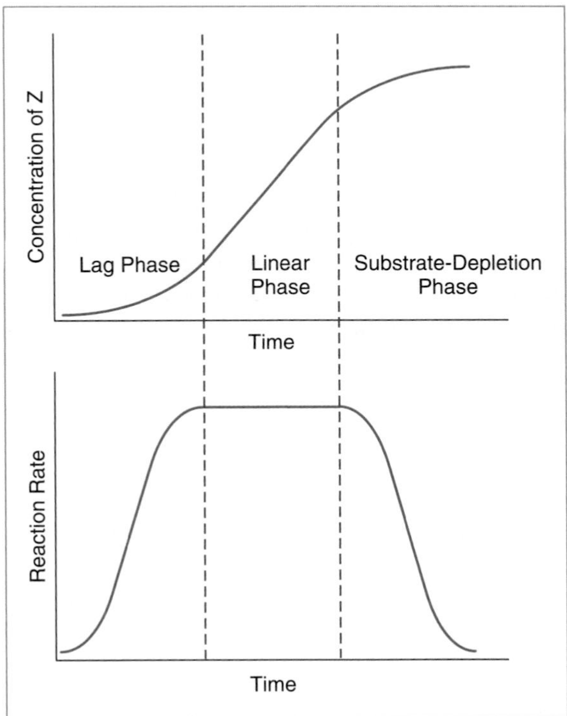

■ **FIGURE 9-5** Typical phases of an enzyme-catalyzed reaction. *Lag phase*: the enzyme is undergoing activation by cofactors and coenzymes in the reaction mixture. *Linear phase*: the concentration of product **Z** is directly proportional to time, and the reaction rate is, therefore, constant. *Substrate-depletion phase*: the reaction has proceeded so long that the substrate has been consumed and the concentration of **Z** has stopped changing (i.e., the rate goes back down to zero).

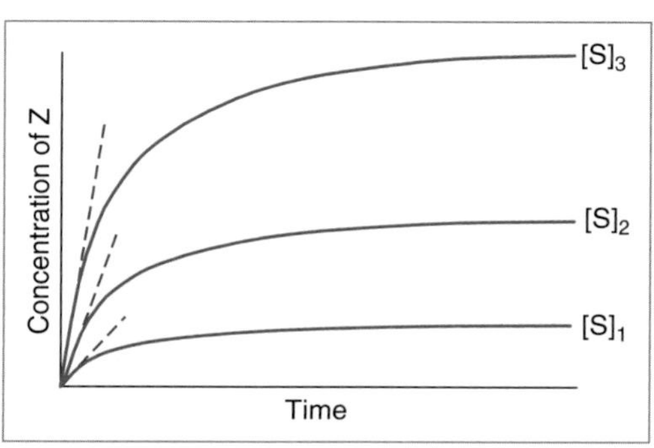

FIGURE 9-6 Initial rates of the enzyme-catalyzed reaction A → Z at three starting substrate concentrations, $[S]_x$. The initial rate (v) at each [S] is the slope of the linear part (broken blue line) of the curve.

concentration at the beginning of the reaction. Each initial rate is the slope of its line, which, of course, can be described by an equation of the form $y = mx + b$.

The initial rate (v) can be plotted against the starting substrate concentration ([S]), giving a curve like that in Figure 9-7. At low [S], v increases almost linearly with [S]. As [S] continues increasing, however, v rises more slowly, eventually entering a plateau where it nearly stops rising even though [S] continues going up. The value that the rate approaches at very high [S] is known as the **maximal velocity**, symbolized as $\mathbf{V_{max}}$. In this region of the graph, where the rate does not respond appreciably to further increases in substrate concentration, the enzyme is said to be *saturated* because it cannot bind substrate any faster. (The V_{max} is an asymptote, a line that a curve approaches without ever merging with it.) The value of [S] at half of V_{max} is defined as $\mathbf{K_M}$.

In 1913, Leonor Michaelis and Maude Menten proposed a model to explain this behavior. In their model, the enzyme binds the substrate, executes the necessary chemical changes, and then releases the product; after this last step, the enzyme is ready to repeat the process. Emerging from this model is the **Michaelis-Menten equation**, which describes the curve in Figure 9-7:

EQUATION 2

$$v = \frac{V_{max}[S]}{K_M + [S]}$$

Appendix 9-2
"Models of Enzyme Catalysis"
www.myhealthprofessions.kit.com
PEARSON myhealthprofessionskit

Appendix 9-2 on the website lays out their model in detail and derives Equation 2.

Figure 9-7 shows us that when [S] is very large, v is V_{max}. Moreover, when $v = {}^1/_2\, V_{max}$, the substrate concentration, [S], is defined as K_M. K_M reflects the affinity of enzyme for substrate, or, in a sense, the strength of binding between enzyme and substrate. As affinity rises, therefore, the concentration of substrate necessary to bring v to ${}^1/_2\, V_{max}$ falls because the enzyme can bind the same number of substrate molecules even with fewer of them present. As affinity falls, however, the concentration of substrate necessary to bring v to ${}^1/_2\, V_{max}$ rises because the enzyme can bind the same number of

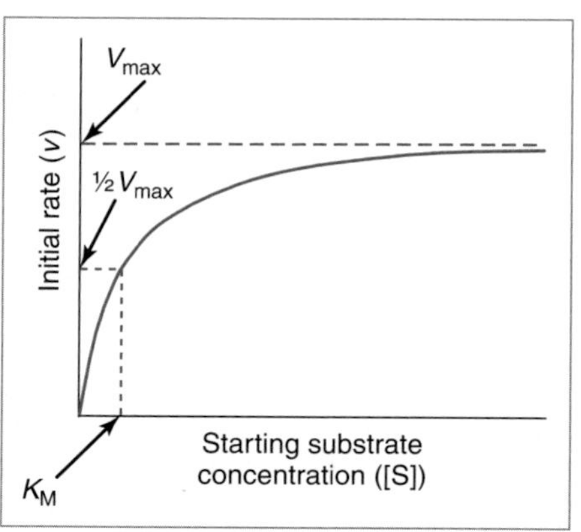

FIGURE 9-7 A graph of the Michaelis-Menten equation (Equation 2).

molecules *only* when more of them are present. Thus, as affinity increases, K_M decreases; as affinity decreases, K_M increases.

At low [S], the initial rate is close to linearity. In this part of the curve, the reaction is called *first-order* because its initial rate is directly proportional to substrate concentration. At high [S], however, the initial rate does not depend on substrate concentration. In this part of the curve, the reaction is said to be *zero-order* because its rate does not change with further increases in [S]. Appendix 9-1 on the website discusses reaction order in greater depth.

Appendix 9-1
"Elementary Chemical Kinetics"
www.myhealthprofessions.kit.com
PEARSON myhealthprofessionskit

Physiological Significance of K_M

As Figure 9-7 illustrates, the initial rate can increase with a substrate concentration that is slightly below, at, or slightly above K_M. Consider an example of this property at work in a biochemical pathway.

There are two enzymes that catalyze the phosphorylation of glucose in the cell: hexokinase and glucokinase. Their K_M values are about 0.1 mmol/L and 10 mmol/L, respectively (Figure 9-8 ■). What this means is that, as the glucose concentration gradually rises from about 4 mmol/L after several hours of fasting to about 20 mmol/L after a meal, the rate of the glucokinase-catalyzed reaction can increase, but that of the hexokinase-catalyzed reaction cannot. This is so because hexokinase is already functioning at or near its V_{max} when glucose is present at 4 mmol/L, whereas glucokinase is functioning well below its V_{max}. Glucokinase, therefore, is the enzyme that responds to changes in the concentration of circulating glucose. After a meal, this acceleration of glucose phosphorylation translates into faster glycogen storage in the liver, release of insulin by the pancreas, and removal of excess glucose from the blood. Appendix 9-3 on the website presents another example of the physiological significance of K_M, this one focusing on ethanol metabolism in the liver.

Appendix 9-3
"An Example of the Physiological Significance of K_M"
www.myhealthprofessions.kit.com
PEARSON myhealthprofessionskit

Significance of K_M in the Clinical Laboratory

Enzymes in patient specimens are typically assayed at saturating substrate concentrations so that v is at V_{max}. This ensures that only the concentration of enzyme in the specimen affects the observed rate. To achieve this condition *in vitro*, the substrate concentration is set at 20–100 times the K_M.

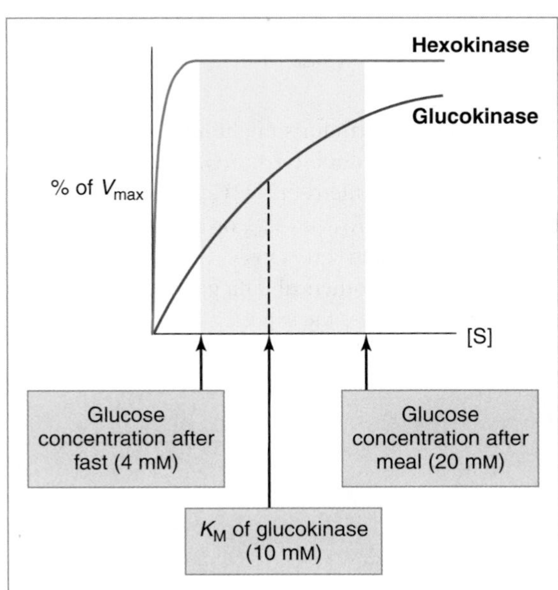

■ **FIGURE 9-8** Physiological significance of K_M, exemplified by two enzymes that phosphorylate glucose. As the glucose concentration rises from 4 mM after a fast to 20 mM after a meal (yellow area), only the glucokinase-catalyzed reaction (blue curve) goes faster. Hexokinase (pink curve) cannot increase its rate because it is already operating at its own V_{max}. Acceleration of the glucokinase-catalyzed reaction in the liver and pancreas ultimately leads to removal of excess glucose from the blood.

Linear Transformations

Generating enough data points to draw an accurate curve of *v* versus [S] (Figure 9-7) is quite difficult. Even when there are enough data points, though, gleaning accurate values for V_{max} and then K_M is a bit perilous because visually evaluating an asymptote is a matter of human judgment.

To circumvent this obstacle, various linear transformations of the Michaelis-Menten equation (Equation 2) have been developed over the years. Straight lines, of course, are easier both to draw and to interpret than are curves. Nevertheless, as Chapter 8 explains, high-speed computers have nearly obviated these techniques. In fact, linear transformations are almost obsolete, *except* that (1) they display data in such a way that makes visual interpretation easy and quick and (2) they expose features of the data that curves obscure.

Lineweaver-Burk Plots

The most widely used linear transformation of the Michaelis-Menten equation (Equation 2) has been

EQUATION 3

$$\frac{1}{v} = \left(\frac{K_M}{V_{max}}\right)\frac{1}{[S]} + \frac{1}{V_{max}}$$

This linear equation emerges from straightforward rearrangement of Equation 2:

$$v = \frac{V_{max}[S]}{K_M + [S]}$$

$$\frac{1}{v} = \frac{K_M + [S]}{V_{max}[S]}$$

$$\frac{1}{v} = \frac{K_M}{V_{max}[S]} + \frac{[S]}{V_{max}[S]}$$

$$\frac{1}{v} = \left(\frac{K_M}{V_{max}}\right)\frac{1}{[S]} + \frac{1}{V_{max}}$$

Equation 3 fits the slope-intercept form for straight lines, $y = mx + b$, where y is $1/v$ and x is $1/[S]$. A graph of this equation is known as a **double-reciprocal** or **Lineweaver-Burk plot** (Figure 9-9 ■). The slope of this line is K_M/V_{max} and the y-intercept is $1/V_{max}$. The x-intercept is $-1/K_M$. Clearly, when visual inspection is the method, evaluating K_M and V_{max} on a Lineweaver-Burk plot is much easier than it is on a direct plot of the Michaelis-Menten equation.

Consider an example involving hypothetical data gathered on an enzyme-catalyzed reaction (Table 9-1 ★). A direct plot of the data gives the expected Michaelis-Menten curve (Figure 9-10A ■) and a plot of the reciprocals gives a straight line (Figure 9-10B).

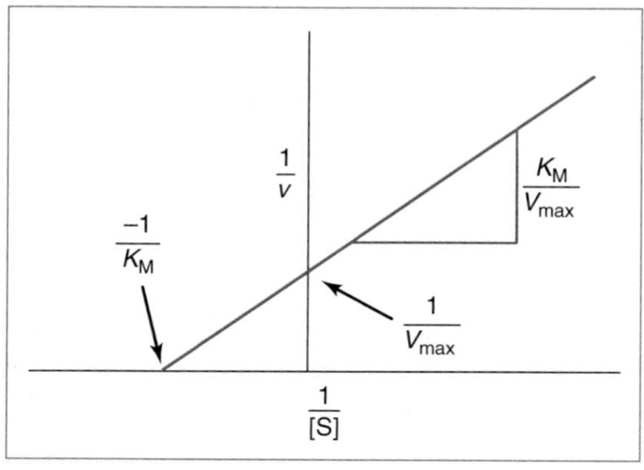

■ **FIGURE 9-9** A typical Lineweaver-Burk plot.

★ TABLE 9-1 Hypothetical Data for Enzyme Kinetics

Raw Data		Reciprocals	
[S] (nmol/mL)	v (pmol/second)	1/[S] (mL/nmol)	1/v (seconds/pmol)
2	3.1	0.500	0.323
5	7.2	0.200	0.139
10	12.9	0.100	0.078
20	22.0	0.050	0.045
40	33.0	0.025	0.030
70	40.2	0.014	0.025
100	42.1	0.010	0.024

For the data in Table 9-1, the V_{max} is the reciprocal of the *y*-intercept on the Lineweaver-Burk plot (Figure 9-10B). Because the line crosses the *y*-axis at 0.02 seconds/pmol, the value of V_{max} is 50 pmol/second:

$$\frac{1}{V_{max}} = y\text{-intercept}$$

$$\frac{1}{V_{max}} = \frac{0.02 \text{ seconds}}{\text{pmol}}$$

$$V_{max} = \frac{50 \text{ pmol}}{\text{second}}$$

The K_M is the negative reciprocal of the *x*-intercept. Because the line crosses the *x*-axis at −0.03 mL/nmol, the value of K_M is 33 nmol/mL:

$$\frac{-1}{K_M} = x\text{-intercept}$$

$$\frac{-1}{K_M} = \frac{-0.03 \text{ ml}}{\text{nmol}}$$

$$K_M = \frac{33 \text{ nmol}}{\text{mL}}$$

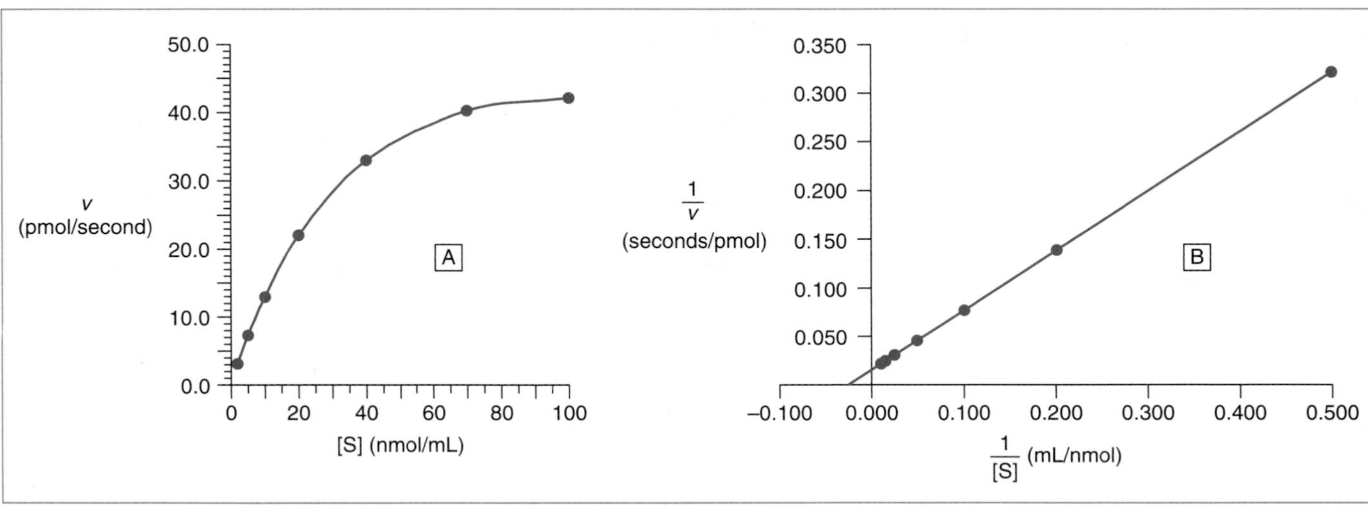

FIGURE 9-10 Plots of hypothetical data in Table 9-1. (**A**) Direct plot of the raw data. (**B**) Lineweaver-Burk plot of the reciprocals of the data.

In this example, we used only our eyes to estimate the values of V_{max} and K_M. Chapter 8 details rigorous mathematical procedures for fitting a line to data points and for finding the best equation to describe that line.

Our example in Figure 9-10B illustrates a major drawback of the Lineweaver-Burk transformation. Because it plots reciprocals of the raw data, the spacing is not uniform across the range of concentrations used. The data points are compressed at low values of 1/[S], which correspond to high values of [S]. Consequently, drawing an accurate line through them poses a challenge to the naked eye, a challenge that carries less risk only when proven statistical methods are brought to bear on the data.

There is, however, another major drawback of the Lineweaver-Burk transformation. Experimental uncertainty in the data is not uniform, being larger at low values of [S], which correspond to high values of 1/[S]. We might ask how significant such uncertainty can be in evaluating V_{max} and K_M on a double-reciprocal plot.

To answer this question, let us consider a reaction whose true rate at $[S]_1$ is 2.00 mM/min. If the uncertainty in the measurement is ± 0.10 mM/min, then the observed rate might be as high as 2.10 mM/min. Thus, the observed value of $1/v$ would be 0.48 min/mM, as opposed to the true $1/v$ of 0.50 min/mM. The difference is $0.50 - 0.48$, or 0.02 min/mM. At a higher substrate concentration, $[S]_2$, where the true rate is 10.0 mM/min, the same uncertainty in the measurement would generate a difference of 0.001 min/mM between the observed and true values of $1/v$.

On a double-reciprocal plot, therefore, these two data points would have uncertainties that differ by a factor of 20! Even using proper statistical procedures, one cannot with high confidence draw a line through data points whose uncertainties differ so much from each other.

Despite obsolescence and disadvantages, there are at least three reasons that the clinical laboratory scientist should be comfortable constructing and reading Lineweaver-Burk plots: (1) they are still commonly used, (2) they abound in the older literature, and, as mentioned above, (3) they display data in a uniquely effective way. The last of these reasons is especially valuable in the context of enzyme inhibition. Appendix 9-4 on the website discusses linear transformations in greater depth.

Appendix 9-4
"Linear Transformations of the Michaelis-Menten Equation"
PEARSON myhealthprofessionskit

*p*H BUFFERING

As Chapter 5 explains, *p*H affects many chemical reactions in the laboratory and nearly all physiological processes in the human body. Therefore, maintaining proper *p*H, whether in a test tube or in a living cell, is vital. In a test tube, for example, the *p*H of a solution can decrease as CO_2 from the air dissolves into it and generates carbonic acid. But the *p*H can be higher than expected if a trace of detergent remains on the glassware in which a solution is prepared. In a living cell, the *p*H would drop fast as the acidic products of ordinary metabolism accumulate.

However, when the *p*H of a solution is **buffered**, it does not change significantly when acid (H^+) or base (OH^-) enters the system in a small amount. What carries out the buffering are certain chemical substances present in the solution that remove excess H^+ or OH^- as either of these appears, thereby keeping the *p*H about the same.

The Acid Dissociation Constant

An acid (HA) is a substance that dissociates in water to give a hydrogen ion (H^+) and a base (A^-). In fact, A^- is considered the **conjugate base** of HA, and HA the **conjugate acid** of A^-. The two together are a *conjugate acid-base pair*:

$$HA \rightleftharpoons H^+ + A^-$$

Strong acids dissociate completely, whereas weak acids dissociate only partially, establishing an equilibrium among HA, H^+, and A^-. That equilibrium is quantified by the constant K_a:

$$K_a = \frac{[H^+][A^-]}{[HA]}$$

where each pair of brackets represents molarity.

The constant "$\boldsymbol{K_a}$" goes by several names, the most common being **acid dissociation constant**. It puts a number on the strength of an acid. As that strength increases, the acid dissociates more;

consequently, $[H^+]$ and $[A^-]$ go up, [HA] goes down, and the value of K_a rises. Conversely, as the strength of an acid decreases, less dissociation occurs; consequently, $[H^+]$ and $[A^-]$ go down, [HA] goes up, and the value of K_a falls. Thus, K_a parallels acid strength. If, for example, the K_a of acid **X** is 1.0×10^{-5} and the K_a of acid **Y** is 4.0×10^{-6}, then acid **X** is the stronger.

Recall that *p*H simplifies expression of the concentration of H^+ in a solution:

$$pH = -\log [H^+]$$

Similarly, $\boldsymbol{pK_a}$ simplifies expression of the dissociation constant of an acid:

$$pK_a = -\log K_a$$

Just as *p*H and $[H^+]$ move in opposite directions, so do pK_a and K_a. A stronger acid has a high K_a and a low pK_a, whereas a weaker acid has a low K_a and a high pK_a. Therefore, using the example above, we see that the pK_a of acid **X** is 5.0 and the pK_a of acid **Y** is 5.4. Having the lower pK_a, acid **X** is the stronger.

How a Buffering System Works

When *p*H is buffered, as mentioned earlier, a chemical substance present in the solution removes excess H^+ or OH^- as either of these arises, thereby keeping the *p*H about the same. The buffering chemical substance is itself a weak acid (HA) in equilibrium with its conjugate base (A^-). If H^+ enters the system, then the conjugate base, A^-, reacts with it to generate HA:

$$H^+ + A^- \rightarrow HA$$

Consequently, H^+ does not accumulate as fast as it would otherwise, and the *p*H stays close to its original value. If OH^- enters the system, however, then HA reacts with it to generate water and A^-:

$$HA + OH^- \rightarrow H_2O + A^-$$

As long as there is sufficient A^- present to take up new H^+, along with sufficient HA to eliminate new OH^-, the *p*H is buffered. We can prepare *p*H-buffered solutions (commonly called "buffers") by dissolving HA and a salt of A^- in known amounts. To do so, we employ a special equation that relates [HA], $[A^-]$, *p*H, and pK_a.

The Henderson-Hasselbalch Equation

To prepare a buffer at a selected *p*H, use the **Henderson-Hasselbalch equation:**

$$pH = pK_a + \log\frac{[A^-]}{[HA]}$$

This equation tells us the ratio of the base concentration $[A^-]$ to that of the conjugate acid [HA] in a solution at any *p*H, when the pK_a of HA is known. A conjugate acid-base pair buffers most effectively at a *p*H that is within about 1 unit of the acid's pK_a. In other words, an acid-base pair is most suitable as a buffer when

$$pH = pK_a \pm 1$$

It is in this range that the concentrations of HA and A^- are about equal and buffering capacity is at its highest.

Suppose we want to prepare 1.0 L of a buffer at *p*H 5.0, with a total concentration of 0.10 M for the conjugate acid-base pair. We select an acid with a pK_a between 4.0 and 6.0. Acetic acid qualifies with a pK_a of 4.76. Of course, there are other considerations in choosing the acid-base pair, such as reactivity in the system being studied, but those are beyond the scope of this book.

For the buffer solution we are preparing, let us now calculate the required concentrations of acetic acid (HA) and its conjugate base, acetate (A^-). First, we use the Henderson-Hasselbalch equation to give us the ratio of [A^-] to [HA]:

$$5.0 = 4.76 + \log\frac{[A^-]}{[HA]}$$

$$0.24 = \log\frac{[A^-]}{[HA]}$$

$$\text{antilog } 0.24 = 10^{0.24} = \frac{[A^-]}{[HA]}$$

$$1.74 = \frac{[A^-]}{[HA]}$$

This means that the solution must have 1.74 times as much A^- as it does HA. Because we know the total of A^- and HA is 0.10 M, we can calculate their individual concentrations in the solution. We start with the ratio:

$$1.74 = \frac{[A^-]}{[HA]}$$

$$1.74 \times [HA] = [A^-]$$

The total concentration is 0.10 M:

$$[HA] + [A^-] = 0.10 \text{ M}$$

Substitution gives

$$[HA] + (1.74 \times [HA]) = 0.10 \text{ M}$$

Solving for [HA] gives

$$2.74 \times [HA] = 0.10 \text{ M}$$

$$[HA] = 0.0365 \text{ M}$$

Therefore, [A^-] is

$$0.10 \text{ M} - 0.0365 \text{ M} = [A^-]$$

$$0.0635 \text{ M} = [A^-]$$

What this all means is that, if we prepare a solution of acetic acid at 0.0365 M with a salt of its conjugate base, such as sodium acetate, at 0.0635 M, then the *p*H will be 5.0. Furthermore, the *p*H will be buffered. The actual *p*H, of course, may deviate slightly from 5.0, depending on factors such as (1) the purity of our chemicals and (2) the accuracy of our measuring the volumes, weights, and *p*H; but we can adjust the *p*H by adding a strong acid or base in a negligibly tiny volume.

Now that we know the final concentrations of the acid-base pair, we can calculate the amounts of acetic acid and sodium acetate to measure out. We then dissolve the substances in water and dilute the solution to a final volume of 1.0 L. The mathematical techniques laid out in Chapter 4 are useful for this purpose. To see the rest of this calculation in detail, consult Appendix 9-5 on the website.

Appendix 9-5
"Sample Calculation of an Acetic Acid/Acetate Buffer"
www.myhealthprofessions.kit.com
PEARSON myhealthprofessionskit

Physiological Acid-Base Calculations

The kidneys and lungs act to keep the *p*H of the blood between 7.35 and 7.45. However, when the *p*H of the blood falls below 7.35, there is too much acid; this state is called **acidosis**, which may be seen in uncontrolled diabetes mellitus, lung disease, and kidney disease. When the *p*H of the blood rises above 7.45, there is too little acid (too much base); this state is called **alkalosis**, which can result from vomiting, hyperventilating, or moving to a higher altitude.

The primary *p*H-buffering system in the blood involves the conjugate acid-base pair of carbonic acid (H_2CO_3) and bicarbonate (HCO_3^-):

$$CO_2 + H_2O \rightleftharpoons H_2CO_3 \rightleftharpoons H^+ + HCO_3^-$$

The concentration of H_2CO_3 in the blood is negligibly small, about 1000 times less than that of CO_2:

$$dCO_2 = 1000 \times [H_2CO_3]$$

where dCO_2 is the concentration of dissolved carbon dioxide in the blood. Therefore, we delete $[H_2CO_3]$ from the chemical equation, which then becomes

$$CO_2 + H_2O \rightleftharpoons H^+ + HCO_3^-$$

which treats CO_2, rather than H_2CO_3, as the acid. This equilibrium is catalyzed by the enzyme carbonic anhydrase, in the absence of which the reaction would proceed too slowly to sustain life.

As a metabolic waste product, CO_2 assumes three forms in the blood:

1. a dissolved gas,
2. bicarbonate ion from the reaction $CO_2 + H_2O \rightleftharpoons H_2CO_3 \rightleftharpoons H^+ + HCO_3^-$, and
3. carbaminohemoglobin, in which the CO_2 has attached covalently to hemoglobin in the erythrocytes.

The *p*H of blood is 7.4 and the relevant pK_a is 6.1. Applying the Henderson-Hasselbalch equation to the carbon dioxide / bicarbonate buffering system gives

$$7.4 = 6.1 + \log\frac{[HCO_3^-]}{dCO_2}$$

$$1.3 = \log\frac{[HCO_3^-]}{dCO_2}$$

$$20 = \frac{[HCO_3^-]}{dCO_2}$$

What this ratio says is that, in the blood, the HCO_3^- concentration is 20 times the CO_2 concentration. To see the reason this ratio has a value of 20, consult Appendix 9-8 on the website.

Appendix 9-8
"The Bicarbonate Buffer System of Blood"
www.myhealthprofessions .kit.com
PEARSON myhealthprofessionskit

Physiological Buffering

The pK_a of this buffering system, 6.1, violates the guideline stated earlier that a conjugate acid-base pair is suitable as a buffer only when the *p*H is within 1 unit of the pK_a. Nevertheless, the Henderson-Hasselbalch equation tells us that, as long as the ratio of bicarbonate to dissolved carbon dioxide remains about 20, the *p*H stays about 7.4. Under normal conditions, the lungs and the kidneys maintain that ratio and, therefore, the proper *p*H.

The lungs respond to a drop in *p*H (excess acid) by hyperventilating, which removes more CO_2 from the blood, thereby lowering the concentration of carbon dioxide and raising the *p*H. However, an increase in *p*H (too little acid) causes the lungs to hypoventilate, which allows CO_2 to accumulate in the blood, thereby raising the concentration of carbon dioxide and lowering the *p*H. Changes in the breathing rate can affect blood *p*H in just a few seconds.

The kidneys regulate *p*H by controlling the reabsorption of HCO_3^- from the urine into the blood. As *p*H falls, the kidneys reabsorb more HCO_3^- to react with the excess H^+ and remove it from circulation. As *p*H rises, the kidneys reabsorb less HCO_3^-, allowing more H^+ to accumulate and the *p*H to go back down. Unlike changes in the rate of respiration, these processes can take hours or days to affect blood *p*H.

CO_2 as a Dissolved Gas

When there are several gases above a solution, each one has its own pressure, called **partial pressure**. In discussing the CO_2/HCO_3^- buffering system, we use the CO_2 concentration, not only because the H_2CO_3 concentration is so low, but also because what we actually measure in the laboratory is the partial pressure of CO_2. Henry's law says that the solubility of a gas is directly proportional to its partial pressure in equilibrium with the solution:

$$S = kP_{gas}$$

where *S* is the mass of a gas that dissolves, P_{gas} is the partial pressure of that gas above the solution, and *k* is the Henry's law constant for the gas (at a fixed temperature).

We can easily rationalize this equation by realizing that, to dissolve in a liquid, gas atoms or molecules must strike the liquid's surface. Increasing the pressure of a gas in contact with a liquid increases the collision rate with the surface; more gas dissolves, and its concentration in the solution goes up. The solubility has increased with pressure.

Therefore, the concentration of CO_2 dissolved in a solution is related to the partial pressure of CO_2 above the solution by this equation:

$$dCO_2 = \alpha \times PCO_2$$

where α is the solubility coefficient (0.0301 mmol/L/mmHg). So, we substitute "dCO_2," which is "$\alpha \times PCO_2$," into the Henderson-Hasselbalch equation:

$$pH = pK_a + \log \frac{[HCO_3^-]}{\alpha \times PCO_2}$$

In the clinical laboratory, we directly measure *p*H and PCO_2. From these two values, we can calculate the bicarbonate concentration by means of the Henderson-Hasselbalch equation, although methods do exist for quantifying it directly.

ACID-BASE DISORDERS

As defined above, *acidosis* ($pH < 7.35$) is the condition in which too much acid is present, and *alkalosis* ($pH > 7.45$) is the condition in which too little acid (too much base) is present. As explained above, the lungs respond to acidosis by exhaling more CO_2 and to alkalosis by exhaling less. The kidneys respond to acidosis by reabsorbing more HCO_3^- and to alkalosis by reabsorbing less. (Note that there are actually two sets of terms for these conditions. Technically, "acidosis" and "alkalosis" do not specify a fluid or a tissue in which the condition is occurring. However, the terms "acidemia" and "alkalemia" refer, respectively, to the states of excess acid and excess base *in the blood*. Medical professionals often interchange the "-osis" and "-emia" terms, unless a patient has both acidosis and alkalosis, one of which dominates the other to cause a net rise or fall in blood *p*H.)

Each condition, acidosis and alkalosis, is categorized by its cause: *respiratory* or *metabolic*. Respiratory acid-base disorders result from abnormal breathing, whether caused by lung disease, airway obstruction, hyperventilation, or another condition. By contrast, metabolic acid-base disorders arise from changes in the bicarbonate concentration; such changes can be caused by kidney disease, diabetes, vomiting, poisoning, or some other condition. See Table 9-2 ★.

Respiratory Acidosis

Hypoventilation (from airway obstruction, certain drugs, head injury, emphysema, asthma, etc.) can lead to an increase in the CO_2 concentration in the blood ("hypercapnia"), which decreases the ratio of HCO_3^- to CO_2 below 20 and pushes the *p*H down below 7.35 ("acidemia"). The body compensates for this condition by (1) buffering the excess H^+ within cells and (2) reabsorbing more bicarbonate from the urine. Therefore, the laboratory findings in compensated respiratory acidosis are (1) a low *p*H, (2) a high PCO_2, and (3) an increased concentration of HCO_3^-.

Respiratory Alkalosis

Hyperventilation (from anxiety, certain drugs, high altitude, fever, etc.) can lead to a decrease in the CO_2 concentration in the blood ("hypocapnia"), which increases the ratio of HCO_3^- to CO_2 and raises the

★ **TABLE 9-2** The Four General Acid-Base Disorders

Disorder	pH	Primary Abnormality	Compensation
Respiratory acidosis	↓	↑CO_2	Renal reabsorption of HCO_3^-
Respiratory alkalosis	↑	↓CO_2	Renal excretion of HCO_3^-
Metabolic acidosis	↓	↓HCO_3^-	Hyperventilation
Metabolic alkalosis	↑	↑HCO_3^-	Hypoventilation

*p*H above 7.45 ("alkalemia"). The body compensates for this condition by (1) releasing H^+ ions from intracellular buffers, (2) reabsorbing less bicarbonate from the urine, and (3) excreting less H^+ in the urine. Therefore, the laboratory findings in compensated respiratory alkalosis are (1) a high *p*H, (2) a low PCO_2, and (3) a decreased concentration of HCO_3^-. There is also an increase in the Cl^- concentration to maintain electrical neutrality in the plasma.

Metabolic Acidosis

When the concentration of HCO_3^- is too low, either through direct loss or through the buffering of excess acid, the ratio of HCO_3^- to CO_2 is also too low, and the *p*H can fall below 7.35. Among the many causes are uncontrolled diabetes, diarrhea, prolonged exercise, kidney disease, and certain poisons. The body compensates for this condition by (1) extracellular buffering of excess H^+ with HCO_3^-, (2) intracellular buffering with proteins and with carbonates and phosphates in bone, (3) acceleration of respiration, and (4) greater excretion of H^+ in the urine. Therefore, the laboratory findings in compensated metabolic acidosis are (1) a low *p*H, (2) a low PCO_2, and (3) a decreased concentration of HCO_3^-.

Metabolic Alkalosis

The direct loss of H^+ ions or the accumulation of HCO_3^- ions can lead to an increase in the ratio of HCO_3^- to CO_2. This, in turn, can nudge the *p*H above 7.45. Such a loss of H^+ can occur through vomiting or through abnormally high urinary excretion. The accumulation of HCO_3^- can result from the loss of extracellular water (often because of a diuretic agent) as bicarbonate is retained; the retained HCO_3^- then reacts with H^+ to form CO_2, thereby raising the *p*H.

Metabolic alkalosis also arises when extracellular potassium levels are low. As potassium ions leave the cells in response to this condition, H^+ ions replace them in order to maintain electrical neutrality. This shift of H^+ ions from plasma into cells raises blood *p*H. Another cause of alkalosis is the immoderate use of alkalotic agents, such as antacids.

The body compensates for metabolic alkalosis by (1) releasing H^+ from intracellular buffers, (2) reabsorbing less HCO_3^- from the urine, and (3) hypoventilating. The additional CO_2 in the blood from hypoventilation generates more CO_2, which brings down *p*H. The laboratory findings in compensated metabolic alkalosis are (1) a high *p*H, (2) a high concentration of HCO_3^-, and (3) a high PCO_2.

ANION GAP

For electrical neutrality, the total concentration of all positive charges in the plasma must equal the total concentration of all negative charges. As Chapter 5 explains, we normally express the concentration of an electrolyte as "mEq/L." Therefore, when expressed as "mEq/L," the total concentration of all cations in the plasma must equal the total concentration of all anions. Some of these ions are quantified routinely in the laboratory, whereas others are not:

	Cations	Anions
Routinely quantified	Na^+, K^+	Cl^-, HCO_3^-
Not routinely quantified (a.k.a. "unquantified ions" or "unmeasured ions")	Mg^{2+}, Ca^{2+}, Zn^{2+}, γ-globulins	lactate, sulfate, phosphate, β-hydroxybutyrate, metabolites of poisons

The following equation expresses the relationship among the cations and anions in the plasma. Figure 9-11 ■ depicts this relationship.

$$[Na^+] + [K^+] + [UC] = [Cl^-] + [HCO_3^-] + [UA]$$

UC = unquantified cations (Ca^{2+}, Mg^{2+}, Zn^{2+}, γ-globulins, etc.)

UA = unquantified anions (lactate, sulfate, phosphate, β-hydroxybutyrate, albumin, metabolites of poisons, etc.)

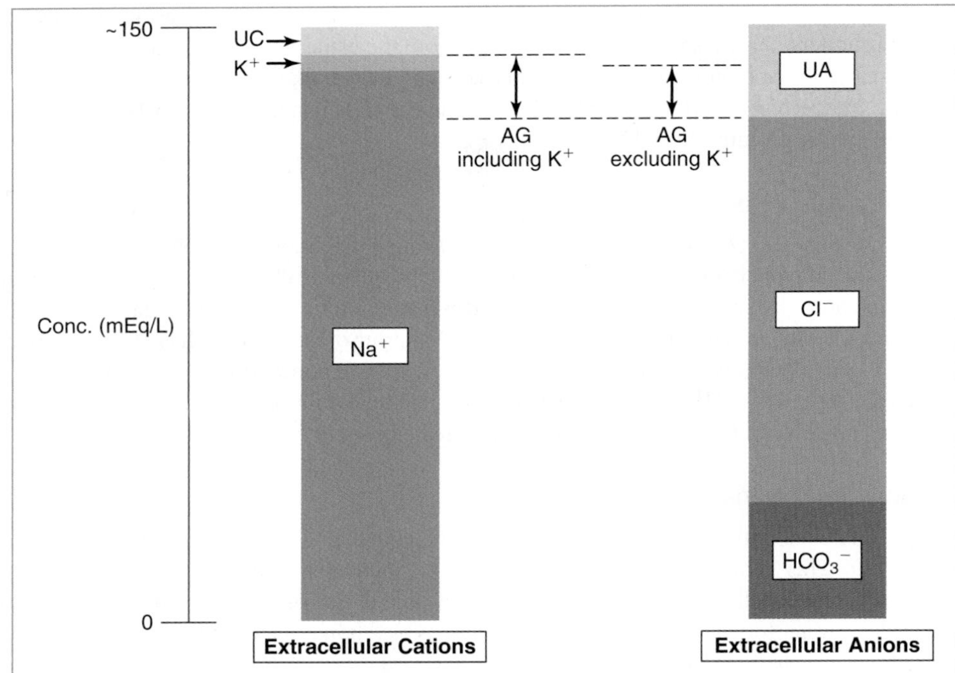

FIGURE 9-11 The anion gap (AG) is the approximate concentration of unquantified anions (UA) that are not balanced by unquantified cations (UC). The reference range for the AG is typically 8–12 mEq/L.

Rearrangement of this equation gives

$$[Na^+] + [K^+] - [Cl^-] - [HCO_3^-] = [UA] - [UC] = AG$$

where "AG" is the **anion gap** (Figure 9-11). It is the difference between the concentrations of the unquantified anions and the unquantified cations, representing the approximate concentration of unquantified anions in the plasma that are not balanced by unquantified cations. As a single number, the anion gap provides useful information about the cause of metabolic acidosis in a given patient.

The [UC] is comparatively low. Even when it does change, its impact on the AG is only minor. Therefore, we drop it from the equation:

EQUATION 4

$$AG = [Na^+] + [K^+] - [Cl^-] - [HCO_3^-] = [UA]$$

Because $[K^+]$ also is comparatively low, we often omit it from the formula.

EQUATION 5

$$AG = [Na^+] - [Cl^-] - [HCO_3^-]$$

In practical terms, therefore, the AG is the difference between the concentration of the major cation in the plasma (Na^+) and the total concentration of the major quantified anions (Cl^- and HCO_3^-). For Equation 5, the reference range is 6–10 mEq/L. Although Equation 5 is used more often than Equation 4, there are sometimes clinical reasons to include potassium in the formula. Nephrologists, for example, often prefer Equation 4 because of fluctuations in the potassium concentration during kidney disease.

During metabolic acidosis, an unquantified anion (e.g., lactate) accumulates with its accompanying H^+ ions. Those H^+ ions are immediately buffered by HCO_3^- to produce CO_2, which the lungs then exhale. The net result is a *decrease* in the concentration of HCO_3^-, along with an *increase* in the concentration of the unquantified anion. Thus, the anion gap widens (its value goes up).

OSMOLARITY AND OSMOLALITY

Consider two solutions of unequal concentrations separated by a semipermeable membrane (Figure 9-12). The membrane allows water, but not solutes, to pass through it. In a process called **osmosis**, water moves across the membrane from the solution of low solute concentration (the **hypotonic** side) to the solution of high solute concentration (the **hypertonic** side). The high

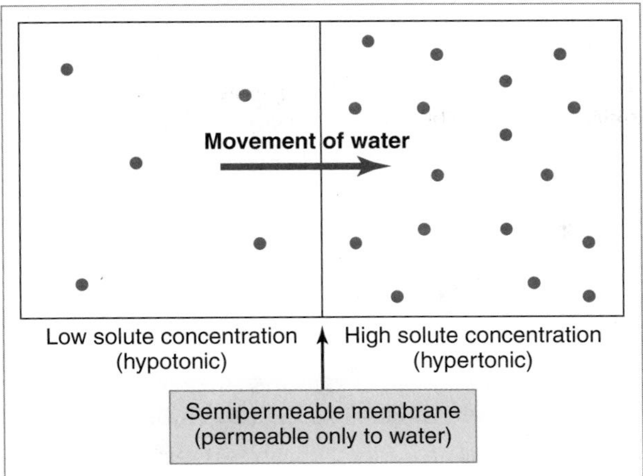

■ FIGURE 9-12 Osmosis. Water moves across a semipermeable membrane from the solution of low concentration to the solution of high concentration, thereby reducing the difference between them.

concentration is exerting an **osmotic pressure** that holds water on its side of the membrane, while drawing water from the other side. As water moves across the membrane, the concentration on the hypotonic side increases, and the concentration on the hypertonic side decreases. Thus, osmosis reduces the difference in concentration between the two solutions.

An **osmole** ("Osm") is a mole of osmotically active particles (dissolved particles that cannot cross the membrane). One mole of sodium chloride dissociates into two moles of ions ($NaCl \rightarrow Na^+ + Cl^-$). Therefore, a NaCl solution at a concentration of 1 mol/L has a concentration of 2 Osm/L. Likewise, a potassium sulfate solution at 1 mol/L has a concentration of 3 Osm/L because one mole dissociates into three moles:

$$K_2SO_4 \rightarrow 2K^+ + SO_4^{2-}$$

For substances that do not dissociate, such as sucrose and urea, molarity equals osmolarity.

The **osmolarity** of a solution is the number of osmoles of particles per liter of solution. By contrast, **osmolality** is the number of osmoles of particles per kilogram of solvent. This distinction is the same as it is for their counterparts, molarity and molality. The reason the clinical laboratory favors osmolarity less is that its value depends on the volume of water, which, in turn, depends on temperature.

The osmolality of plasma or urine is measured directly in an osmometer. Osmolarity, however, is calculated from the concentrations of the major osmotically active solutes (sodium, glucose, and urea) determined routinely by other analytical methods. If the concentrations of glucose and BUN are in "mg/dL," as they sometimes are, then the formula is

$$\text{plasma osmolarity} = 2[Na^+] + \frac{[\text{glucose}]}{18} + \frac{[\text{BUN}]}{2.8}$$

EQUATION 6

Appendix 9-6 on the website explains the rationale behind this formula.

Appendix 9-6
"The Formula for Calculating Plasma Osmolarity"
www.myhealthprofessions.kit.com
PEARSON myhealthprofessionskit

OSMOLALITY GAP/OSMOLARITY GAP

The difference between the measured osmolality (MO) and the calculated osmolality (CO) is the **osmolality gap** (OG):

$$OG = MO - CO$$

For most patients, this value is between −10 and +10. The calculated osmolality comes from a slight modification of Equation 6 that corrects for the difference between mola*R*ity and mola*L*ity:

$$\text{calculated osmolality} = 2[Na^+] + \frac{1.15 \times [\text{glucose}]}{18} + \frac{[\text{BUN}]}{2.8}$$

EQUATION 7

A high OG (> 14) suggests either of two possibilities: (1) the abnormal presence of a solute such as ethanol, methanol, or ethylene glycol, or (2) a condition, such as hyperlipidemia or kidney failure, that raises the concentrations of endogenous substances. However, because ethanol is so often the cause of an elevated OG, its concentration can be inserted directly into Equation 7:

$$\text{calculated osmolality} = 2[\text{Na}^+] + \frac{1.15 \times [\text{glucose}]}{18} + \frac{[\text{BUN}]}{2.8} + \frac{1.2 \times [\text{ethanol}]}{4.6}$$

Therefore, when the osmolality gap remains high even after correction for ethanol, one should consider the possibility that another toxic alcohol is present.

☑ CHECKPOINT 9-2

Calculate the osmolality gap for a patient whose test results are the following:

Na = 143 mEq/L Gluc = 104 mg/dL BUN = 4 mg/dL

Measured osmolality = 301 mOsm/kg

The first step is to calculate the osmolality using Equation 7:

$$\text{CO} = 2(143) + \frac{1.15 \times 104}{18} + \frac{4}{2.8}$$

$$= 294 \text{ mOsm/kg}$$

The second step is to calculate the difference between the measured and calculated osmolalities:

$$\text{OG} = \text{MO} - \text{CO}$$

$$\text{OG} = 301 \text{ mOsm/kg} - 294 \text{ mOsm/kg}$$

$$\text{OG} = 7 \text{ mOsm/kg}$$

LIPID CALCULATIONS

Triglycerides (more correctly called "triacylglycerols") are fats, which function as energy storage. Cholesterol, however, is a steroid alcohol that serves as a precursor of steroid hormones and bile acids and that helps stabilize cell membranes.

Because they are insoluble in water, triglycerides and cholesterol are transported in the blood associated with proteins; these complexes are called **lipoproteins**, and we classify them by their density. The major lipoproteins are *high-density lipoprotein* (**HDL**), *low-density lipoprotein* (**LDL**), and *very-low-density lipoprotein* (**VLDL**).

In the clinical laboratory, total cholesterol, HDL cholesterol, and triglycerides are all quantified directly, usually by automated methods. Although LDL cholesterol is sometimes quantified by those methods, they are time-intensive and expensive, and they require special equipment not often available. Consequently, many laboratories calculate the LDL value from the other concentrations by means of the **Friedewald equation:**

EQUATION 8

$$[\text{LDL}] = [\text{Cholesterol}]_{\text{total}} - [\text{HDL}] - \frac{[\text{TG}]}{5}$$

Equation 8 is based on the fact that the total concentration of cholesterol is the sum of the cholesterol concentrations in HDL, LDL, and VLDL:

$$[\text{Cholesterol}]_{\text{total}} = [\text{Cholesterol}]_{\text{HDL}} + [\text{Cholesterol}]_{\text{LDL}} + [\text{Cholesterol}]_{\text{VLDL}}$$

or, more simply,

$$[\text{Cholesterol}]_{\text{total}} = [\text{HDL}] + [\text{LDL}] + [\text{VLDL}]$$

Therefore,

$$[\text{LDL}] = [\text{Cholesterol}]_{\text{total}} - [\text{HDL}] - [\text{VLDL}]$$

EQUATION 9

Furthermore, the VLDL concentration is generally about one-fifth of the triglyceride concentration:

$$[\text{VLDL}] = \frac{[\text{TG}]}{5}$$

EQUATION 10

Substitution of Equation 10 into Equation 9 gives Equation 8 above.

Beware, however, that there are at least three conditions in which we should not apply the Friedewald equation: hypertriglyceridemia (i.e., when [TG] > 400 mg/dL), chylomicronemia, and dysbetalipoproteinemia. Underlying these limitations are two assumptions that the Friedewald equation makes and that are not strictly true: (1) that nearly all the circulating TG is in VLDLs and (2) that the ratio of [TG] to $[\text{cholesterol}]_{\text{VLDL}}$ is constant at 5. In lipid disorders such as those listed above, these assumptions lose even more of their validity, and either the concentration of LDL cholesterol must be determined directly by a laboratory method or special correction factors must be included in the calculation.

☑ CHECKPOINT 9-3

From the following laboratory results, calculate the LDL concentration by means of the Friedewald equation.

Total cholesterol = 269 mg/dL

Triglycerides = 185 mg/dL

HDL = 30 mg/dL

$[\text{VLDL}] = [\text{TG}] \div 5 = (185\text{ mg/dL}) \div 5 = 37\text{ mg/dL}$

$[\text{LDL}] = 269\text{ mg/dL} - 30\text{ mg/dL} - 37\text{ mg/dL} = 202\text{ mg/dL}$

CREATININE CLEARANCE

A **creatinine clearance** test determines the rate at which the kidneys remove creatinine from the blood. As a breakdown product of creatine phosphate in muscle cells, creatinine enters the bloodstream at a fairly constant rate, and the kidneys clear it from the blood with little reabsorption. Therefore, the concentrations of creatinine in the blood and urine can be used to estimate the **glomerular filtration rate** (GFR), which is the rate at which the kidneys are filtering blood through the glomeruli. This information is valuable in the assessment of kidney function, particularly in ascertaining whether the GFR is normal and whether it is stable over time.

Creatinine is not the only substance useful for measuring GFR. There are clearance tests for several others, some *intrinsic* and others *extrinsic* to the human body. Intrinsic clearance tests use endogenous substances, most commonly creatinine and urea; extrinsic tests, by contrast, employ exogenous substances, such as inulin, iohexol, *p*-aminohippurate, and radiolabeled isothalamate. Extrinsic tests are uncommon because the substance must be introduced into the blood by intravenous infusion and because the analytical methods are expensive and time-consuming.

Advanced Topic V "Estimation of Glomerular Filtration Rate by Means of Exogenous Tracers"

PEARSON myhealthprofessionskit

The creatinine clearance test requires a 24-hour urine specimen (all the urine the patient voids within a 24-hour period) and a blood specimen drawn at either the beginning or end of that 24-hour period. Creatinine in the urine and blood is then quantified, and the GFR is calculated. The calculation, however, includes the surface area of the patient's body because the rate of creatinine production and excretion depends on lean-muscle mass. The equation for the clearance rate is

$$C_{\text{creatinine}} = \left(\frac{U_{\text{creatinine}} \times V_{\text{urine}}}{P_{\text{creatinine}}}\right) \times \left(\frac{1.73\text{ m}^2}{A}\right)$$

EQUATION 11

where $C_{\text{creatinine}}$ is the creatinine clearance rate (mL/min), $U_{\text{creatinine}}$ is the urinary concentration of creatinine (mg/dL), V_{urine} is the volume of urine excreted per minute (mL/min), $P_{\text{creatinine}}$ is the plasma concentration of creatinine (mg/dL), and A is the surface area of the patient's body (m^2). The reference range is 82–140 mL/min for men and 75–128 mL/min for women.

We compute the value of V_{urine} from the total volume of the 24-hour urine specimen. For example, if the patient passed 1500 mL of urine in 24 hours (and collected it all), then the volume excreted per minute is

$$V_{urine} = \left(\frac{1500 \text{ mL}}{24 \text{ h}}\right) \times \left(\frac{1 \text{ h}}{60 \text{ min}}\right) = 1.04 \text{ mL/min}$$

The second term in the equation, 1.73 m^2/A, is a correction factor for the patient's body surface area that allows for comparison of the patient's clearance rate with the rates for other patients. The numerator of 1.73 m^2 is the average body surface area for an adult. We can calculate the value of A from a formula or we can glean it from a nomogram (widely available in printed and electronic resources). The formula is

EQUATION 12

$$A = 0.007184 \times W^{0.425} \times H^{0.725}$$

or the equivalent,

$$A = \frac{W^{0.425} \times H^{0.725}}{139.2}$$

where A is the body surface area, W is weight (kg), and H is height (cm). To convert "pounds" to "kilograms," multiply by 0.45; to convert "inches" to "centimeters," multiply by 2.54. To examine Equation 11 in depth, consult Appendix 9-7 on the website.

Appendix 9-7
"Making Sense of the Equation for Creatinine Clearance"
www.myhealthprofessions.kit.com

PEARSON myhealthprofessionskit

Shortcomings of the Test

Creatinine is not the ideal substance for a clearance test. Although its concentration in the blood is approximately constant, the renal tubules secrete creatinine in small amounts, thereby increasing its concentration in the urine and falsely elevating the clearance rate. Furthermore, the method for quantifying creatinine can affect the result, as can certain drugs, exercise, diurnal variation in the GFR, inadequate hydration during the 24-hour collection period, and failure to collect the urine properly.

Summary

1. Solutions of some chemical substances absorb light that is directed through them. The fraction of light that passes through the substance is the *transmittance:*

$$T = \frac{I}{I_0}$$

where I_0 is the intensity of the light entering the solution and I is the intensity of the light emerging from the solution.

2. *Absorbance* is related to transmittance by the equation

$$A = -\log \frac{I}{I_0} = -\log T$$

3. Absorbance is directly proportional to (a) the concentration of the absorbing chemical substance, (b) the length of the path the light takes passing through the solution, and (c) the *molar absorptivity*, which represents the inherent ability of the chemical substance to absorb light of a given wavelength.

4. The *Beer-Lambert law* relates absorbance to the above three factors:

$$A = \epsilon \, c \, l$$

where ϵ is the molar absorptivity, c is the concentration, and l is the path length.

5. *Enzymes* are biomolecules that catalyze reactions in living systems.

6. *Enzyme kinetics* is the quantitative study of enzyme catalysis.

7. In an *end-point assay*, absorbance is measured at a fixed time point, and the rate is calculated from a standard curve, a single standard, or molar absorptivity. In a *two-point assay*, absorbance is measured at each of two time points, and the rate between them is calculated. In a *kinetic assay*, absorbance is measured at each of several time points, and the rate is calculated from all of them. The kinetic assay is the most reliable.

8. An enzyme-catalyzed reaction typically has three phases: (a) *lag phase*, in which the rate is not yet linear, (b) *linear phase*, in which concentration is directly proportional to time, and (c) *substrate-depletion phase*, in which the rate goes to zero.
9. The Michaelis-Menten model of enzyme catalysis is described by the equation

$$v = \frac{V_{max}[S]}{K_M + [S]}$$

where v is the observed reaction rate, [S] is the starting substrate concentration, V_{max} is the *maximal velocity* (the highest reaction rate possible under the circumstances), and K_M is the substrate concentration at half of V_{max}. K_M can be considered a measure of the affinity of an enzyme for its substrate.
10. We can use linear transformations of the Michaelis-Menten equation to simplify evaluation of K_M and V_{max}. They have major weaknesses and are no longer necessary because curve-fitting computer programs can now evaluate the constants directly from the original data. Nevertheless, linear transformations are still uniquely effective for displaying data.
11. When *buffered*, the pH of a solution does not change significantly when acid or base enters the system in small amounts.
12. A *conjugate acid* and a *conjugate base* are converted into each other by losing or accepting a hydrogen ion.
13. The *acid dissociation constant*, represented as K_a, is a measure of the strength of an acid, rising and falling in parallel with it. The negative logarithm of K_a, represented as pK_a, decreases with increasing strength of an acid and increases with decreasing strength:

$$pK_a = -\log K_a$$

14. The *Henderson-Hasselbalch equation* relates pH, pK_a, and the concentrations of conjugate acid and conjugate base. It is particularly useful for preparing solutions at selected pH values:

$$pH = pK_a + \log\frac{[A^-]}{[HA]}$$

where [HA] is the concentration of the acid and $[A^-]$ is the concentration of its conjugate base.
15. *Acidosis* and *alkalosis* are the conditions in which, respectively, there is too much acid and too little acid in body fluids. Acidemia is the condition in which the pH of the blood is below 7.35, and alkalemia is that when it is above 7.45.
16. The primary pH-buffering system in the blood is the conjugate acid-base pair of carbon dioxide and bicarbonate:

$$CO_2 + H_2O \rightleftharpoons H_2CO_3 \rightleftharpoons H^+ + HCO_3^-$$

17. The pK_a of the carbon dioxide / bicarbonate pair is 6.1. The lungs and the kidneys normally function to keep the ratio of $[HCO_3^-]$ to $[CO_2]$ at 20 such that the pH of the blood remains at 7.4.
18. In the laboratory, we directly measure the PCO_2 rather than the concentration of H_2CO_3.
19. Henry's law states that the solubility of a gas is directly proportional to its *partial pressure* in equilibrium with the solution:

$$S = kP_{gas}$$

where S is the mass of a gas that dissolves, P_{gas} is the partial pressure of that gas above the solution, and k is the Henry's law constant for the gas (at a fixed temperature).
20. We can calculate the concentration of bicarbonate in a specimen from the measured pH and PCO_2 by means of the Henderson-Hasselbalch equation:

$$pH = pK_a + \log\frac{[HCO_3^-]}{\alpha \times PCO_2}$$

where α is the solubility coefficient (0.0301 mmol/L/mmHg).
21. We can differentiate the four compensated acid-base disorders of respiratory and metabolic acidosis and alkalosis from each other by pH, PCO_2, and bicarbonate concentration.
22. The *anion gap*, which provides useful information about the cause of a metabolic acidosis, is the difference between the concentration of the major cation in the plasma (Na^+) and the total concentration of the major quantified anions (Cl^- and HCO_3^-):

$$\text{anion gap} = [Na^+] - [Cl^-] - [HCO_3^-]$$

Sometimes potassium is included in the equation:

$$\text{anion gap} = [Na^+] + [K^+] - [Cl^-] - [HCO_3^-]$$

23. *Osmosis* is the phenomenon in which water moves across a semipermeable membrane from a solution of low solute concentration (the *hypotonic* side) to a solution of high solute concentration (the *hypertonic* side).
24. *Osmotic pressure* is the force with which the hypertonic solution holds water in itself and draws water from the hypotonic solution.
25. An *osmole* ("Osm") is a mole of osmotically active particles.
26. *Osmolarity* is the number of osmoles of particles per liter of solution. *Osmolality* is the number of osmoles of particles per kilogram of solvent.
27. We measure osmolality directly. We calculate osmolarity from the concentrations of sodium, glucose, and BUN:

$$\text{plasma osmolarity} = 2[Na^+] + \frac{[\text{glucose}]}{18} + \frac{[\text{BUN}]}{2.8}$$

where [glucose] and [BUN] are in "mg/dL."
28. The *osmolality gap* is the difference between the measured osmolality (MO) and the calculated osmolality (CO):

$$OG = MO - CO$$

For most patients, this value is between −10 and +10. A high value suggests the abnormal presence of a solute or a condition that raises the concentrations of endogenous substances.

29. We calculate osmolality from this equation:

$$\text{calculated osmolality} = 2[\text{Na}^+] + \frac{1.15 \times [\text{glucose}]}{18} + \frac{[\text{BUN}]}{2.8}$$

30. We can correct the calculated osmolality for the presence of ethanol by this equation:

$$\text{calculated osmolality} = 2[\text{Na}^+] + \frac{1.15 \times [\text{glucose}]}{18} + \frac{[\text{BUN}]}{2.8} + \frac{1.2 \times [\text{ethanol}]}{4.6}$$

31. We can calculate the concentration of *LDL* cholesterol by means of the *Friedewald equation:*

$$[\text{LDL}] = [\text{Cholesterol}]_{\text{total}} - [\text{HDL}] - \frac{[\text{TG}]}{5}$$

where [HDL] is the concentration of *HDL* cholesterol and [TG] is the triglyceride concentration.

32. The Friedewald equation should not be used when [TG] $>$ 400 mg/dL or when chylomicronemia or dysbetalipoproteinemia is present.

33. *Creatinine clearance* is used to estimate the *glomerular filtration rate* (GFR), which is the rate at which the kidneys are filtering blood through the glomeruli. This information is valuable in the assessment of kidney function. The rate of creatinine clearance is

$$C_{\text{creatinine}} = \left(\frac{U_{\text{creatinine}} \times V_{\text{urine}}}{P_{\text{creatinine}}}\right) \times \left(\frac{1.73\ \text{m}^2}{A}\right)$$

where $C_{\text{creatinine}}$ is the creatinine clearance rate (mL/min), $U_{\text{creatinine}}$ is the urinary concentration of creatinine (mg/dL), V_{urine} is the volume of urine excreted per minute (mL/min), $P_{\text{creatinine}}$ is the plasma concentration of creatinine (mg/dL), and A is the surface area of the patient's body (m^2).

34. We calculate body surface area from the equation

$$A = 0.007184 \times W^{0.425} \times H^{0.725}$$

where A is the body surface area, W is weight (kg), and H is height (cm).

Practice and Contextual Problems

1. (LO 3) Supply the missing value for each of the following solutions. Assume linearity.

Solution	A	ε (L · mol^{-1} · cm^{-1})	c (mol/L)	l (cm)
a	0.446	7020		1
b	0.917	13,400		1
c	0.205		0.00031	1
d	0.822	51,500	3.19×10^{-5}	
e	0.506	29,700		0.5
f		800	0.00050	1
g	1.123		6.7×10^{-4}	1
h	0.174	662		1

2. (LO 2, 3) At 624 nm, substance **Q** has a molar absorptivity of 13,280 M^{-1} cm^{-1}, and the absorbance is linear with concentration only from 1.0×10^{-5} up to 6.8×10^{-5} M. Consider three solutions of **Q**, each at a unique concentration. Under the same conditions of solvent, temperature, and so forth, the three solutions have these absorbance values at 624 nm (assume l = 1.0 cm):

   #1: 0.239 #2: 0.478 #3: 0.956

   (a) What is the concentration of #2 relative to that of #1?

   (b) Is the concentration of #3 four times that of #1? Explain.

3. (LO 3, 4) You have a solution at a concentration of 4.6×10^{-5} M. At a wavelength of 305 nm, its absorbance is 0.339. There is another solution of the same chemical substance under the same conditions, but its concentration is unknown. If the second solution's absorbance is 0.502 at 305 nm, then what is its concentration? The path length is 1.0 cm, and the absorbance is known to be linear from 0 to 1.00.

4. (LO 3, 4) You have a solution at a concentration of 2.8×10^{-6} M. At a wavelength of 260 nm, its absorbance is 0.872. There is another solution of the same chemical substance under the same conditions, but its concentration is unknown. If the second solution's absorbance is 0.077 at 260 nm, what is its concentration? The path length is 1.0 cm and the absorbance is known to be linear from 0 to 1.00.

5. (LO 1, 2, 3) Evaluate each of the following statements as true or false.

   (a) If the transmittance of a substance at 10 mM is 0.40, then its transmittance at 5 mM must be 0.20.

   (b) If the transmittance of a substance at 10 mM is 0.40, then its transmittance at 5 mM must be 0.80.

   (c) If the transmittance is 0.52, then the absorbance is 0.284.

   (d) If the molar absorptivity is 855 M^{-1} cm^{-1}, the path length is 1.0 cm, and the concentration is 0.00036 M, then the absorbance is 0.308. Assume linearity.

   (e) If the molar absorptivity is 29,000 M^{-1} cm^{-1}, the path length is 1.0 cm, and the absorbance is 0.188, then the concentration is 6.48×10^{-6} M. Assume linearity.

(f) If the path length is 0.5 cm, the absorbance is 0.388, and the concentration is 9.2×10^{-5} M, then the molar absorptivity is 8435 M^{-1} cm^{-1}, Assume linearity.

(g) If the transmittance is 0.39, then the absorbance is 0.409.

(h) All else being constant, absorbance decreases as transmittance increases.

(i) All else being constant, absorbance decreases as path length increases.

6. (LO 2, 3) You have the following data for a chemical substance in solution. (Assume the path length to be 1 cm.)

Concentration (μmol/L)	A_{380}
10	0.041
50	0.205
100	0.410
200	0.821
300	1.230
400	1.394

(a) Construct a standard curve from the data above.

(b) Calculate the molar absorptivity.

(c) If a solution of this substance has an absorbance of 1.080, what is the concentration?

(d) If a solution of this substance has an absorbance of 1.500, should Beer's law be used to calculate its concentration? Explain.

(e) If a solution of this substance has an absorbance of 1.647, describe a laboratory procedure for determining its concentration from the standard curve.

(f) Suppose you have a solution of absorbance 1.8. You mix 1.0 mL of the solution with 2.0 mL of appropriate solvent, and then you measure the absorbance of the resulting solution. If that absorbance is 0.757, what is the concentration of the original solution?

7. (LO 9) The following set of data was collected in an enzyme kinetics experiment. Plot *v* as a function of [S] and 1/*v* as a function of 1/[S]. From the Lineweaver-Burk plot, estimate V_{max} and K_M.

[S] (μmol/L)	v (nmol/L/s)
0	0
10	30
20	53
40	85
80	123
120	144
160	159

8. (LO 9) The following set of data was collected in an enzyme kinetics experiment. Plot *v* as a function of [S] and 1/*v* as a function of 1/[S]. From the Lineweaver-Burk plot, estimate V_{max} and K_M.

[S] (μmol/L)	v (nmol/L/s)
0	0
2	0.061
4	0.110
8	0.186
12	0.240
16	0.281
20	0.314

9. (LO 6) You work for a manufacturer of clinical assays that bases their reagents on enzymes.

(a) Your company is developing an assay for uric acid in serum. In this assay, an enzyme converts uric acid to a product that absorbs light, which the instrument measures.

In the procedure, serum is pipetted into the reaction mixture, in which the uric acid concentration ranges from 1 μmol/L up to 5 μmol/L, depending on the patient's condition. Your task is to select an enzyme appropriate for the assay; there are two that catalyze the desired reaction. On the basis of their K_M values (all else being equal), identify the enzyme more suitable for incorporation into the assay. Explain.

Enzyme	K_M (μmol/L)
1	0.2
2	50

(b) Your company is developing an assay for an enzyme in serum. The K_M of the enzyme for its substrate is 9 mM. Therefore, how high or low should the concentration of substrate be in the reaction mixture?

10. (LO 3, 6) The amount of enzyme present in a specimen is often expressed as "international units per liter" (IU/L). An IU is defined as the amount of enzyme in a specimen that catalyzes the reaction of 1 μmol of substrate per minute under specific conditions, such as pH and temperature.

The enzyme alkaline phosphatase in serum is assayed in 1.0 mL of a reaction mixture containing 25 μL of serum. The colorless substrate, *p*-nitrophenylphosphate, undergoes reaction to *p*-nitrophenol, which is bright yellow because it absorbs light at 405 nm with a molar absorptivity of 18,450 $L \cdot mol^{-1} \cdot cm^{-1}$. Incubation of the reaction mixture is carried out at 37°C. In the following run, the absorbance of the reaction mixture at 405 nm (A_{405}) was read every 20 seconds (s) (path length = 1 cm). From the data gathered, calculate the amount of enzyme (in "IU/L") present in the serum.

Incubation time (seconds)	A_{405}
20	0.033
40	0.114
60	0.195
80	0.276
100	0.357
120	0.438

11. (LO 6, 8, 9) The following data were collected for an enzyme kinetics experiment. At each of five starting substrate concentrations ($[S]_x$), the concentration of product was determined at six time points.

	Concentration of Product (μmol/L)				
Time (s)	$[S]_1$ (1 mM)	$[S]_2$ (2 mM)	$[S]_3$ (4 mM)	$[S]_4$ (10 mM)	$[S]_5$ (40 mM)
0	0	0	0	0	0
10	5	10	18	38	80
20	10	20	36	76	160
40	20	39	72	152	320
80	40	78	144	304	640
120	60	118	216	456	960

(a) On a single graph, plot the data for the five starting substrate concentrations.

(b) Plot the initial rate as a function of starting substrate concentration.

(c) Plot a Lineweaver-Burk transformation of the curve in part *b*.

(d) Evaluate K_M and V_{max} from both the curve and the line. Comment on the accuracy of the values.

12. (LO 11) Calculate the pK_a for each of the following five weak acids and rank the acids in order of descending strength.

Acid	K_a
acetic	1.74×10^{-5} M
lactic	8.32×10^{-4} M
formic	1.78×10^{-4} M
salicylic	1.05×10^{-3} M
valproic	2.51×10^{-5} M

13. (LO 12) Calculate the mass of KH_2PO_4 and of K_2HPO_4 required to prepare 1.0 L of a 0.10 M phosphate buffer at *p*H 7.0. The relevant acid dissociation is

$$H_2PO_4^- \rightleftharpoons H^+ + HPO_4^{2-}$$

and the $pK_a = 7.2$. The formula weights are 136.09 g/mol for KH_2PO_4 and 174.18 g/mol for K_2HPO_4.

14. (LO 12) Calculate the mass of KH_2PO_4 and of K_2HPO_4 required to prepare 500 mL of a 50 mM phosphate buffer at *p*H 7.4. The relevant acid dissociation is

$$H_2PO_4^- \rightleftharpoons H^+ + HPO_4^{2-}$$

and the $pK_a = 7.2$. The formula weights are 136.09 g/mol for KH_2PO_4 and 174.18 g/mol for K_2HPO_4.

15. (LO 12) Calculate the mass of KH_2PO_4 and of K_2HPO_4 required to prepare 100 mL of a 150 mM phosphate buffer at *p*H 7.2. The relevant acid dissociation is

$$H_2PO_4^- \rightleftharpoons H^+ + HPO_4^{2-}$$

and the $pK_a = 7.2$. The formula weights are 136.09 g/mol for KH_2PO_4 and 174.18 g/mol for K_2HPO_4.

16. (LO 12) Calculate the volume of acetic acid (CH_3CO_2H) and the mass of sodium acetate (CH_3CO_2Na) required to prepare 1.0 L of a 200 mM acetate buffer at *p*H 4.5. The relevant acid dissociation is

$$CH_3CO_2H \rightleftharpoons H^+ + CH_3CO_2^-$$

Pure acetic acid (called "glacial") is a liquid at room temperature, with a density of 1.049 g/mL and a formula weight of 60.05 g/mol. Sodium acetate is a solid, with a formula weight of 82.03 g/mol.

17. (LO 14) For the test results shown on the following four blood specimens, calculate the corresponding bicarbonate concentrations.

Specimen	PCO_2 (mmHg)	pH	$[HCO_3^-]$ (mmol/L)
1	40	7.40	
2	42	7.37	
3	36	7.44	
4	33	7.42	

18. (LO 13) Calculate the *p*H of a blood specimen with $PCO_2 = 37$ mmHg and $[HCO_3^-] = 21$ mmol/L.

19. (LO 13) Calculate the *p*H of the following buffer solution. The pK_a of HCO_2H is 3.75.

$$\underset{0.060\text{ M}}{HCO_2H} \rightleftharpoons H^+ + \underset{0.040\text{ M}}{HCO_2^-}$$

20. (LO 15) For each of the following patients, tell (a) whether the condition is acidosis or alkalosis, (b) whether the origin is respiratory or metabolic, and (c) whether compensation is present.

Patient	pH	PCO_2 (mmHg) Normal: 35–45	$[HCO_3^-]$ (mmol/L) Normal: 22–28
1	7.51	49	38
2	7.25	59	25
3	7.30	21	10

21. (LO 16) For each of the following patients, calculate the anion gap with and without potassium.

Patient	$[Na^+]$ (mEq/L)	$[K^+]$ (mEq/L)	$[Cl^-]$ (mEq/L)	$[HCO_3^-]$ (mEq/L)
1	140	4.6	103	25
2	136	5.1	108	22
3	148	5.0	101	19

22. (LO 17) Calculate the osmolarity of each of the following solutions.

(a) 0.1 M NaCl

(b) 10 mM $CaCl_2$

(c) 50 mM KI

(d) 0.25 M glucose

23. (LO 18, 19) Use the data in the following table to solve the problems below.

Specimen	$[Na^+]$ (mmol/L)	[glucose] (mg/dL)	[BUN] (mg/dL)	Measured Osmolality
1	142	80	16	304
2	136	135	14	299
3	148	220	19	310

(a) Calculate the plasma osmolarity and osmolality for each specimen.

(b) Calculate the osmolality gap for each specimen.

24. (LO 20) Using the Friedewald equation, calculate the concentration of LDL cholesterol for each of the following specimens.

Specimen	[HDL] (mg/dL)	[TG] (mg/dL)	[Cholesterol] (mg/dL)
1	60	188	210
2	38	260	180
3	49	190	300

25. (LO 21) Calculate the creatinine clearance rate for the following four patients.

Patient	*H* (in)	*W* (lb)	24-Hour Urine Volume (mL)	Plasma Creatinine Conc. (mg/dL)	Urine Creatinine Conc. (mg/dL)
1	59	155	1600	1.2	140
2	74	210	1830	1.9	128
3	70	183	1360	1.5	162
4	66	131	1780	2.3	155

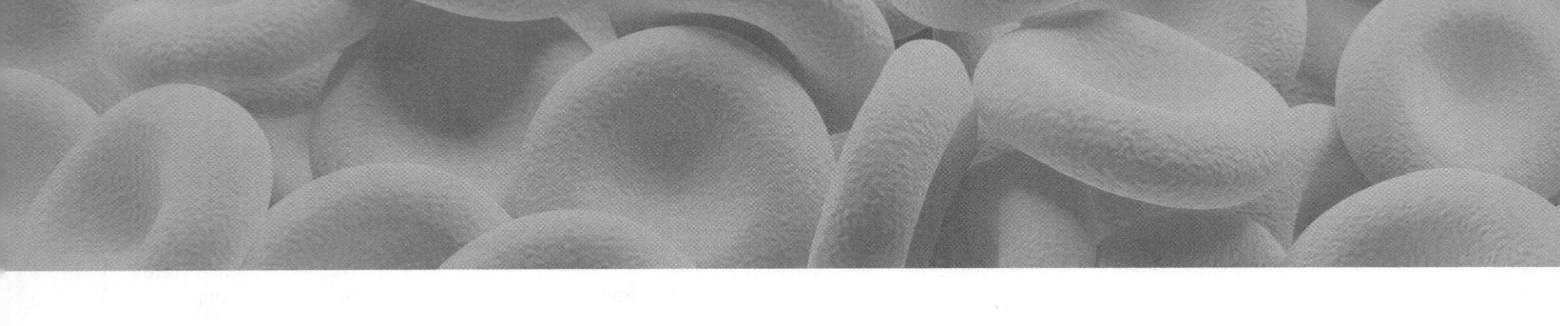

10 Hematology

Learning Objectives

At the end of this chapter, the student should be able to do the following:

1. Calculate cell counts from hemacytometer data
2. Calculate RBC indices from appropriate hematology data
3. Verify the hemoglobin concentration, hematocrit, and RBC count by the Rule of Three
4. Calculate the reticulocyte index
5. Calculate the reticulocyte production index
6. Calculate the reticulocyte percentage from data obtained by the slide method or by the Miller disk
7. Plot osmotic fragility data and interpret the curves
8. Calculate the International Normalized Ratio from appropriate data
9. Explain the advantages in using a thromboplastin reagent with an International Sensitivity Index close to 1.0
10. Correct the WBC count for the presence of nucleated RBCs

Key Terms

hemacytometer
hematocrit
International Normalized Ratio (INR)
International Sensitivity Index (ISI)
mean cell hemoglobin (MCH)
mean cell hemoglobin concentration (MCHC)
mean cell volume (MCV)
osmotic fragility
prothrombin time (PT)
red-cell distribution width (RDW)
reticulocyte index (RI)
reticulocyte production index (RPI)

Chapter Outline

MANUAL CELL ENUMERATION

Although counting blood cells is now largely automated, we still perform manual enumeration occasionally. In short, this procedure consists of diluting the blood with a special diluent, transferring a small volume of the diluted blood onto a ruled glass platform (a hemacytometer), and counting the cells under a microscope. We report the final result as the number of cells per mm^3.

Figure 10-1 ■ shows a **hemacytometer**. It comprises two identical ruled glass platforms separated by an H-shaped moat. On each platform is a 3 mm × 3 mm ruled square, subdivided into nine large squares, each being 1 mm × 1 mm. The four corner squares (labeled "W") are each subdivided into 16 squares; these are used for counting white blood cells (WBCs).

We use the large square in the center, containing five "R"s, for counting red blood cells (RBCs) and platelets. This square is itself subdivided into 25 squares, each of which has an area of 0.04 mm^2. There is further subdivision of the 25 squares into 16 squares each, creating 400 tiny squares in total. We use the five squares bearing "R"s for counting red blood cells, whereas we use the entire center square for counting platelets.

Flanking the ruled glass platforms are two raised ridges on which the cover glass rests. There is a distance of exactly 0.1 mm between the cover glass and the surface of the ruled counting area. Because the counting area measures 3 mm × 3 mm × 0.1 mm, its volume is 0.9 mm^3.

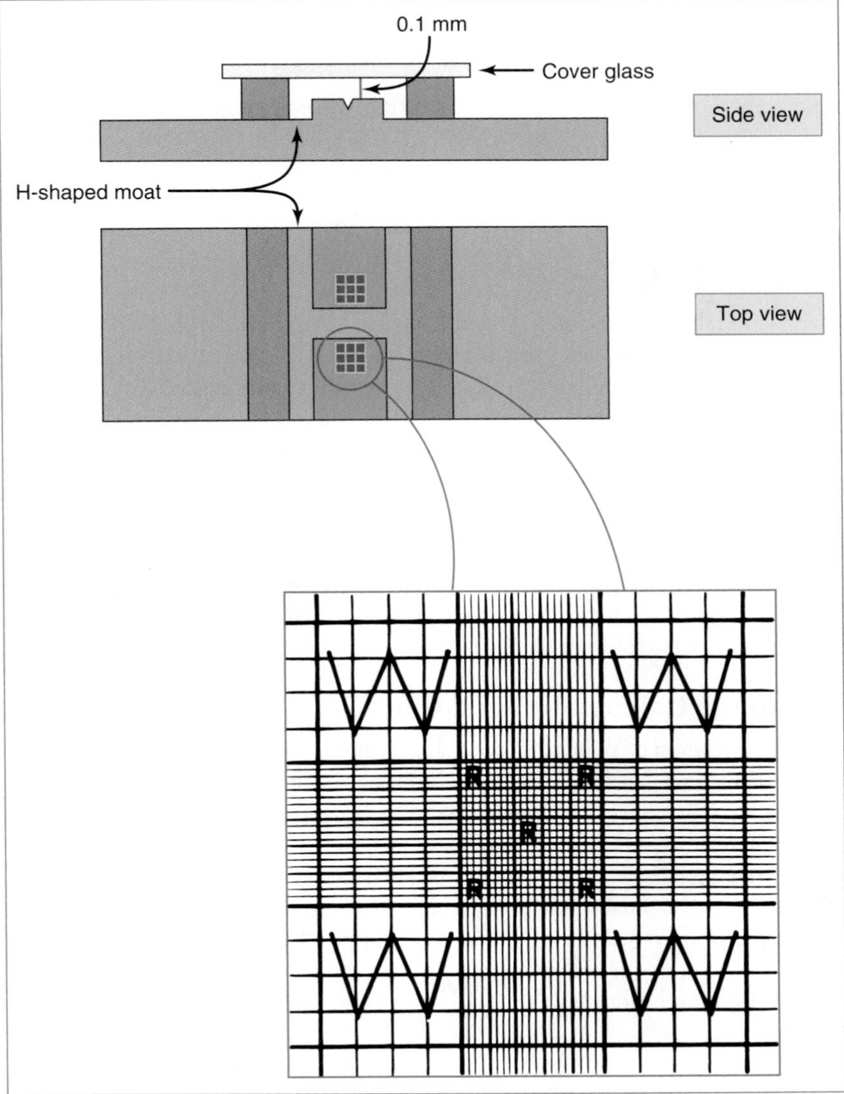

■ FIGURE 10-1 Hemacytometer with Neubauer ruling.

Source: McKenzie, Shirlyn B., *Clinical Laboratory Hematology, 2nd Ed.*, c 2010. Reprinted and electronically reproduced by permission of Pearson Education, Inc., Upper Saddle River, New Jersey.

Through the V-shaped indentation, diluted blood enters the hemacytometer by capillary action into the counting area, where the cells are enumerated microscopically. Afterward, the procedure is repeated on the other side of the hemacytometer, and the two counts are averaged.

Enumerating Leukocytes

To count WBCs, whole blood is diluted 1:20 in a weak acid, which lyses (ruptures) the non-nucleated red blood cells. After the hemacytometer is charged with the diluted blood, cells are counted microscopically in the four large corner squares labeled "W."

Suppose the four corner squares on one side of the hemacytometer give WBC counts of 25, 24, 28, and 22. The four counts from the other side of the hemacytometer are 26, 30, 31, and 28. The difference between any two of these counts should be less than 10, and the difference between the highest and lowest counts should be less than 15. Both conditions are satisfied in this case. The total count from the first side is 99 and that from the second is 115. Their average is 107. Now let us reason from this number to the final result before arriving at a general formula.

The 107 WBCs were all present in the four corner squares. Because each of those squares has a volume of 0.1 mm^3 (1 mm $\times$ 1 mm $\times$ 0.1 mm), the total volume is 0.4 mm^3 (4 $\times$ 0.1 mm^3). Thus, the total count is 267.5 per mm^3 (107 $\div$ 0.4 mm^3). To correct for the 1:20 dilution, however, this value must be multiplied by 20, giving a final result of 5350 WBCs per mm^3 (or per μL).

Here is the formula:

EQUATION 1

$$\text{cell count (per mm}^3) = \frac{\text{number of cells counted}}{\text{total volume (mm}^3)} \times \text{dilution factor}$$

An equivalent formula that bypasses calculating the total volume first is

$$\text{cell count (per mm}^3) = \frac{\text{number of cells counted} \times \dfrac{1}{\text{depth (mm)}}}{\text{total area (mm}^2)} \times \text{dilution factor}$$

Enumerating Erythrocytes

To count red blood cells, whole blood is diluted 1:200 in 0.85% (w/v) saline both to prevent lysis and to bring the number of cells into a range suitable for counting. After the hemacytometer is charged with the diluted blood, cells are counted microscopically in the five squares labeled "R."

Equation 1 is used to calculate the final result, but the total volume and dilution factor have different values than do their counterparts in leukocyte counting. On each side of the hemacytometer, the total area is 0.2 mm^2 (5 $\times$ 0.04 mm^2), and the dilution factor is 200.

Enumerating Platelets

To count platelets, whole blood is diluted 1:100. On the hemacytometer, cells are counted in all 25 squares within the central square, which means that the total volume is 0.1 mm^3 (0.04 mm^2 $\times$ 25 $\times$ 0.1 mm). Again, Equation 1 is used to calculate the final result.

Shortcuts to the Calculated Final Cell Count

If we perform enumeration of WBCs, RBCs, and platelets *exactly* in accord with standard procedure, as outlined above, then we can simply multiply the absolute number of cells counted on the hemacytometer by a single factor to give the same final count as Equation 1 would have given. If, however, any part of the procedure is *not* standard, we must use Equation 1.

If WBCs are counted in all four corner squares and if the dilution is 1:20, then the raw count can be multiplied by 50 to give the final count. For example, if the raw count is 100, then multiplying it by 50 gives a final count of 5000 WBCs per mm^3. This is the same as Equation 1 returns:

$$\text{WBC count (per mm}^3) = \frac{\text{100 WBCs}}{0.4 \text{ mm}^3} \times 20 = \text{5000 WBCs per mm}^3$$

For RBCs, the single factor is 10,000, but only if we count the cells in all five "R" squares and if the dilution is 1:200. For platelets, the single factor is 1000, but only if we count the cells in all 25 squares within the central square and if the dilution is 1:100. Table 10-1 summarizes the factors and the constraints for using them.

★ TABLE 10-1 Single Factors for Calculating Cell Counts Obtained by Standard Procedure

Cell	Single Factor	Constraints
WBC	50	Cells must be counted in all four corner squares. Dilution must be 1:20.
RBC	10,000	Cells must be counted in all five "R" squares. Dilution must be 1:200.
Platelets	1000	Cells must be counted in all 25 squares within central square. Dilution must be 1:100.

HEMATOCRIT

The **hematocrit** (Hct) is the volume of whole blood occupied by packed RBCs. To ascertain this value, blood is loaded into a capillary tube and centrifuged; the resulting volume taken by the RBCs is expressed as a percentage of the total volume. For example, an Hct of 42% means that RBCs take up 42 of every 100 mL of whole blood. Hct may also be expressed as "L/L."

ERYTHROCYTE INDICES

For differentiating among anemias and for detecting analytical errors, three simple calculated indices were developed long ago. We compute these "RBC indices" from the RBC count, hematocrit, and hemoglobin (Hb) concentration.

- **Mean cell volume (MCV):** the average size of an erythrocyte
- **Mean cell hemoglobin (MCH):** the amount of hemoglobin per erythrocyte
- **Mean cell hemoglobin concentration (MCHC):** the amount of hemoglobin relative to the erythrocyte's size

Mean Cell Volume (MCV)

MCV is the average volume, in "fL", of the RBCs. We calculate it using this formula:

$$\text{MCV (fL)} = \frac{\text{Hct (\%)}}{\text{RBC count } (\times 10^6/\mu\text{L})} \times 10$$

EQUATION 2

For example, if a blood sample has an Hct of 38% and an RBC count of $4.0 \times 10^6/\mu$L, then the MCV is

$$\text{MCV} = \frac{38}{4.0} \times 10 = 95$$

The MCV's unit is "fL" ("femtoliters"), which is 1×10^{-15} liters. To prove this, calculate the volume per cell directly, given that (1) RBCs occupy 38% of any volume of this sample of whole blood and (2) there are 4.0×10^6 cells in a μL:

$$\text{MCV} = \frac{\text{volume}}{\text{cell}} = \frac{38\% \text{ of } 1\ \mu\text{L}}{4.0 \times 10^6 \text{ cells}} = \frac{0.38 \times 1\ \mu\text{L}}{4.0 \times 10^6 \text{ cells}} = 9.5 \times 10^{-8}\ \mu\text{L/cell}$$

The volume of $9.5 \times 10^{-8}\ \mu$L is equal to 95 fL because $1\ \mu\text{L} = 10^9$ fL:

$$\frac{1\ \mu\text{L}}{10^9 \text{ fL}} = \frac{9.5 \times 10^{-8}\ \mu\text{L}}{x}$$

$$x = \frac{(9.5 \times 10^{-8}\ \mu\text{L})(10^9 \text{ fL})}{1\ \mu\text{L}} = 95 \text{ fL}$$

Mean Cell Hemoglobin (MCH)

The concentration of Hb, which is the oxygen-carrying protein in RBCs and which renders them red, is usually expressed as "g/dL" but may also appear as "g/L." MCH is the average mass, in "pg," of hemoglobin in an individual RBC. We calculate it using this formula:

$$\text{MCH (pg)} = \frac{\text{Hb (g/dL)}}{\text{RBC count } (\times 10^6/\mu\text{L})} \times 10$$

EQUATION 3

Mean Cell Hemoglobin Concentration (MCHC)

Finally, MCHC is the average concentration, in "g/dL," of hemoglobin in the RBCs themselves. We calculate it using this formula:

EQUATION 4

$$\text{MCHC (g/dL)} = \frac{\text{Hb (g/dL)}}{\text{Hct (\%)}} \times 100$$

RULE OF THREE

The "Rule of Three" is a simple but effective check on the integrity of the measurements and calculations that went into the hemoglobin concentration, hematocrit, and RBC count:

$$3 \times [\text{Hb}] = \text{Hct} \pm 3$$

$$3 \times \text{RBC count} = [\text{Hb}]$$

This rule applies only to normocytic, normochromic erythrocytes. Let us consider an example.

	Actual	Expected (From Rule of Three)
RBC count ($\times 10^6$ cells/μL)	4.0	
Hb concentration (g/dL)	12.4	$3 \times 4.0 = 12$
Hct (%)	36.9	$3 \times 12.4 = 37.2$

When a set of results fails the Rule of Three, an investigation should follow immediately. If the failure is not due to a pathological condition, then the cause is probably interference in the specimen or a preanalytical, analytical, or postanalytical error.

RED-CELL DISTRIBUTION WIDTH

Red-cell distribution width, abbreviated "RDW," is a measure of the variation in RBC size in a given blood specimen. It answers this question: how much of the MCV does one standard deviation encompass? The formula, therefore, is

$$\text{RDW (\%)} = \frac{\text{standard deviation of MCV}}{\text{MCV}} \times 100\%$$

The normal range is 11–15%. A result above this range indicates anisocytosis (a state of unequal RBC sizes), which raises the possibility of several disorders. Moreover, the RDW and the MCV together can help diagnose deficiencies of iron, vitamin B_{12}, and folate.

The word ***width*** in the name does not refer to the width of the cells themselves. Rather, it refers to the width of the distribution curve that relates RBC volume to the frequency of occurrence in a given blood specimen:

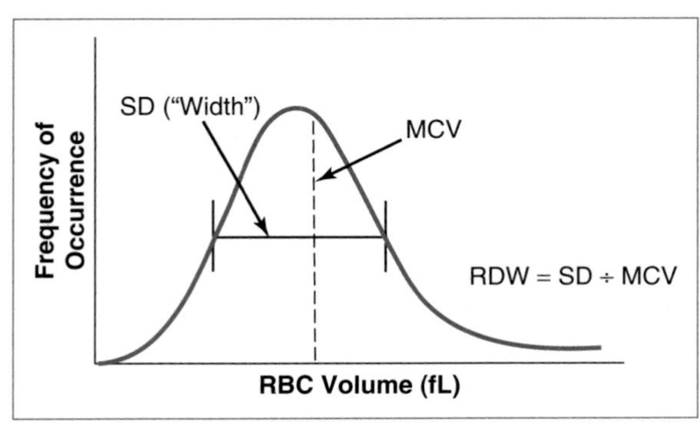

RETICULOCYTE PRODUCTION INDEX

Reticulocytes are immature RBCs that contain residual ribosomal RNA that one can stain and view under a microscope. Because reticulocytes represent the final stage in the maturation of RBCs, counting them is a simple means of monitoring the effectiveness of erythrocyte production.

When hematopoiesis is normal, reticulocytes account for about 1% (40,000–50,000 cells/μL) of the peripheral RBC population. An increase in this percentage, of course, can follow from an increase in the number of circulating reticulocytes, but it can also result from a decrease in the number of circulating RBCs. Therefore, to use the reticulocyte count as a measure of erythropoiesis, we must correct it for the severity of anemia that may be present.

There are two ways to carry out this correction. The first way is to calculate the **reticulocyte index (RI)**, which adjusts the count to the patient's actual hematocrit:

$$\text{Reticulocyte Index} = \text{Reticulocyte Count (\%)} \times \frac{\text{Actual Hct}}{\text{Normal Hct}}$$

EQUATION 5

The normal hematocrit is taken to be 45. The second way to correct it is to convert the reticulocyte percentage into an absolute count for comparison with the normal count:

$$\text{Absolute Reticulocyte Count} = (\text{\% Reticulocytes}) \times (\text{Actual RBC Count})$$

EQUATION 6

Consider this example. An anemic patient's hematocrit is 23%, reticulocyte count 15%, and RBC count 2.6×10^6 cells/μL. Equation 5 gives the reticulocyte index as

$$\text{RI} = 15\% \times \frac{23}{45} = 8\%$$

Equation 6 returns the absolute count:

$$\text{Absolute Count} = 15\% \times (2.6 \times 10^6) = 390{,}000$$

If we take 50,000 as normal, then our patient's absolute count is 7.8 times higher—about the same multiple as the RI:

$$\frac{390{,}000}{50{,}000} = 8$$

When erythropoiesis is being stimulated, as in anemia, maturation time for reticulocytes in the bone marrow goes down, and immature reticulocytes are released earlier into the bloodstream, where they circulate and continue maturing. The result of this early release is an increase in the reticulocyte count, although what that increase represents is a premature shifting into the circulation rather than an acceleration of RBC production in the marrow. Reticulocytes in circulation normally mature (i.e., lose their RNA) in 24 hours. But when anemia is present, the hematocrit falls, shifting occurs sooner, and maturation time in the circulation rises.

The blood of an anemic patient may have circulating reticulocytes that take 2 or 3 days to mature. Therefore, some of them will be counted on more than one day. To correct for this, we divide the RI by the expected maturation time, which we glean from Table 10-2 ★. The quotient is called the **reticulocyte production index (RPI):**

$$\text{Reticulocyte Production Index} = \frac{\text{Reticulocyte Index}}{\text{Expected Maturation Time}}$$

EQUATION 7

★ **TABLE 10-2** Correction Factors for RPI Calculation

Hct (%)	Expected Maturation Time (days)
36–45	1.0
26–35	1.5
16–25	2.0
≤15	2.5

For our anemic patient in the example above (Hct = 23%, reticulocyte count = 15%, RBC count = 2.6 × 10^6, RI = 8%), the RPI value is

$$\text{RPI} = \frac{8\%}{2.0} = 4\%$$

We get the same multiple by comparing absolute counts:

$$\frac{\left(\dfrac{390{,}000}{2.0}\right)}{50{,}000} = 4$$

The principal reason for obtaining an RPI is assessment of the marrow's response to the patient's anemia. In this case, what the value of 4 means is that the patient's RBC production is about four times normal. In other words, erythropoiesis is proceeding about four times faster than it would be in the absence of anemia. In general, an RPI value greater than 3 indicates an adequate response, implying that the marrow is well supplied with raw materials, the kidneys are releasing erythropoietin appropriately, and the cause of the anemia is probably RBC loss. By contrast, an RPI value less than 2 suggests ineffective erythropoiesis, such as that occurring in anemia of chronic disease, renal failure, or iron deficiency.

ENUMERATING RETICULOCYTES

We can manually count reticulocytes by the slide method or by use of a Miller disk. The slide method entails incubating whole blood with new methylene blue, preparing a smear, letting it dry, and then counting under oil immersion. We count 1000 RBCs while noting the number of reticulocytes. The subsequent calculation is straightforward:

EQUATION 8

$$\text{Reticulocyte Percentage} = \frac{\text{Number of Reticulocytes per 1000 RBCs}}{\text{1000 RBCs}} \times 100\%$$

For example, if we see 14 reticulocytes per 1000 RBCs, then the reticulocyte percentage is

$$\text{Reticulocyte Percentage} = \frac{14}{\text{1000 RBCs}} \times 100\% = 1.4\%$$

The Miller disk is a special glass insert for the microscope ocular, and its use in counting reticulocytes improves the precision. The disk comprises two squares (Figure 10-2 ■), the smaller one having one-ninth the area of the larger.

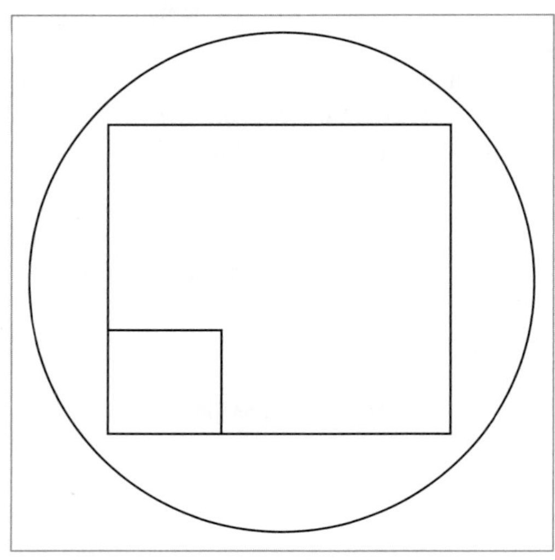

■ **FIGURE 10-2** The Miller disk insert for counting reticulocytes.

In consecutive fields, we count RBCs in the smaller square while counting the reticulocytes in both squares. At the end, we calculate the number of reticulocytes as a percentage of the total RBCs:

$$\text{Reticulocyte Percentage} = \frac{\text{Number of Reticulocytes in Both Squares}}{\text{Number of RBCs in Smaller Square} \times 9} \times 100\%$$

EQUATION 9

OSMOTIC FRAGILITY

When an RBC is immersed in a hypotonic solution, water moves into the cell by osmosis in order to achieve a concentration equilibrium across the membrane. As this process goes forward, the cell swells until it is no longer able to withstand the pressure, at which point it lyses. Spherocytes, which we see in hereditary spherocytosis (HS) and a few other conditions, are spherical RBCs that have a lower ratio of surface area to volume than do normal biconcave RBCs. Consequently, they have a greater **osmotic fragility** and lyse at a higher concentration of NaCl. By contrast, target cells, which we see in thalassemia and iron-deficiency anemia, have a *lower* osmotic fragility, which is to say that they lyse at a lower concentration of NaCl than do normal RBCs. Therefore, we use the test for osmotic fragility to confirm the presence of spherocytes and target cells. This test does not, however, differentiate HS from other causes of spherocytosis or thalassemia from iron-deficiency anemia.

To perform the osmotic fragility test, we prepare a series of hypotonic solutions, ranging in concentration from 0% to 0.85% NaCl (w/v). To each we add a small amount of heparin-anticoagulated blood. After a room-temperature incubation, each solution is centrifuged, and the absorbance of the supernate at 540 nm is measured. This wavelength represents a peak in the absorption spectrum of hemoglobin, which RBCs release into solution as they lyse. The patient's specimen and a normal specimen are run in parallel so that a comparison of the results becomes possible.

For each tube, we calculate the percent lysis from this equation:

$$\text{Percent lysis} = \frac{A_{\text{tube}} - A_{0.85\%}}{A_{0\%} - A_{0.85\%}}$$

We plot the percent lysis as a function of NaCl concentration, giving a curve that is roughly sigmoidal (Figure 10-3 ■). For a normal specimen, lysing begins at about 0.50% NaCl and is complete by 0.30%. If a specimen's curve has shifted to the right of the normal curve (Figure 10-3B), then its RBCs lysed at higher NaCl concentrations; thus, the specimen's RBCs are more osmotically fragile, a finding

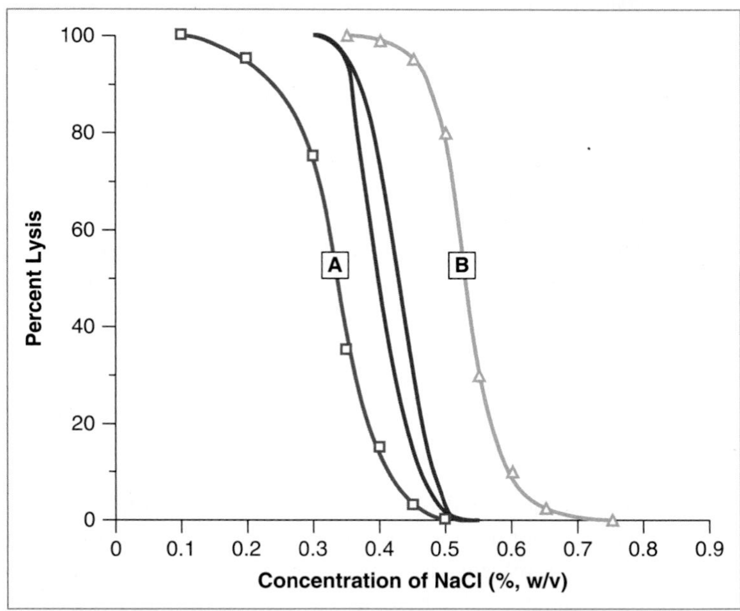

■ FIGURE 10-3 Typical osmotic fragility curves for (**A**) thalassemia and (**B**) hereditary spherocytosis. The normal range lies between the two blue curves.

consistent with the presence of spherocytes. However, if the curve has shifted left (Figure 10-3A), then its RBCs lysed at lower NaCl concentrations, indicating lower osmotic fragility, which is consistent with the presence of target cells.

Some patients with mild HS will show normal results in the osmotic fragility test, as described above, when the blood used in the procedure is fresh. Revealing a difference between normal and abnormal results becomes possible by incubating the blood at 37°C for 24 hours before running the test. During this longer incubation, spherocytes become more susceptible to lysis. Increased osmotic fragility after the 24-hour incubation is characteristic of mild HS, whereas normal fragility nearly rules out HS as a diagnosis.

INTERNATIONAL NORMALIZED RATIO

We employ the **prothrombin time (PT)** to screen for certain coagulation disorders and to monitor anticoagulant therapy. In short, it represents the amount of time required for a plasma specimen to clot *in vitro* when mixed with a commercial reagent containing thromboplastin, which initiates the coagulation cascade. The reference range for this test is 10–13 seconds.

Because of marked variation in the commercial preparations of thromboplastin used by laboratories around the world, as well as differences in instrumentation and controls, the PT result is usually standardized. This is especially important for a patient who takes a vitamin K antagonist (e.g., warfarin) and has this routine test run at various laboratories, depending on his or her whereabouts at the time. Standardization gives what is known as the **International Normalized Ratio (INR):**

EQUATION 10

$$INR = \left(\frac{PT_{patient}}{PT_{normal}}\right)^{ISI}$$

Appendix 8-7 "Arithmetic Means, Geometric Means, and Log-Normal Distributions" www.myhealthprofessions.kit.com

PEARSON myhealthprofessionskit

where $PT_{patient}$ is the PT for the patient (in "seconds"), PT_{normal} is the *geometric* mean of normal PT values (in "seconds"), and ISI is the **International Sensitivity Index**. ISI is a laboratory standard for thromboplastins used to determine the PT. The geometric mean is used rather than the arithmetic mean because the INR relies on a linear relationship between logarithms. For more information on geometric means, consult Appendix 8-7 on the website.

For a normal patient not on anticoagulant therapy, the INR is about 1.0 (0.8–1.2). For a patient on warfarin, the INR should fall between 2.0 and 3.0, which means that the patient's clotting time is about two or three times normal. An INR of 5 or greater implies an unacceptably high risk of bleeding.

In patients on anticoagulant therapy, the ISI represents the average sensitivity, or responsiveness, of a given thromboplastin preparation to the deficiency of clotting factors being induced by the drug. It attempts to correct the prothrombin ratio for the variations mentioned above. The reagent manufacturer calculates the ISI for every lot of thromboplastin reagent, and automated instruments request this value as input from the user.

The ISI standardization system is based on the first World Health Organization (WHO) international reference preparation of thromboplastin. That preparation, called "67/40," was established in 1976 but is no longer available; its ISI value was defined as 1.0. Each new reference preparation of thromboplastin issued by the WHO was, and is, calibrated against the previous one—a process that ultimately compares it with 67/40. Likewise, commercial reagents are calibrated against those reference preparations and, therefore, also against 67/40.

Appendix 10-1 "International Sensitivity Index" www.myhealthprofessions.kit.com

PEARSON myhealthprofessionskit

Theoretically, the value of the INR represents what the prothrombin ratio would have been if the WHO reference preparation of thromboplastin had been used as the reagent and if the manual technique had been employed. A thromboplastin reagent is considered highly sensitive if its ISI is about 1.0. A less sensitive preparation would have a greater ISI. For an explanation of how the ISI is calculated, see Appendix 10-1 on the website.

A thromboplastin preparation selected for use should have an ISI close to 1.0. The reason for this is that a less sensitive reagent—one with a higher ISI—can return an INR value outside the target range of 2.0–3.0 (Table 10-3 ★). When the reagent is less sensitive, the dose of the drug required to achieve a PT ratio in the middle of the target range (e.g., 2.5) would have to be markedly higher than the dose required

★ **TABLE 10-3** Influence of ISI on INR.

Observed Prothrombin Time Ratio $\left(\frac{PT_{patient}}{PT_{normal}}\right)$	International Normalized Ratio (INR)		
	ISI = 1.0	ISI = 1.4	ISI = 1.8
1.30	1.30	1.44	1.60
1.72	1.72	2.14	2.65
2.16	2.16	2.94	4.00
2.95	2.95	4.55	7.01

when the reagent is sensitive. Consequently, the clinician might raise the dose and unintentionally impair the patient's clotting response to a dangerous degree.

CORRECTION OF WBC COUNT FOR NUCLEATED RBCS

Nucleated RBCs (nRBCs) represent the stage in the erythrocyte maturation sequence right before that of reticulocytes. In fact, an nRBC, also called a *metarubricyte* or *orthochromatic normoblast*, expels its nucleus to become a reticulocyte. Though usually seen only in the bone marrow, nRBCs can appear in the blood of patients who have bone marrow disorders and in the blood of normal infants for a few days after birth. We may inadvertently include nRBCs among WBCs whether the method is manual or automated (the dilution medium in the manual technique does not lyse them). Therefore, their presence may falsely elevate the WBC count.

To correct for the presence of nRBCs, we identify and enumerate them in a blood smear. Then, the number of nRBCs goes into this formula:

$$\text{corrected WBC count} = \frac{\text{uncorrected WBC count}}{1 + \dfrac{\text{nRBCs per 100 WBCs}}{\text{100 WBCs}}} = \frac{\text{uncorrected WBC count} \times 100}{100 + \text{nRBCs per 100 WBCs}}$$

EQUATION 11

For example, if the uncorrected WBC count is 14,500 and if 16 nRBCs were seen per 100 WBCs, then the corrected WBC count is

$$\text{corrected WBC count} = \frac{14{,}500 \times 100}{100 + 16} = \frac{1{,}450{,}000}{116} = 12{,}500$$

The reasoning behind this formula is straightforward. The denominator, which is

$$1 + \frac{\text{nRBCs per 100 WBCs}}{\text{100 WBCs}}$$

reflects the fractional increase in the WBC count due to nRBCs. If there are no nRBCS, then this denominator is simply "1," and the corrected count is the same as the uncorrected count. However, if there are, say, 200 nRBCs per 100 WBCs, then the denominator becomes

$$1 + \frac{200}{100} = 3$$

This means that the uncorrected count is actually three times higher than it would have been in the absence of nRBCs. Therefore, it must be *divided* by three to bring it back down to the correct value.

Summary

1. We carry out manual enumeration of blood cells microscopically on a *hemacytometer*, which is a ruled glass platform subdivided into squares of known dimensions.
2. WBCs are counted in the four squares labeled "W," after 1:20 dilution of the blood. The total volume of the square is 0.4 mm^3. We count RBCs in the five squares labeled "R," after 1:200 dilution of the blood. The total volume of the squares is 0.2 mm^3. We count platelets in all 25 squares within the central square. The total volume is 0.1 mm^3. We then calculate the cell count from either of these two equations:

$$\text{cell count (per mm}^3) = \frac{\text{number of cells counted}}{\text{total volume (mm}^3)} \times \text{dilution factor}$$

$$\text{cell count (per mm}^3) = \frac{\text{number of cells counted} \times \dfrac{1}{\text{depth (mm)}}}{\text{total area (mm}^2)} \times \text{dilution factor}$$

3. The *hematocrit* (Hct) is the volume of whole blood occupied by packed RBCs. We express the volume taken by the RBCs as a percentage of the total blood volume.
4. There are three calculated RBC indices used for differentiating among anemias and for detecting analytical errors:
   (a) *Mean cell volume (MCV)*, the average size of an erythrocyte

$$\text{MCV (fL)} = \frac{\text{Hct (\%)}}{\text{RBC count } (\times 10^6/\mu\text{L})} \times 10$$

   (b) *Mean cell hemoglobin (MCH)*, the amount of hemoglobin per erythrocyte

$$\text{MCH (pg)} = \frac{\text{Hb (g/dL)}}{\text{RBC count } (\times 10^6/\mu\text{L})} \times 10$$

   (c) *Mean cell hemoglobin concentration (MCHC)*, the amount of hemoglobin relative to the erythrocyte's size

$$\text{MCHC (g/dL)} = \frac{\text{Hb (g/dL)}}{\text{Hct (\%)}} \times 100$$

5. The "Rule of Three" is a check on the integrity of the measurements and calculations that went into the hemoglobin concentration, hematocrit, and RBC count. It applies only to normocytic, normochromic erythrocytes:

$$3 \times [\text{Hb}] = \text{Hct}$$

$$3 \times \text{RBC count} = [\text{Hb}]$$

6. The *red-cell distribution width (RDW)* is a measure of the variation in RBC size in a given blood specimen. The normal range is 11–15%:

$$\text{RDW (\%)} = \frac{\text{standard deviation of MCV}}{\text{MCV}} \times 100$$

7. Reticulocytes are immature RBCs that contain residual ribosomal RNA that one can stain and view under a microscope.
8. When hematopoiesis is normal, reticulocytes account for about 1% (40,000–50,000 cells/μL) of the peripheral RBC population.
9. When anemia is present, the reticulocyte count rises as the RBC count falls (if kidney and marrow function are normal), pushing the reticulocyte percentage up. Therefore, the count must be corrected for this misleading increase.
10. The *reticulocyte index (RI)* corrects the reticulocyte count for the presence of anemia (the normal hematocrit is taken to be 45):

$$\text{Reticulocyte Index} = \text{Reticulocyte Count} \times \frac{\text{Actual Hct}}{\text{Normal Hct}}$$

11. The *reticulocyte production index (RPI)* corrects the reticulocyte count for the early release of reticulocytes into the blood. The formula is used in conjunction with a table of predetermined values:

$$\text{Reticulocyte Production Index} = \frac{\text{Reticulocyte Index}}{\text{Expected Maturation Time}}$$

Hct (%)	Expected Maturation Time (days)
36–45	1.0
26–35	1.5
16–25	2.0
≤15	2.5

12. There are two methods for counting reticulocytes. The slide method entails incubating whole blood with new methylene blue, preparing a smear, letting it dry, and then counting under oil immersion. With this method, one counts 1000 RBCs while noting the number of reticulocytes:

$$\text{Reticulocyte Percentage} = \frac{\text{Number of Reticulocytes per 1000 RBCs}}{\text{1000 RBCs}} \times 100\%$$

13. The second method for counting reticulocytes involves the Miller disk, a special glass insert for the microscope ocular that comprises two squares, the smaller one having one-ninth the area of the larger. In consecutive fields, we count RBCs in the smaller square while counting the reticulocytes in both squares. At the end, we calculate the number of reticulocytes as a percentage of the total RBCs:

$$\text{Reticulocyte Percentage} = \frac{\text{Number of Reticulocytes in Both Squares}}{\text{Number of RBCs in Smaller Square} \times 9} \times 100\%$$

14. The test for *osmotic fragility* confirms the presence of spherocytes, which lyse at higher NaCl concentrations than do normal RBCs, and target cells, which lyse at lower

concentrations. Heparin-anticoagulated blood is added to a series of hypotonic solutions (0–0.85% NaCl). After centrifugation, the A_{540} of each supernate is measured and the percent lysis is calculated:

$$\text{Percent lysis} = \frac{A_{tube} - A_{0.85\%}}{A_{0\%} - A_{0.85\%}}$$

15. The percent lysis is then plotted against NaCl concentration. Right-shifting relative to the normal curve indicates greater osmotic fragility, which is consistent with the presence of spherocytes. Left-shifting indicates lower osmotic fragility, which is consistent with the presence of target cells.
16. The *International Normalized Ratio (INR)* corrects prothrombin-time results for variations among laboratories, instruments, thromboplastin preparations, and so forth. The reference ranges for this test are 0.8–1.2 if the patient is not on anticoagulant therapy and 2.0–3.0 if the patient is taking an anticoagulant:

$$\text{INR} = \left(\frac{PT_{patient}}{PT_{normal}}\right)^{ISI}$$

where $PT_{patient}$ is the PT for the patient (in "seconds"), PT_{normal} is the geometric mean of normal PT values (in "seconds"), and ISI is the *International Sensitivity Index*.

17. The ISI represents the average sensitivity, or responsiveness, of a given thromboplastin preparation to the deficiency of clotting factors being induced by an anticoagulant. The manufacturer calculates the ISI for every lot of reagent. As sensitivity rises, ISI falls.
18. The WBC count must be corrected for the presence of nucleated RBCs (nRBCs), which can appear in the peripheral blood of patients who have bone marrow disorders and of normal infants for a few days after birth:

$$\text{corrected WBC count} = \frac{\text{uncorrected WBC count}}{1 + \dfrac{\text{nRBCs per 100 WBCs}}{\text{100 WBCs}}}$$

$$= \frac{\text{uncorrected WBC count} \times 100}{100 + \text{nRBCs per 100 WBCs}}$$

Practice and Contextual Problems

1. (LO 1) An automated cell counter found 6620 WBCs per mm^3 in a particular blood sample. How many WBCs, therefore, would be present in a space measuring 1 mm × 1.5 mm × 0.1 mm?
2. (LO 1) The RBCs are counted in a blood specimen according to the standard procedure outlined in the main text. If a total of 200 RBCs are found in the five squares on one side of the hemacytometer, what is the number of RBCs per cubic millimeter of blood?
3. (LO 1) The WBCs are counted in a blood specimen according to the standard procedure outlined in the main text. If a total of 57 WBCs are counted in the four corner squares on one side of the hemacytometer, what is the number of WBCs per cubic millimeter of blood?
4. (LO 1) A blood specimen is suspected of having a WBC count of about 20,000 per mm^3. What dilution would bring the count to 50 cells per "W"-labeled square on the hemacytometer?
5. (LO 1) The RBCs are counted in a blood specimen according to the standard procedure outlined in the main text, except that the dilution is 100-fold. If a total of 166 RBCs are found in the five squares on one side of the hemacytometer, what is the number of RBCs per cubic millimeter of blood?
6. (LO 1) The WBCs are counted in a blood specimen according to the standard procedure outlined in the main text, except that the dilution is 10-fold. If a total of 36 WBCs are counted in the four corner squares on one side of the hemacytometer, what is the number of WBCs per cubic millimeter of blood?
7. (LO 2) Calculate the MCV of a blood specimen with Hct = 38% and RBC count = 4.7 × 10^6/mm^3.
8. (LO 2) Calculate the MCV of a blood specimen with Hct = 44% and RBC count = 5.1 × 10^6/mm^3.
9. (LO 2) Calculate the MCV of a blood specimen with Hct = 47% and RBC count = 6.0 × 10^{12}/L.
10. (LO 2) Calculate the MCH of a blood specimen with Hb = 15.2 g/dL and RBC count = 5.4 × 10^6/mm^3.
11. (LO 2) Calculate the MCHC of a blood specimen with Hb = 13.9 g/dL and Hct = 41%.
12. (LO 2) If Hct is expressed as "L/L," how does Equation 2 change?
13. (LO 8) Complete the following table.

PT_{norm}	$PT_{patient}$	ISI	INR
12	21	1.22	
12	16	1.91	
12	21	2.0	
12	24	1.5	
11	19	1.35	
11	30	1.1	
11	23	2.2	
11	10	1.0	

14. (LO 1) The platelets are counted in a blood specimen according to the standard procedure outlined in the main text. If a total of 91 platelets are found in the 25 squares on one side of the hemacytometer, what is the number of platelets per cubic millimeter of blood?

15. (LO 1) The platelets are counted in a blood specimen according to the standard procedure outlined in the main text. If a total of 137 platelets are counted in the 25 squares on one side of the hemacytometer, what is the number of platelets per cubic millimeter of blood?

16. (LO 1) The platelets are counted in a blood specimen according to the standard procedure outlined in the main text. If a total of 208 platelets are counted in the 25 squares on one side of the hemacytometer, what is the number of platelets per cubic millimeter of blood?

17. (LO 6) Calculate the reticulocyte percentage from each of the following raw counts obtained by the slide method.

Reticulocytes per 1000 RBCs	Reticulocyte Percentage
37	
106	
9	
22	
64	

18. (LO 6) Calculate the reticulocyte percentage from each of the following raw counts obtained from a Miller disk.

Reticulocytes in Both Squares	RBCs in Smaller Square	Reticulocyte Percentage
40	260	
18	194	
105	297	
26	174	
88	213	

19. (LO 4) Calculate the reticulocyte index for each of the following specimens.

Reticulocyte Count (%)	Hematocrit (%)	Reticulocyte Index (%)
3.3	31	
10.0	28	
2.6	19	
8.3	21	
1.1	35	

20. (LO 5) Calculate the reticulocyte production index for each of the following specimens.

Reticulocyte Index (%)	Hematocrit (%)	Reticulocyte Production Index (%)
1.7	32	
9.0	28	
2.0	25	
0.9	30	
7.8	18	

21. (LO 3) Tell whether each of the following sets of data satisfies the Rule of Three.

	RBC Count ($\times 10^6$ cells/μL)	Hb Concentration (g/dL)	Hematocrit (%)
(a)	4.9	14.6	42.8
(b)	6.0	17.9	52.0
(c)	3.7	11.4	39.2
(d)	5.1	15.1	47.1
(e)	4.6	14.0	40.5

22. (LO 7) Plot the following osmotic fragility data and decide whether the patient results are consistent with the presence of spherocytes.

	Percent Lysis	
NaCl Concentration (%)	Normal Specimen	Patient Specimen
0.85	0	0
0.75	0	0
0.65	0	0
0.60	0	1
0.55	0	30
0.50	2	75
0.45	20	96
0.40	60	99
0.35	95	100
0.30	98	100
0.20	100	100
0.10	100	100

23. (LO 10) Correct each of the following WBC counts for the presence of nRBCs.

	Uncorrected WBC Count (cells/μL)	nRBCs per 100 WBCs	Corrected WBC Count (cells/μL)
(a)	18,500	14	
(b)	5600	28	
(c)	2200	47	

24. (LO 1) Cells were counted by standard procedure on a hemacytometer. From the following raw counts, calculate the final counts.

	Raw Count			Final Count		
	RBCs (total in 5 squares on one side)	WBCs (total in 4 corner squares on one side)	Platelets (total in all 25 squares on one side)	RBCs (cells/mm^3)	WBCs (cells/mm^3)	Platelets (cells/mm^3)
(a)	193	72	136			
(b)	467	112	200			
(c)	250	400	61			
(d)	590	231	277			

25. (LO 1) Cells were counted on a hemacytometer but with nonstandard dilutions. From the following raw counts, calculate the final counts.

	Raw Count			Final Count		
	RBCs (total in 5 squares on one side)	WBCs (total in 4 corner squares on one side)	Platelets (total in all 25 squares on one side)	RBCs (cells/mm^3)	WBCs (cells/mm^3)	Platelets (cells/mm^3)
(a)	550 (dil. = 1:300)	200 (dil. = 1:30)	80 (dil. = 1:50)			
(b)	360 (dil. = 1:100)	310 (dil. = 1:40)	95 (dil. = 1:50)			
(c)	242 (dil. = 1:50)	95 (dil. = 1:10)	427 (dil. = 1:200)			
(d)	498 (dil. = 1:400)	400 (dil. = 1:30)	341 (dil. = 1:200)			

PEARSON myhealthprofessionskit™

Go to www.myhealthprofessionskit.com <http://www.myhealthprofessionskit.com/> to access the Companion Website created for this textbook. Simply select "Clinical Laboratory Science" from the choice of disciplines. Find this book and log in using your username and password to access additional practice problems, answers to the practice and contextual problems, additional information, and more

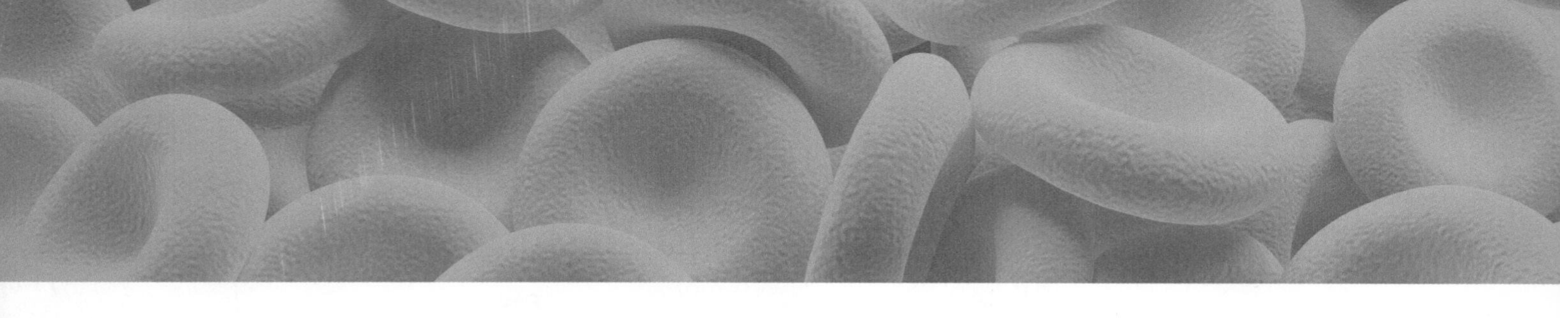

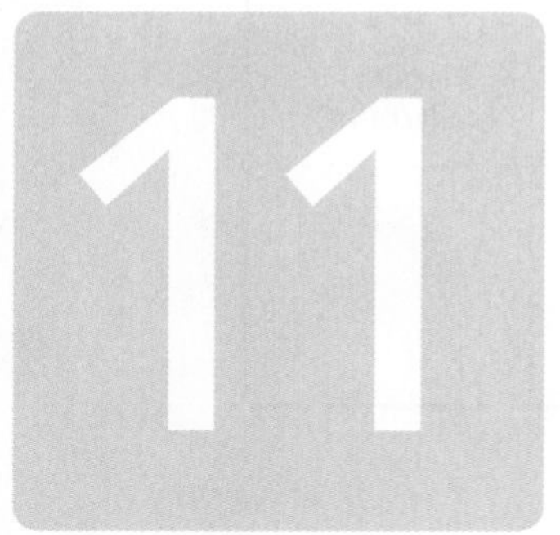

11 Quality Control

Learning Objectives

At the end of this chapter, the student should be able to do the following:

1. Explain the purpose of quality control and the general strategy for performing it
2. Explain the role of the standard deviation in quality control decisions
3. Construct and interpret Levey-Jennings charts
4. Identify outliers, trends, and shifts in a Levey-Jennings chart
5. Explain the purpose of multirule systems
6. Apply Westgard multirules to evaluate a control run
7. Identify random, systematic, constant systematic, and proportional systematic errors

Key Terms

constant systematic error
controls
in range, in control
Levey-Jennings chart
multirules
out of range, out of control
outlier
proportional systematic error
quality control
random error
shift
systematic error
trend

Chapter Outline

To help ensure the accuracy of laboratory results, we employ **quality control**, a process for verifying the performance characteristics of a testing system, which includes reagents, electronics, and robotics. In short, the process consists of running special quality-control materials in the test we are checking and then comparing the results with previous results in which we have confidence. If the current results are acceptably close to the previous results, we conclude that our testing system is functioning properly and that we may proceed to run patient specimens. If, however, the current results are too far from the previous results, we suspect a malfunction somewhere in the analysis, in which case we do not run patient samples until the situation has been rectified and acceptable control results have been obtained.

The materials we use to generate quality control data are called **controls**. We might purchase these controls from vendors or make them ourselves in the laboratory. In either case, controls should simulate, both chemically and physically, the patient specimens we typically run in the test.

The Clinical Laboratory Improvement Act (Sect. 493.1256) requires laboratories to run, at least once per day, two controls at different concentrations when the assay is quantitative, and a positive and negative control when qualitative. It is customary to run controls with two or three different levels of the result, such as low, medium, and high. For example, controls for glucose might have concentrations of 30, 90, and 250 mg/dL because the reference range for glucose in healthy adults is 70–100 mg/dL. Thus, running these three controls would reveal whether our method for quantifying glucose is reliable below, within, and above the reference range.

But how do we decide whether the actual result from a given control is acceptably close to the previous result? Chapter 8 discusses the role of the standard deviation in the acceptance and rejection of quality control runs (see Figure 8-3); those two paragraphs are reproduced here.

> Suppose, for example, that your laboratory runs a test for ferritin in serum. Before running any patient specimens, you must ensure that your analytical method is functioning properly. You run your ferritin control solution and compare the result (147 ng/mL) to the mean (151 mg/dL) for the 60 other ferritin control results that have been recorded for the previous 6 weeks. If the standard deviation of those control results is 3 ng/mL, then 68% of the data fall between 148 and 154 ng/mL, or between $\bar{x} - 1s$ and $\bar{x} + 1s$ (i.e., between 151 − 3 and 151 + 3). Moreover, 95% of the data would fall between 145 and 157 ng/mL, or between $\bar{x} - 2s$ and $\bar{x} + 2s$ (i.e., between 151 − 6 and 151 + 6).
>
> Your result of 147 ng/mL falls between one and two standard deviations below the mean. At this point, the question is whether your result is close enough to the mean to conclude that the analytical method is functioning properly and, therefore, whether to proceed with patient specimens. Laboratories have policies governing this decision based on the deviation of a given result from the mean. If your laboratory's established limit for the ferritin assay is $\pm 2s$, then your result of 147 ng/mL passes the standard-deviation test, and you proceed to run patient samples. However, if the limit is $\pm 1s$, then your result fails, and you do not run patient samples until the malfunction is rectified.

A control result that falls within the defined limits of acceptability is said to be **in range** or **in control**, whereas a result that falls outside those limits is said to be **out of range** or **out of control**.

LEVEY-JENNINGS CHARTS

To simplify the review of quality control data, most clinical laboratories plot them on a **Levey-Jennings chart**, which is a graphical representation of the results over a certain period of time. A Levey-Jennings chart makes it easy to spot outliers, trends, and shifts in the data, with the ultimate goal of showing whether an analytical method is working properly. Consider, for example, 20 consecutive runs of a glucose control (Figure 11-1 ■).

The 20 hypothetical results are averaged (87.8 mg/dL) and the standard deviation is calculated (2.6 mg/dL). Then the data are plotted on a chart with seven horizontal lines, one indicating the mean and the other six indicating the values at 1 SD, 2 SD, and 3 SD above and below the mean. As Figure 11-1 illustrates, it takes only a quick glance at the chart to see that all 20 results fall within two standard deviations of the mean ($\bar{x} \pm 2s$).

Typically, we examine the chart for **outliers**, which are points that lie outside the acceptable range (Figure 11-2A ■), whether that range is $\bar{x} \pm 1s$, $\bar{x} \pm 2s$, or $\bar{x} \pm 3s$. We also look for **trends**.

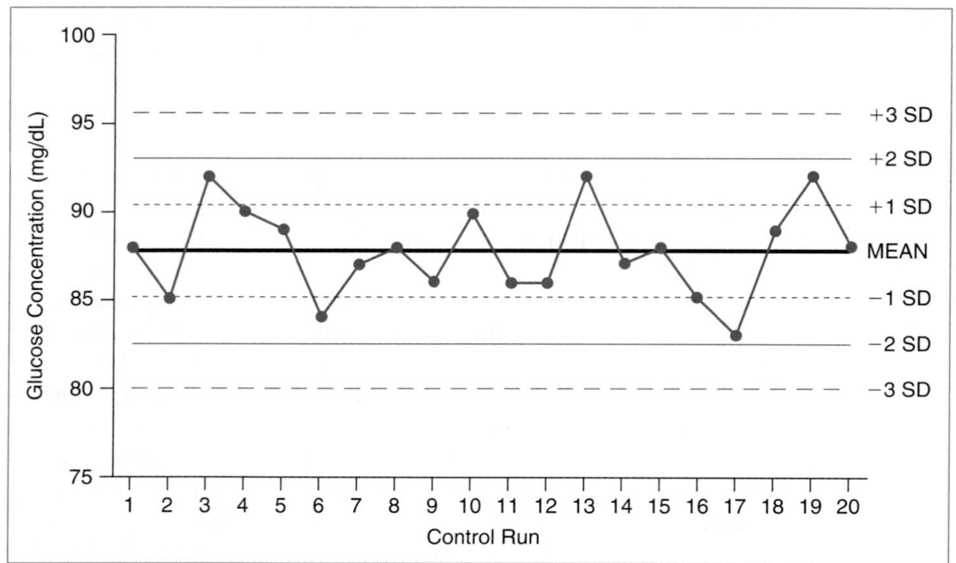

■ **FIGURE 11-1** A typical Levey-Jennings chart. All results for 20 consecutive runs are within 2 SD of the mean ($\bar{x} \pm 2s$).

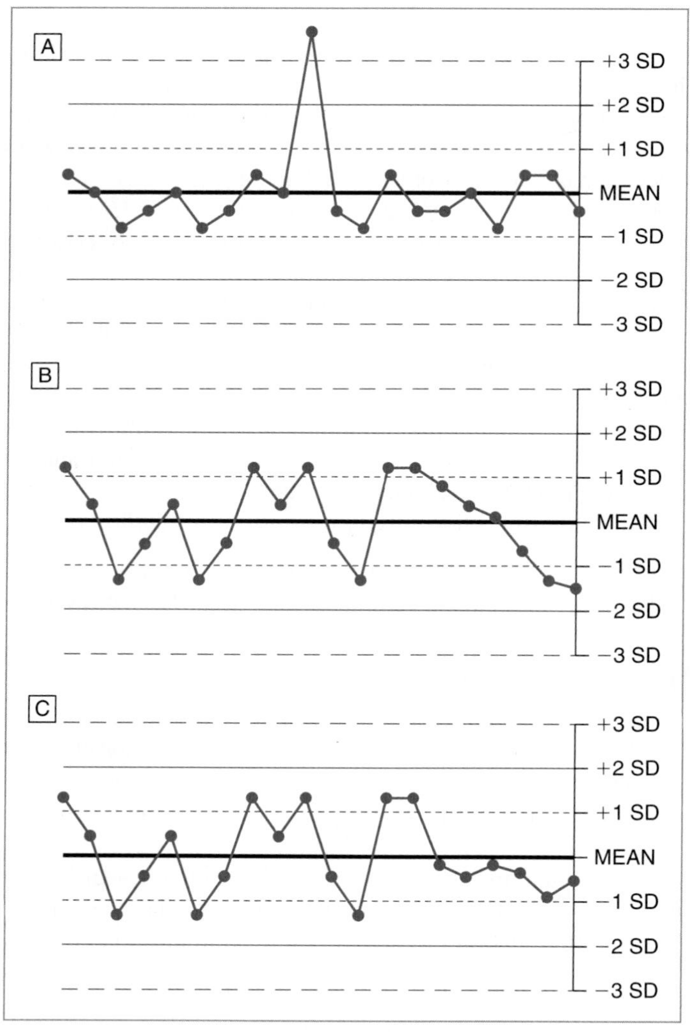

■ **FIGURE 11-2** Hypothetical Levey-Jennings chart showing (*A*) an outlier, (*B*) a trend, and (*C*) a shift.

A trend is a gradual movement in one direction, either upward or downward, by a set of six or more consecutive data points (Figure 11-2B). Finally, we look for **shifts**, an abrupt move in which six or more consecutive data points all occur above or below the mean (Figure 11-2C). When one of these aberrations appears on a Levey-Jennings chart, there is an investigation to search for an incipient problem in the assay.

WESTGARD MULTIRULES

This single rule that control values must fall within two standard deviations of the mean ($\bar{x} \pm 2s$) succeeds in detecting error. However, because the rule is also rather rigid, it can trigger false alarms that cause rejection of acceptable runs and waste the laboratory's time and money.

To lower the rate of false rejection, we can widen the control limits to $\bar{x} \pm 3s$. This change, however, also lowers the rate of error detection. Single rules often force an unacceptable compromise between error detection and false rejection. Consequently, systems of multiple rules, or **multirules**, have been developed to keep the rate of error detection high and the rate of false rejection low. The Westgard system of multirules is perhaps the most commonly used in clinical laboratories. The following section defines each Westgard rule and depicts it in a Levey-Jennings chart. Keep in mind, however, that these multirules are most successful when we use two control materials in a run. When we use three control materials, other multirules may be superior (see the next section). Figure 11-3 ■ summarizes the decision criteria for the acceptance and rejection of a run.

Rule 1_3 One data point falls outside the range $\bar{x} \pm 3s$. The run is rejected.

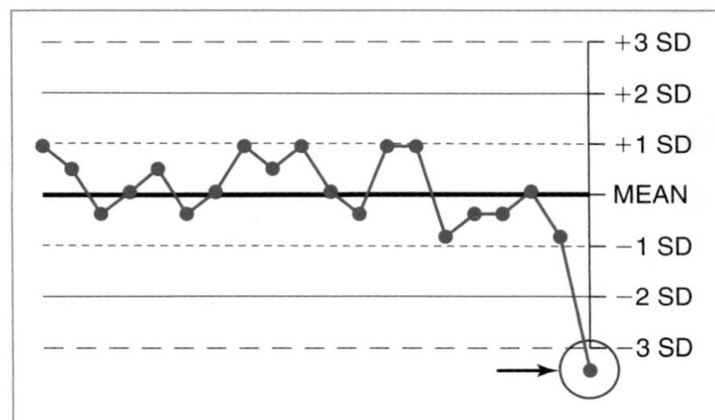

Rule 1_2 One data point falls outside the range $\bar{x} \pm 2s$. This rule is only a *warning* that we should examine the control data in light of the other rules.

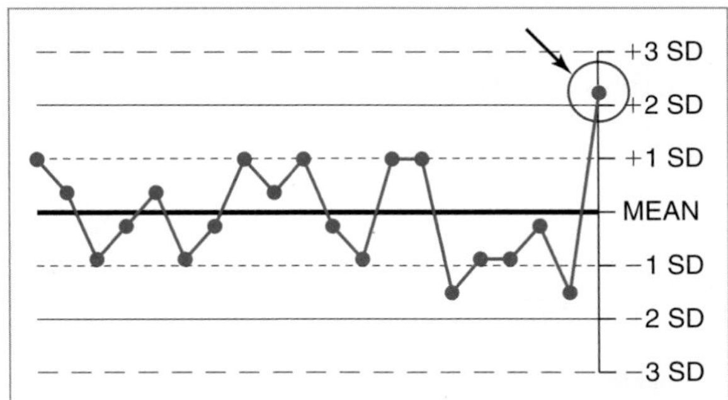

Rule 2_2 Two consecutive data points, from the same control material, exceed $\bar{x} \pm 2s$ but not $\bar{x} \pm 3s$. The two points must lie on the same side of the mean. This rule also applies across two different control levels in corresponding runs, that is, when one result from each of two different controls exceeds $\bar{x} \pm 2s$. In either case, the run is rejected.

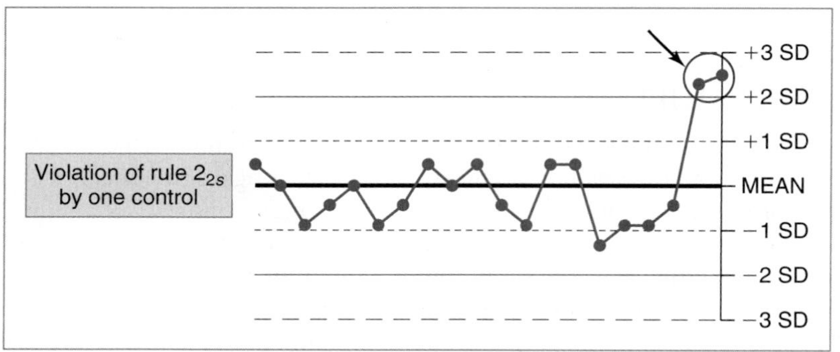

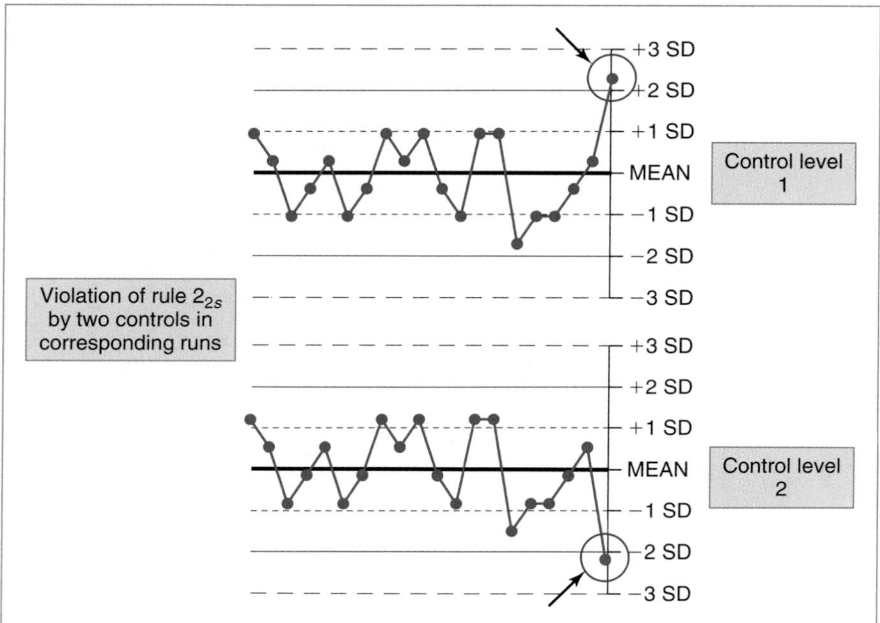

Rule R_{4s}. The difference between two consecutive data points is at least 4 SD, with one data point lying above $\bar{x} + 2s$ and another below $\bar{x} - 2s$. This rule also applies across two different control levels in corresponding runs, that is, when the result from one of two different controls is greater than $\bar{x} + 2s$ and the other is less than $\bar{x} - 2s$. In either case, the run is rejected.

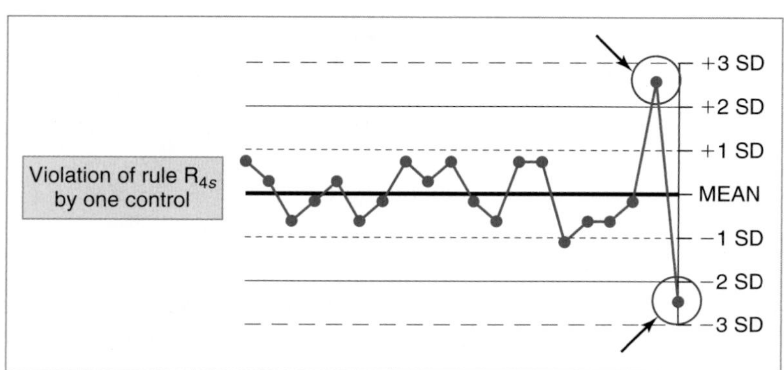

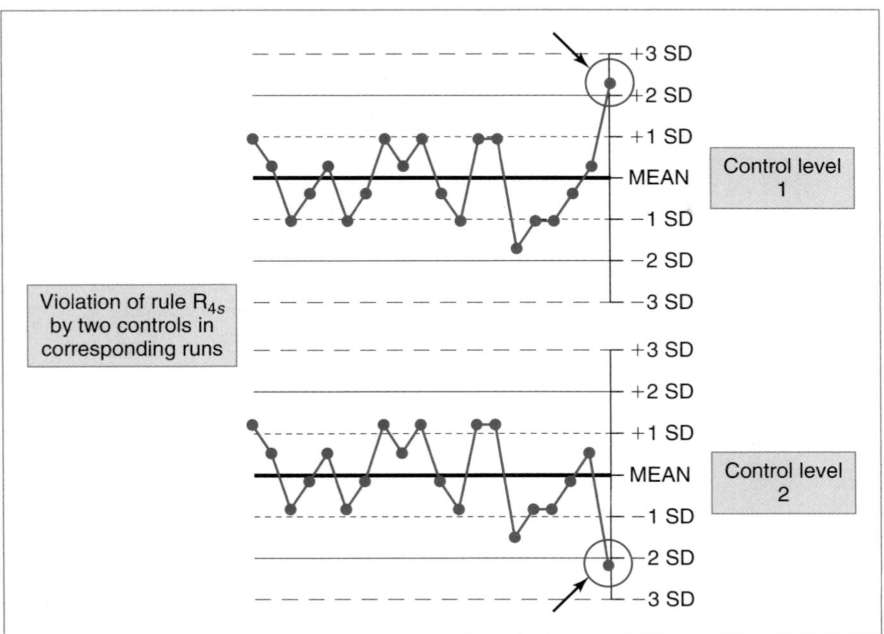

Rule 4_{1s}. Four consecutive data points exceed $\bar{x} \pm 1s$. All four points lie on the same side of the mean. This rule also applies across two different control levels, that is, when two consecutive corresponding runs of two different controls together satisfy these conditions. In either case, the run is rejected.

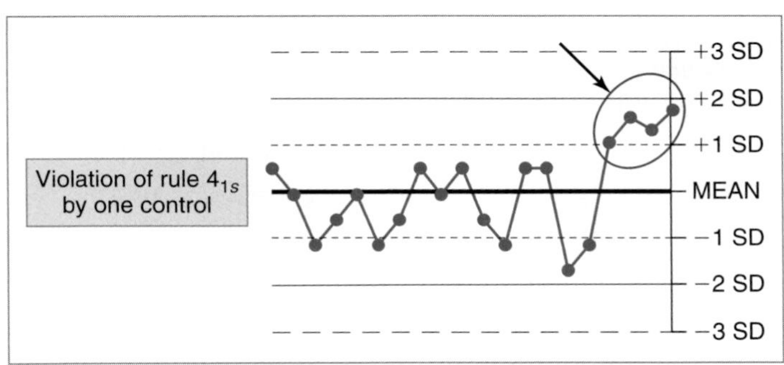

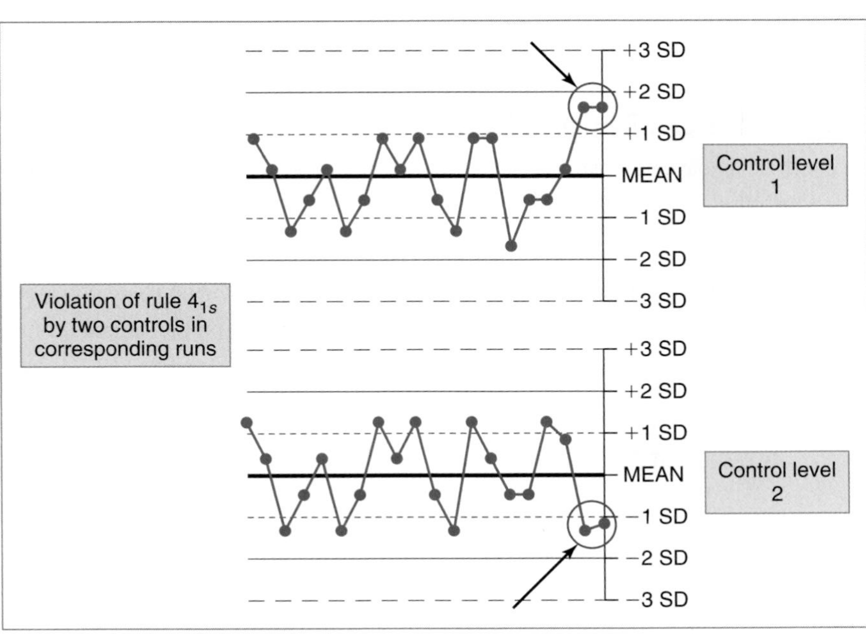

Rule $10_{\bar{x}}$. Ten consecutive data points all fall on the same side of the mean. This rule also applies across two different control levels in corresponding runs when five consecutive points from one control and five from the other satisfy this condition. In either case, the run is rejected.

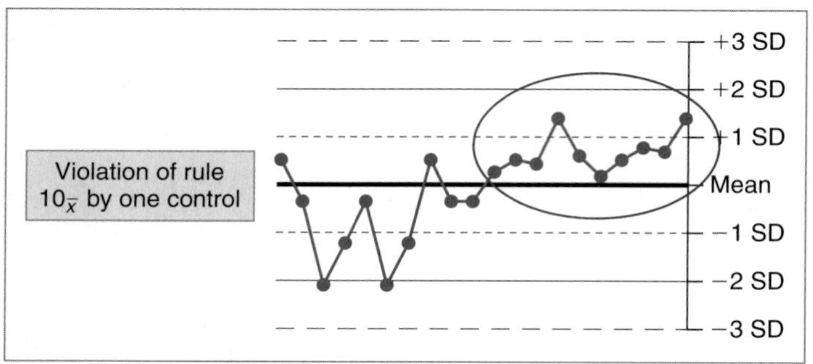

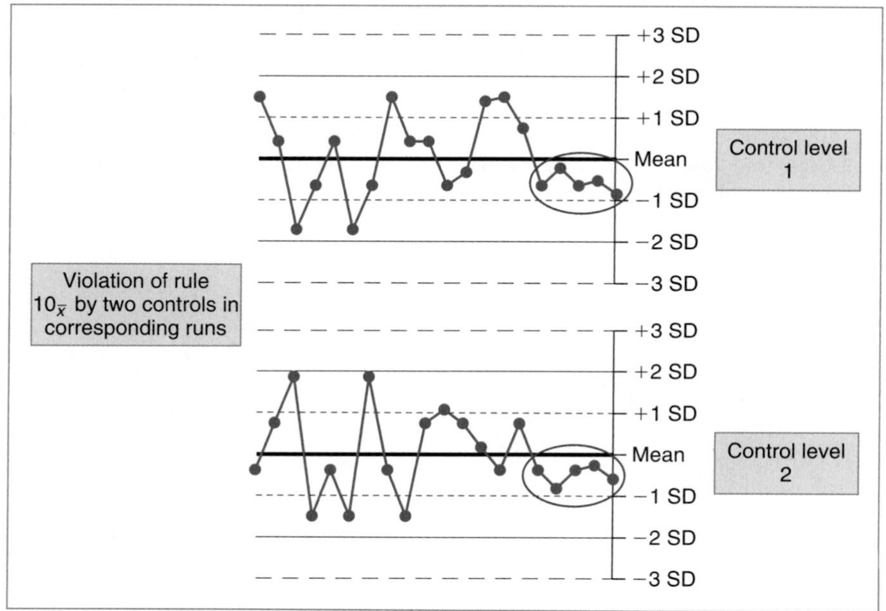

MULTIRULES FOR THREE CONTROLS

For three controls, we have multirules that are preferable to those for two controls. There are various rules and combinations of rules suitable for three controls. What follows is one such combination.

Rules 1_{3s} and R_{4s}. These are the same as they are in the use of two controls, discussed previously.

Rule 2-of-3_{2s}. Two of three control values lie outside the range $\bar{x} \pm 2s$, on the same side of the mean. Violation of this rule triggers rejection of the run.

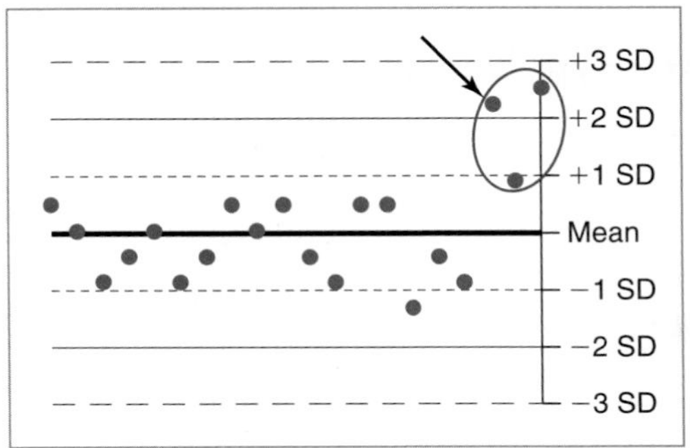

Rule 3_{1s}. Three consecutive control values lie outside the range $\bar{x} \pm 1s$, on the same side of the mean. Violation causes rejection.

Rule $6_{\bar{x}}$. Six consecutive control values lie on the same side of the mean. Violation causes rejection.

RESOLUTION OF OUT-OF-RANGE CONTROLS

When a control is out of range, the action taken depends on the laboratory's policies. If the rule being violated is 1_{2s}, then what sometimes happens is that one repeats the control and, if that result is in range, starts running patient specimens. But this practice, however common it is in laboratories, is controversial because it supplants an internal quality-control procedure that has been designed specifically for the assay in question to minimize the rate of false rejections and maximize the rate of error detection.

In resolving an out-of-range control result, it is best to stop the testing process, try to identify and correct the problem, and then repeat the controls. The error may be due to something as simple as having used the wrong control material, or it may have a more serious cause, such as reagent degradation, software corruption, or hardware failure. Run patient specimens *only* after the controls indicate proper functioning of the assay.

RATIONALE BEHIND THE RULES

Consider the 1_{2s} rule. Because 95% of all the results for a given control fall *within* the range $\bar{x} \pm 2s$, a value *outside* this range is unlikely. Therefore, a violation of this rule warns us that there may be a malfunction somewhere in the assay. Even so, 5% of all the results will exceed two standard deviations even when the assay is functioning properly. In other words, a control will violate the 1_{2s} rule once in every 20 acceptable runs. If, on suspicion of a false rejection, a laboratory just reruns a control whenever the result violates the 1_{2s} rule, then they risk missing a true error.

A value outside the wider range of $\bar{x} \pm 3s$ is even more unlikely, given that this range includes 99.7% of all the results. Therefore, a violation of the 1_{3s} rule probably indicates a true error.

Using only the 1_{2s} rule generates false alarms at the rate of about 9% when two controls are used and 14% when three controls are used.[1] Using only the 1_{3s} rule does lower the risk of falsely rejecting a run but it also lowers the rate of error detection. Thus, even though a multirule system ($1_{3s}/1_{2s}/2_{2s}/R_{4s}/4_{1s}/10_{\bar{x}}$) is more complex than a single rule (1_{2s} or 1_{3s}), it offers a better compromise between false rejection and error detection. Multirules employ single rules that individually have lower rates of false rejection but that collectively raise the rate of error detection.

[1]Westgard, J. O. (2003). Internal quality control: Planning and implementation strategies. *Annals of Clinical Biochemistry, 40*, 593–611.

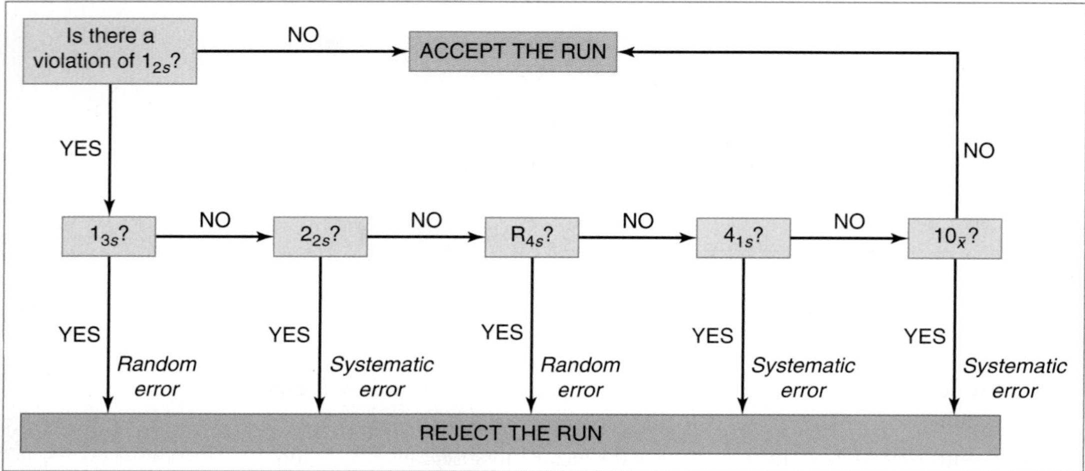

■ FIGURE 11-3 Decision flowchart for the Westgard multirule system.

RANDOM AND SYSTEMATIC ERROR

To determine whether an analytical run is in control or out of control in the Westgard system, use the flowchart in Figure 11-3 ■. As Figure 11-3 also shows, though, one major advantage of multirule systems is their power to differentiate between random and systematic error.

Random error arises from the normal vicissitudes of observation, which have no inherent pattern; these include variations in reading pipets, electronic noise in instruments, fluctuations in room temperature, and so forth. We can minimize random error, or even bring it close to zero, by averaging a large number of results.

Systematic error, by contrast, occurs repeatedly and cannot be minimized by averaging because all the data are wrong in the same direction. For example, the miscalibration of a pipet might cause it to consistently deliver 0.05 mL more than the nominal volume. Similarly, the miscalibration of a balance might cause it to consistently read 20 mg less than the true mass. A malfunctioning automated cell counter might return an erythrocyte count 15% too high. Figure 11-4 ■ depicts random and systematic error.

Systematic error comes in two varieties: constant and proportional (Figure 11-5 ■). **Constant systematic error** is the same regardless of the analyte's concentration. Consider, for example, a hemoglobin assay that has a constant systematic error of +3.0 g/dL because the instrument was not properly zeroed. Observed results of 14.5 and 9.8 g/dL would reflect actual concentrations, respectively, of 11.5 and 6.8 g/dL. At each value, the difference between the actual and observed concentrations is the

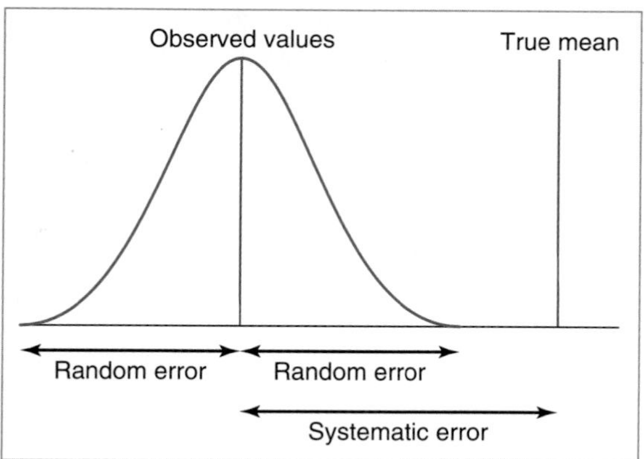

■ FIGURE 11-4 Systematic error, but not random error, changes the mean. Random errors average themselves out to the mean. Systematic errors cannot be averaged out.

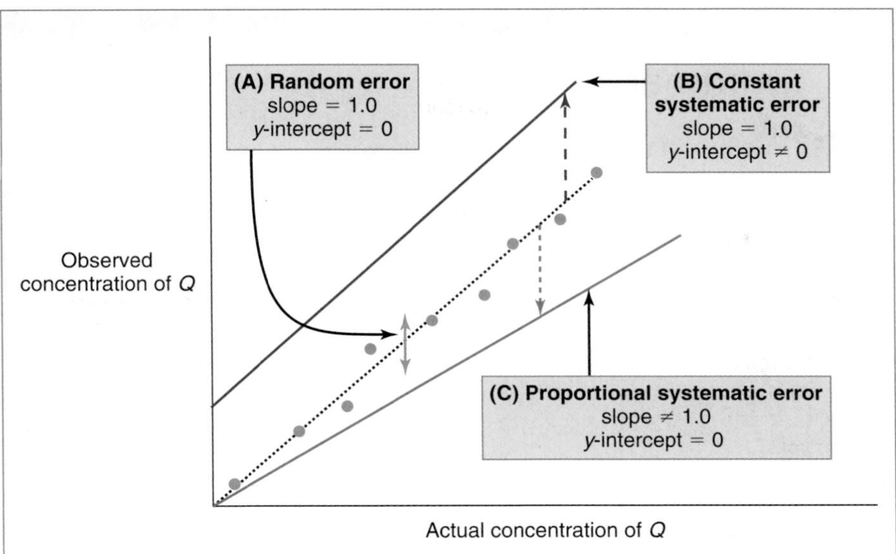

■ **FIGURE 11-5** Random versus systematic error.

(A) Random error only (dotted black line). The observed and actual concentrations agree, and the only error present is random (orange arrow). The regression line has slope = 1.0 and *y*-intercept = 0. Thus, the equation of the line is $y = 1x + 0$.

(B) Constant systematic error (blue line). The observed concentration is higher by a constant amount, regardless of the concentration of Q. Every data point on the regression line is too high by the same amount as every other data point. The *y*-intercept has increased whereas the slope has remained the same. (Constant error can work in either direction; under different circumstances, the values might have been *lower* by a constant amount.)

(C) Proportional systematic error (pink line). The observed concentration is lower by an amount proportional to the concentration of Q. Every data point on the regression line is too low by the same proportion as every other data point. The slope has decreased whereas the *y*-intercept has remained the same. (Proportional error can work in either direction; under different circumstances, the values might have been *higher* by a proportional amount.)

same, 3.0 g/dL. Therefore, constant systematic error changes the *y*-intercept, but not the slope, of the regression line.

Proportional systematic error is, not surprisingly, proportional to the analyte's concentration. Consider, for example, an assay that has two steps: the first for extracting the analyte from blood into a solvent and the second for quantifying the extracted analyte. If the extraction step pulls only 90% of the analyte out of the blood, then an actual concentration of, say, 500 ng/mL in the blood would appear as 450 ng/mL. Moreover, an actual concentration of, say, 1000 ng/mL in the blood would emerge from the assay as 900 ng/mL. At the lower concentration, the difference between the actual and observed results is 500 ng/mL − 450 ng/mL, or 50 ng/mL. At the higher concentration, however, the difference is 1000 ng/mL − 900 ng/mL, or 100 ng/mL. Thus, each observed result is lower than it should be, not by a constant absolute amount but by a constant proportion, 10%. Therefore, proportional systematic error changes the slope, but not the *y*-intercept, of the regression line.

Confirming the presence of constant systematic or proportional systematic error is a matter of constructing the confidence intervals for the slope (Chapter 8, Equation 7) and *y*-intercept (Chapter 8, Equation 9). If the 95% confidence interval for the slope includes 1.0, then the deviation probably carries little significance because that is the slope of the random-error line. If, however, the interval does *not* include 1.0, then the suspected proportional systematic error might be real.

Similarly, if the 95% confidence interval for the *y*-intercept includes 0, then the deviation probably carries little significance because that is the *y*-intercept of the random-error line. If, however, the interval does *not* include 0, then the suspected constant systematic error might be real.

Summary

1. *Quality control* is a process for verifying the performance characteristics of a testing system, which includes reagents, electronics, and robotics.
2. *Controls* are the material we use to generate quality control data. They should simulate, both chemically and physically, the patient specimens we typically run in the test.
3. Laboratories have policies governing the acceptability of control data, based on deviation from the mean. A control result that falls within the defined limits of acceptability is said to be *in range* or *in control*, whereas a result that falls outside those limits is said to be *out of range* or *out of control*.
4. *Levey-Jennings charts* graphically represent quality control data over a certain period of time. They facilitate the detection of outliers, trends, and shifts.
5. An *outlier* is a point that lies outside the range of acceptability.
6. A *trend* is a gradual movement in one direction by a set of six or more consecutive data points.
7. A *shift* is an abrupt move in which six or more consecutive data points all fall above or below the mean.
8. Single rules for accepting control data force a compromise between error detection and false rejection.
9. *Multirules* for accepting control data keep the rate of error detection high and the rate of false rejection low. The most commonly used system of multirules in clinical laboratories is the Westgard system.
10. For two controls, there are six basic Westgard multirules.

Rule 1_{3s}	One data point falls outside the range $\bar{x} \pm 3s$. The run is rejected.
Rule 1_{2s}	One data point falls outside the range $\bar{x} \pm 2s$. This rule is only a warning that the control data should be examined in light of the other rules.
Rule 2_{2s}	Two consecutive data points, from the same control material, exceed $\bar{x} \pm 2s$ but not $\bar{x} \pm 3s$. The two points must lie on the same side of the mean. This rule also applies across two different control levels in corresponding runs. The run is rejected.
Rule R_{4s}	The difference between two consecutive data points is at least 4 SD, with one data point lying above $\bar{x} + 2s$ and another below $\bar{x} - 2s$. This rule also applies across two different control levels in corresponding runs. The run is rejected.
Rule 4_{1s}	Four consecutive data points exceed $\bar{x} \pm 1s$. All four points lie on the same side of the mean. This rule also applies across two different control levels.
Rule $10_{\bar{x}}$	Ten consecutive data points all fall on the same side of the mean. This rule also applies across two different control levels in corresponding runs when five consecutive points from one control and five from the other satisfy this condition. The run is rejected.

11. For three controls, there are various multirules.

Rules 1_{3s} and R_{4s}	These are the same as they are for two controls.
Rule 2-of-3_{2s}	Two of three control values lie outside the range $\bar{x} \pm 2s$, on the same side of the mean. The run is rejected.
Rule 3_{1s}	Three consecutive control values lie outside the range $\bar{x} \pm 1s$, on the same side of the mean. The run is rejected.
Rule $6_{\bar{x}}$	Six consecutive control values lie on the same side of the mean. The run is rejected.

12. In resolving an out-of-range control result, it is best to stop the testing process, try to identify and correct the problem, and then repeat the controls.
13. Even though a multirule system ($1_{3s}/1_{2s}/2_{2s}/R_{4s}/4_{1s}/10_{\bar{x}}$) is more complex than a single rule (1_{2s} or 1_{3s}), it offers a better compromise between false rejection and error detection. Multirules employ single rules that individually have lower rates of false rejection but that collectively raise the rate of error detection.
14. *Random error* has no inherent pattern. We can minimize it by averaging a large number of results.
15. *Systematic error* occurs repeatedly and cannot be minimized by averaging.
16. *Constant systematic error* is the same regardless of concentration. It changes the *y*-intercept but not the slope.
17. *Proportional systematic error* is proportional to concentration. It changes the slope but not the *y*-intercept.

Practice and Contextual Problems

1. (LO 3, 6, 7) Identify the Westgard rules that the following Levey-Jennings charts violate on days 5, 12, and 20. Tell whether each violation implies a random or systematic error.

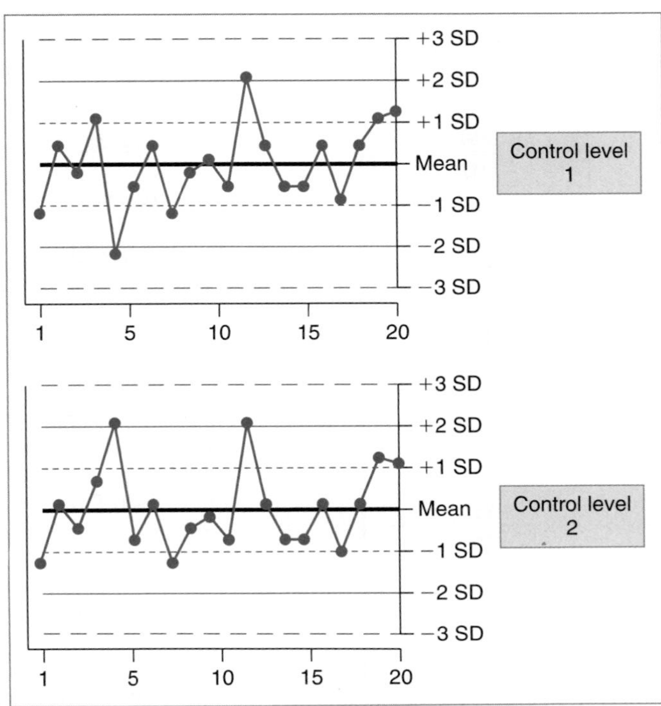

2. (LO 3, 6, 7) Identify the Westgard rules the following Levey-Jennings charts violate on days 12 and 20. Tell whether each violation implies a random or systematic error.

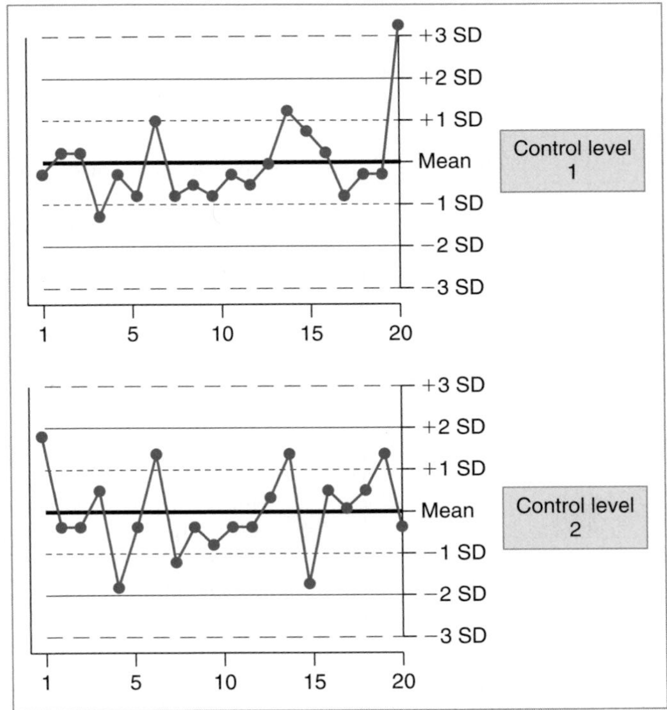

3. (LO 3, 6) Appearing below are data for two levels of cholesterol controls. For each control, calculate the mean and standard deviation and construct a Levey-Jennings chart. Identify any violations of Westgard rules.

Run Number	Control 1 (mg/dL)	Control 2 (mg/dL)
1	180	252
2	175	251
3	187	268
4	186	268
5	176	247
6	177	250
7	191	251
8	175	244
9	179	258
10	175	245
11	181	252
12	181	252
13	180	278
14	191	278
15	180	257
16	176	254
17	178	253
18	179	249
19	178	254
20	174	252

4. (LO 3, 6) For each analyte in the table, construct a Levey-Jennings chart and answer the following two questions. (1) Is the assay currently in control? If not, identify the Westgard violation. (2) Has the assay been in control during the rest of the time period covered by the chart? If not, identify the Westgard violation.

Na^+ (mM)	K^+ (mM)	Glucose (mg/dL)
151	6.6	101
149	6.4	103
148	6.7	97
151	6.5	99
150	6.3	102
150	6.6	100
149	6.5	103
149	6.8	98
150	6.5	100
147	6.4	99
151	6.6	103
148	6.6	91
152	6.7	102
148	6.5	101
147	6.4	100
148	6.7	101
150	6.8	98
152	6.8	99
148	6.9	103
149	6.8	101

5. (LO 3, 4, 6) For each of the following sets of control data, (1) identify any outlier, trend, or shift, if one is present, and (2) explain whether the run should be rejected. Constructing a Levey-Jennings chart is not necessary, but it might be helpful. Assume the range of acceptability to be $\pm$ 2s.

   (a) A control material for serum ammonia is analyzed three times daily for 30 days. The mean is 40 mM and the standard deviation is 2.1 mM. For an additional 3 days, the following data are collected in the order presented.

   39, 41, 41, 36, 34, 39, 45, 40, 39

   (b) A control material for urine chloride is analyzed three times daily for 30 days. The mean is 50 mEq/L and the standard deviation is 2.0 mEq/L. For an additional 3 days, the following data are collected in the order presented.

   47, 50, 51, 48, 50, 51, 53, 54, 57

   (c) A control material for hemoglobin A_{1c} is analyzed once each weekday for 25 days. The result is expressed as a percentage of the total hemoglobin. The mean of the 25 results is 5.0%, and the standard deviation is 0.3 percentage points. For an additional 7 days, the following data are collected in the order presented.

   5.3, 4.9, 4.6, 4.7, 4.8, 4.9, 4.3

6. (LO 2, 6) A control material for valproic acid is analyzed whenever the laboratory receives an order for that test on a patient specimen. There are currently 28 data points for the control. The mean is 130 μg/mL and the standard deviation is 3.0 μg/mL. Consider the following three possible scenarios for the next control result, the 29th in the sequence.

   (a) The next result is 137 μg/mL. If the analyzer flags the result as a violation of Westgard rule 2_{2s} for this single control material, then what are the minimum and maximum possible values of the preceding result?

   (b) The next control result is 134 μg/mL. If the analyzer flags the result as a violation of Westgard rule 4_{1s}, then what is the minimum possible value of each of the preceding three results?

   (c) The next control result is 128 μg/mL. If the analyzer flags the result as a violation of Westgard rule $10_{\bar{x}}$, then what is the minimum possible value of the 19th result in the entire sequence?

7. (LO 2, 6) For assay Q, the means for two different control levels are 60 ng/mL and 200 ng/mL. Their standard deviations, respectively, are 2 ng/mL and 5 ng/mL. Five additional results are gathered for each control in the course of the laboratory routine. Use the Westgard rules to decide whether the most recent run should be accepted.

Run	1	2	3	4	5
Control 1	58	61	63	59	65
Control 2	195	198	203	200	211

8. (LO 2, 6) For assay *X*, the means for two different control levels are 4.5 g/L and 9.2 ng/mL. Their standard deviations, respectively, are 0.22 ng/mL and 0.40 ng/mL. Five additional results are gathered for each control in the course of the laboratory routine. Use the Westgard rules to decide whether the most recent run should be accepted.

Run	1	2	3	4	5
Control 1	4.4	4.2	4.1	4.2	4.2
Control 2	9.3	9.5	9.2	9.1	10.6

9. (LO 2, 6) For assay *J*, the means for two different control levels are 500 IU/mL and 2000 IU/mL. Their standard deviations, respectively, are 20 IU/mL and 100 IU/mL. Five additional results are gathered for each control in the course of the laboratory routine. Use the Westgard rules to decide whether the most recent run should be accepted.

Run	1	2	3	4	5
Control 1	510	488	503	491	518
Control 2	1880	1944	1906	2130	2047

PEARSON
myhealthprofessionskit™

Go to www.myhealthprofessionskit.com <http://www.myhealthprofessionskit.com/> to access the Companion Website created for this textbook. Simply select "Clinical Laboratory Science" from the choice of disciplines. Find this book and log in using your username and password to access additional practice problems, answers to the practice and contextual problems, additional information, and more.

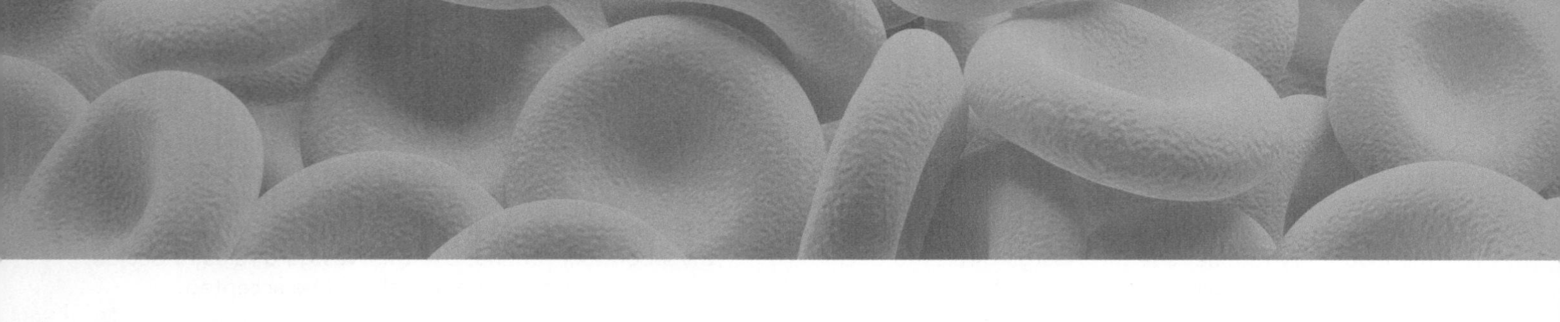

12 Method Evaluation

Learning Objectives

At the end of this chapter, the student should be able to do the following:

1. Calculate and interpret sensitivity, specificity, efficiency, prevalence, and predictive value
2. Explain referent values in the context of binary interpretation of numerical data
3. Predict the effect of moving a referent value on sensitivity and specificity
4. Compare two methods that quantify the same analyte, using linear regression and the *t* test for paired specimens
5. Interpret the results of an interference experiment
6. Interpret the results of a recovery experiment
7. Use the *F* test to compare the precisions of two methods for the same analyte
8. Plan an experiment for determining reportable range
9. Plan, and interpret the results of, an experiment for determining a reference range

Key Terms

bias
cutoff
efficiency
false negative
false positive
interference experiment
negative predictive value (NPV)
positive predictive value (PPV)
prevalence
recovery experiment
referent value
reportable range
sensitivity
specificity
true negative
true positive

Chapter Outline

★ **TABLE 12-1** The Four Possible Outcomes of a Diagnostic Test

	Positive	Negative	TOTAL
Condition present	TP	FN	TP + FN
Condition absent	FP	TN	FP + TN
TOTAL	TP + FP	FN + TN	TP + FP + FN + TN

TP, true positive; FP, false positive; TN, true negative; FN, false negative.

To evaluate a new method or instrument in the laboratory, we must prove not only its accuracy and precision but also its ability to diagnose disorders correctly. Conducting laboratory tests that do not give meaningful results wastes time and money and needlessly confounds a physician's final diagnosis.

DIAGNOSTIC VALUE

A test used to diagnose disorders has four possible outcomes, summarized in Table 12-1 ★.

True positive (TP): a positive result for a patient who has the condition (correct result)

False positive (FP): a positive result for a patient who does not have the condition (wrong result)

True negative (TN): a negative result for a patient who does not have the condition (correct result)

False negative (FN): a negative result for a patient who has the condition (wrong result)

In an ideal world, all "positives" are true, and all "negatives" are true. In reality, however, there are always some false results, whether positive or negative, and a laboratory must factor this inevitability into its decision whether or not to adopt a new test.

Sensitivity

We want a diagnostic test to detect the medical condition in question in every patient who has the condition. **Sensitivity** is a measure of this capability. It is the number of true positives as a percentage of all the results that should have been positive:

$$\text{sensitivity} = \frac{TP}{TP + FN} \times 100\%$$

EQUATION 1

The sensitivity, then, tells us the probability that the test result will be positive when the condition is present. In the notation of conditional probability, this is expressed as

$$P(T+ \mid C+)$$

which symbolizes the probability (P) of a positive test result ($T+$), given the presence of the condition (C+). For example, let us consider the hypothetical study summarized in Table 12-2 ★.

Because the test gave 105 true positives and 15 false negatives, Equation 1 yields a sensitivity of

$$\text{sensitivity} = \frac{105}{105 + 15} \times 100\% = 88\%$$

★ **TABLE 12-2** Hypothetical Data for Illustrating the Diagnostic Properties of a Laboratory Test

	Positive	Negative	TOTAL
Condition present	105	15	120
Condition absent	4	176	180
TOTAL	109	191	300

What this means is that the test will detect the condition in 88 out of every 100 patients who have it.

If there were no false negatives, then *FN* would be 0 and the sensitivity would be 100%; in such a case, the method would detect the condition whenever it is present. Sensitivity, then, reflects the test's ability to rule *out* a particular medical condition because, as sensitivity increases, it is less likely that a person with a negative test result has the condition. Because a highly sensitive test returns few false negatives, a negative result from the test is probably correct.

High sensitivity is desired when the suspected medical condition is serious and treatable and when a false positive does not have harmful consequences. Both the clinic and the laboratory try to detect every case. A false positive does not *necessarily* pose a problem because the test can be repeated and because there are usually other tests the patient can undergo.

Specificity

We want a diagnostic test to detect *only* the medical condition in question. **Specificity** is a measure of this capability. It is the number of true negatives as a percentage of all the results that should have been negative:

EQUATION 2

$$\text{specificity} = \frac{TN}{TN + FP} \times 100\%$$

The specificity, then, tells us the probability of a negative result when the condition is absent. In the notation of conditional probability, this is expressed as

$$\mathrm{P(T-|C-)}$$

which symbolizes the probability (P) of a negative test result (T−), given the absence of the condition (C−).

Consider the same hypothetical data as above (Table 12-2). Because the test gave 176 true negatives and 4 false positives, Equation 2 yields a specificity of

$$\text{specificity} = \frac{176}{176 + 4} \times 100\% = 98\%$$

What this means is that the test will give a negative result in 98 out of every 100 patients who do not have the condition. If there were no false positives, then *FP* would be 0 and the specificity would be 100%; in such a case, the method would detect only the condition of interest. Specificity, then, reflects the test's ability to rule *in* a particular medical condition because, as specificity increases, it is more likely that a person with a positive result actually has the condition. Because a highly specific test returns few false positives, a positive result from the test is probably correct.

We desire high specificity when the suspected medical condition is serious but not treatable, in which case a false positive can cause emotional or financial harm, or even medical harm if a dangerous treatment is attempted. If the diagnosis is accurate (true positive), little or nothing can be done to change the clinical course; if the case is missed (false negative), either new symptoms or a worsening of current symptoms will bring the patient back to the physician for further testing.

Efficiency

The **efficiency** (also called *accuracy*) is a quantity that tells us the probability that a result, whether positive or negative, is correct. It represents the number of correct diagnoses as a percentage of all the diagnoses:

EQUATION 3

$$\text{efficiency} = \frac{TP + TN}{TP + FP + TN + FN} \times 100\%$$

Using the hypothetical data from Table 12-2 above, we see that 94 out of every 100 test results are correct:

$$\text{efficiency} = \frac{105 + 176}{105 + 4 + 176 + 15} \times 100\% = 94\%$$

High efficiency is desired when the condition is both serious and treatable and when a false positive and a false negative are equally injurious. A false positive might lead to needless and harmful intervention, such as surgery, chemotherapy, or radiation, whereas a false negative might delay vital treatment.

Prevalence

The **prevalence** is the frequency of the condition in the population tested at a given time. It is the number of persons who have the condition expressed as a percentage of all people who have similar demographic and clinical characteristics:

$$\text{prevalence} = \frac{\text{persons with condition}}{\text{all people in the population}} = \frac{TP + FN}{TP + FP + TN + FN} \times 100\%$$

EQUATION 4

In the notation of conditional probability, this is expressed as

$$P(C+)$$

which symbolizes the probability (P) of having the condition (C+).

For example, if 6000 individuals have whooping cough in a population of 1,000,000, then the prevalence of whooping cough in that population is

$$\text{prevalence} = \frac{6000}{1{,}000{,}000} \times 100\% = 0.6\%$$

Predictive Value

The predictive value of a positive result, or **positive predictive value (PPV)**, tells us the likelihood that a "positive" result is correct. It is the number of true positives as a percentage of all the positives:

$$\text{positive predictive value (PPV)} = \frac{TP}{TP + FP} \times 100\%$$

EQUATION 5

In the notation of conditional probability, this is expressed as

$$P(C+ \mid T+)$$

which symbolizes the probability (P) of having the condition (C+), given a positive test result (T+).

Using the hypothetical data in Table 12-2, we see that a positive result from this method is correct 96 times out of every 100:

$$\text{positive predictive value (PPV)} = \frac{105}{105 + 4} \times 100\% = 96\%$$

Similarly, the predictive value of a negative result, or **negative predictive value (NPV)**, gives the likelihood that a "negative" result is correct. It is the number of true negatives as a percentage of all the negatives:

$$\text{negative predictive value (NPV)} = \frac{TN}{TN + FN} \times 100\%$$

EQUATION 6

In the notation of conditional probability, this is expressed as

$$P(C- \mid T-)$$

which symbolizes the probability (P) of not having the condition (C−), given a negative test result (T−).

Again using the hypothetical data in Table 12-2, we see that a negative result from this method is correct 92 times out of every 100:

$$\text{negative predictive value (NPV)} = \frac{176}{176 + 15} \times 100\% = 92\%$$

The sensitivity and specificity are measures of a diagnostic test's power to discriminate between the presence and absence of a medical condition. However, to determine the likelihood that a particular patient has a condition after a test result has been reported, the predictive value is determinative. The PPV of 96%, calculated from the hypothetical data in the previous example, tells us that 96 out of every 100 people who test positive actually have the condition in question. High positive predictive value is imperative for conditions in which a false positive might cause harm.

There is a common misconception that a positive result from a test with a high sensitivity means that there is a high probability of having the condition. Consider a population of 100,000 people. If the prevalence of soy-protein allergy in that population is 0.5%, then the condition is present in 500 individuals and absent from the other 99,500. If the sensitivity of the test for this allergy is 92%, then the 500 afflicted persons will give 460 positive results and 40 negative. Moreover, if the specificity of the test is 88%, then the 99,500 persons who do not have the allergy will give 87,560 negative results and 11,940 positive.

Therefore, the probability that a person with a positive test result actually is allergic to soy protein is equal to the positive predictive value:

$$\text{PPV} = \frac{TP}{TP + FP} = \frac{460}{460 + 11{,}940} \times 100\% = 4\%$$

Only four out of every 100 positive test results are true, even though both the sensitivity and specificity of the test are high. What this example demonstrates is that values for sensitivity and specificity alone can be misleading. Although they are properties of a diagnostic test that should be consistent from one patient to the next under similar circumstances, predictive value varies with the prevalence of the condition in question, and it can change between populations even if the sensitivity and specificity of the test remain the same. For example, if the prevalence of allergy to soy protein were 2.5%, not 0.5% as above, then using the same laboratory test with the same sensitivity (92%) and specificity (88%) would yield a PPV of 16%, which is higher by a factor of 4.

The PPV is related to the prevalence, sensitivity, and specificity by this equation:

EQUATION 7

$$\text{PPV} = \frac{(\text{sensitivity})(\text{prevalence})}{(\text{sensitivity})(\text{prevalence}) + \underbrace{(1 - \text{specificity})}_{\substack{\text{fraction of} \\ \text{false positives} \\ P(T+\,|\,C-) \\ = \frac{FP}{TN + FP}}}\underbrace{(1 - \text{prevalence})}_{\substack{\text{probability of not having} \\ \text{the condition} \\ P(C-) \\ = \frac{FP + TN}{TP + FP + TN + FN}}}} \times 100\%$$

in which prevalence, sensitivity, and specificity are expressed as decimals, not as percentages.

Notice that, as the prevalence approaches 1.0 (100%), the influence of the fraction of false positives diminishes. In other words, not surprisingly, if nearly everyone in a population has the condition in question, then false positives become very rare, and the PPV approaches 100%. The upshot of this equation is the fact that, if a test is worth using, then its positive predictive value is greater than the prevalence of the condition. This is so because, if a positive result from the test has no greater power to predict a condition than does merely knowing the frequency of the condition, then the test is no more diagnostically useful than is the prevalence.

Binary Interpretation of Numerical Data

Most clinical questions are binary in that they have a "yes" or "no" answer, whereas most test results are numerical and lie on a continuum. For example, a diagnosis of diabetes, which is a yes-or-no decision, comes from numerical data on the glucose concentration in the blood. At this writing, a fasting blood

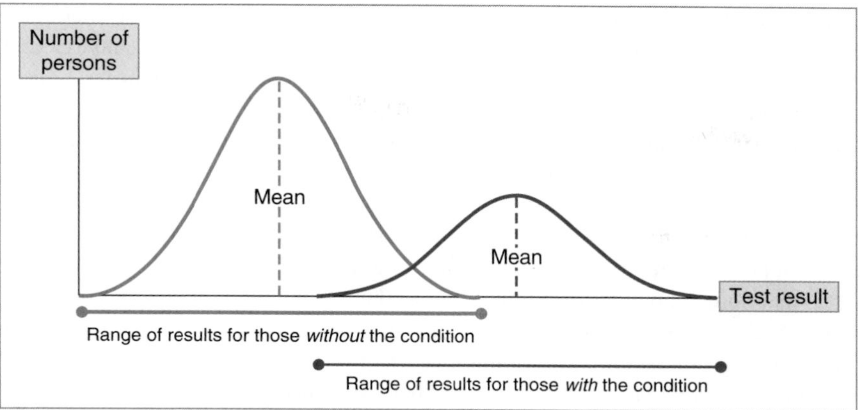

FIGURE 12-1 Classic overlapping distributions of persons with a particular medical condition (blue) and those without it (pink).

glucose concentration of at least 126 mg/dL indicates diabetes (when confirmed on another day).[1] In other words, "126 mg/dL" is the **referent value** or **cutoff**. But how do we go about converting a numerical test result into a yes-or-no clinical diagnosis?

Figure 12-1 depicts the classic overlapping distributions of persons with a given medical condition (blue curve) and of persons without it (pink curve). The mean test result for those with the condition (blue dashed line) is obviously higher than the mean test result for those without the condition (pink dashed line). Nevertheless, results in the low end of the blue curve, which represents persons with the condition, are observed also in the high end of the pink curve, which represents persons without the condition. Thus, there is a range of results in common between those with and those without the condition.

The orange vertical line in Figure 12-2A represents a referent value (a cutoff) for deciding whether a particular patient has the condition in question. If the test result is above the referent value, then the

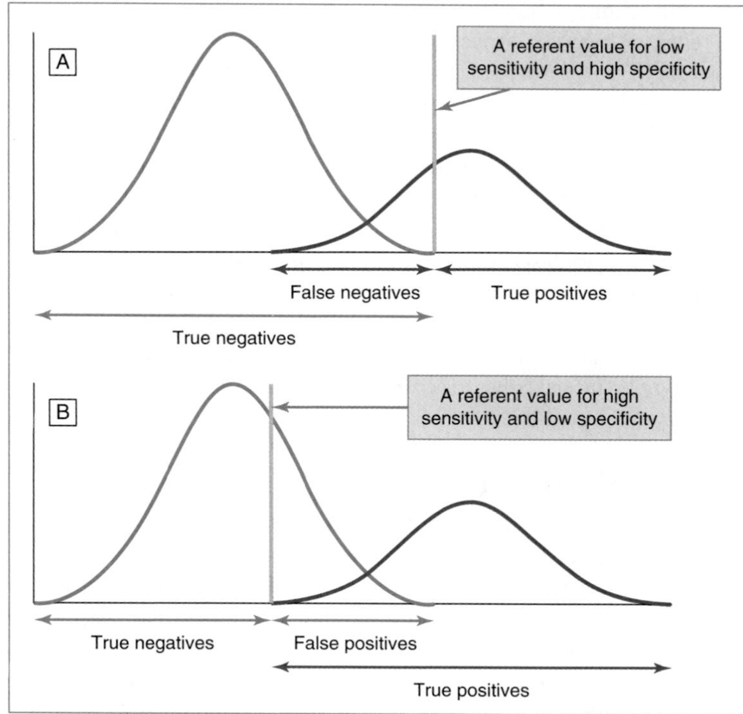

FIGURE 12-2 Effect of shifting the referent value (cutoff) on sensitivity and specificity. (*A*) The chosen cutoff eliminates false positives and maximizes specificity by compromising sensitivity. (*B*) The chosen cutoff eliminates false negatives and maximizes sensitivity by compromising specificity.

[1]National Diabetes Information Clearinghouse (2010). *Diagnosis of diabetes*. Retrieved from http://diabetes.niddk.nih.gov/dm/pubs/diagnosis/.

patient is considered to have the condition; if the result is below the referent value, then the patient is considered not to have the condition. Notice that, because all persons whose test results exceed the cutoff have the condition, we can see there are no false positives; thus, the specificity of the test is high, making it suitable for a serious but untreatable condition, as mentioned previously. In contrast, notice that there are persons who have the condition (blue curve) but whose test results fall below the cutoff. The test gives false negatives, and its sensitivity is accordingly low.

In order to eliminate the false negatives, we might move the referent value to the left, that is, to a lower result. Figure 12-2B shows the effect of such a change. All persons who have the condition (blue curve) now test positive; thus, the sensitivity is high and the test is suitable for a serious and treatable condition, as mentioned above. However, even though there are no longer false negatives, there are now false positives, with many persons who do not have the condition (pink curve) giving test results above the cutoff. Accordingly, the specificity is low.

Establishing a referent value is a compromise between sensitivity and specificity, requiring us to assign relative importance to false positivity and false negativity. False positives carry emotional and financial repercussions, as mentioned earlier, but they also necessitate what may be the difficult removal of a positive diagnosis from a patient's medical history after the mistake is discovered. False negatives, however, may cause a delay in life-saving treatment.

A systematic approach to optimizing referent values and to comparing diagnostic tests involves the use of receiver-operating characteristic curves (ROC curves) and likelihood ratios. Appendix 12-4 on the website discusses these tools in detail.

APPENDIX 12-4
"ROC Curves and Likelihood Ratios"
www.myhealthprofessions.kit.com
PEARSON myhealthprofessionskit

QUALITY ASSURANCE FOR METHODS AND INSTRUMENTS

Quality assurance is a comprehensive program of analyzing preanalytical, analytical, and postanalytical processes for the testing of patient specimens. Quality control, which Chapter 11 discusses, is only one part of a quality-assurance program. Another important part is that of verifying and establishing the performance specifications of methods and instruments that a laboratory employs.

The Clinical Laboratory Improvement Act of 1988 (CLIA 88) standardized the regulations governing all aspects of the clinical laboratory. Since their first publishing in 1992, these regulations have been updated to reflect changes in science and technology. The most recent changes (Sect. 493.1253) obligate the laboratory to *verify* a manufacturer's performance specifications for any test put into use on or after April 24, 2003, if that test has been approved by the FDA and if the laboratory has not modified it. Those specifications consist of (1) accuracy, (2) precision, and (3) reportable range (the highest and lowest results that are accurate). The laboratory also must show that the manufacturer's reference ranges are appropriate for the laboratory's patient population.

However, the laboratory must *establish* performance specifications for FDA-approved tests that the laboratory has modified, for tests not subject to FDA approval (e.g., tests developed in-house), and for tests for which the manufacturer does not provide specifications. Those specifications consist of (1) accuracy, (2) precision, (3) analytical sensitivity, (4) analytical specificity, (5) reportable range, (6) reference ranges, and (7) any other characteristic required for test performance.

The laboratory is not required either to verify or to establish performance specifications for any test that it was using before April 24, 2003.

Verifying or Establishing Accuracy

Chapters 3 and 8 define *accuracy* as the degree of correctness of a result, that is, how close an actual result comes to its true value. For evaluating a new method or instrument, a common approach to determining accuracy is to compare, for two or three dozen specimens, the results obtained by the method under evaluation with the results obtained by an established reference method. Each specimen is divided into two aliquots, one being tested on the new method and the other on the reference method. We then plot the results for the new method against those for the reference method and examine the relationship between the two sets of results. Figures 12-3 ■ and 12-4 ■ depict this kind of experiment: a comparison of two methods for the quantification of serum glucose.

In an ideal scenario (Figure 12-3), the two methods return the same value for every specimen and the data points lie on a straight line described by a very simple equation: $y = x$. The slope is 1, the y-intercept is 0, and the correlation coefficient (r) is 1. By contrast, in a realistic scenario (Figure 12-4), not every point lies on the regression line. The slope of the line differs slightly from 1 and the y-intercept differs slightly from 0. Nevertheless, the correlation coefficient can be high (0.991 in this example).

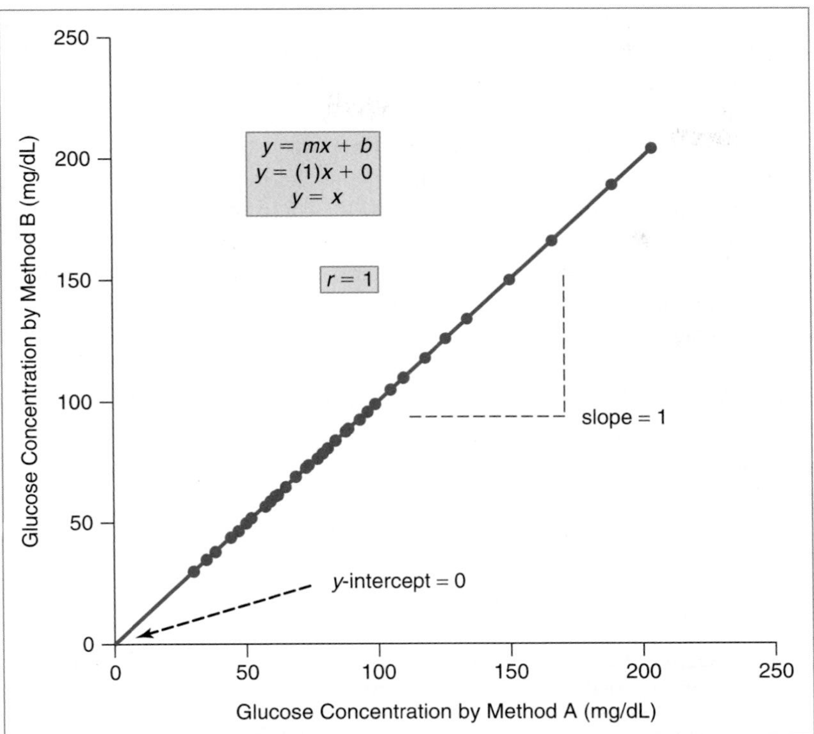

■ **FIGURE 12-3** An idealized comparison of two methods for the quantification of serum glucose. The two methods return the same value for every specimen; thus, the regression lines makes a 45° angle to the origin, every data point lies on the line, and the correlation is perfect. The equation is $y = (1)x + 0$, or $y = x$.

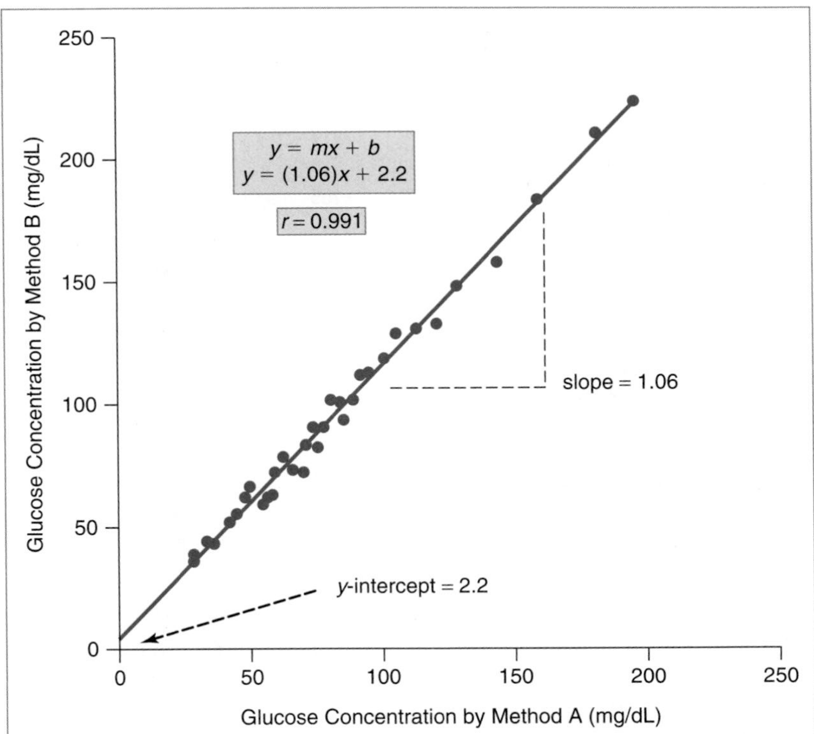

■ **FIGURE 12-4** A realistic comparison of two methods for the quantification of serum glucose. Not all the points lie on the regression line, but the correlation is high ($r = 0.991$). The slope is close to, but not exactly, 1. The *y*-intercept is close to, but not exactly, 0.

As Chapter 8 explained (see Table 8-2 and the corresponding text), the correlation coefficient is an appropriate statistic for method comparison because both variables are measured.

Because each specimen was run under the new method *and* the reference method, the paired *t* test (Equation 14 in Chapter 8) can help us decide whether the two methods differ significantly in the results they give. The example in Chapter 8 compares results from two instruments for the fictitious substance *M*. For the example here, however, let us use the data behind the graph in Figure 12-4.

Table 12-3 ★ summarizes those data. The *t* statistic is **−8.816** and there are 33 degrees of freedom. At $p = 0.01$, therefore, the critical value is between −2.787 (25 d.f.) and −2.678 (50 d.f.). Because the calculated value of *t* is more extreme, we conclude that the two methods differ significantly from each other in the results they return for serum glucose. Therefore, method B has a **bias**, which is defined as the difference between the average result from the new method and the average result from the reference method:

EQUATION 8

$$\text{bias} = \text{mean result from new method} - \text{mean result from reference method}$$

In this case, the bias is

$$\text{bias} = 94.0\text{ mg/dL (method B)} - 86.3\text{ mg/dL (method A)}\ \text{bias} = 7.7\text{ mg/dL}$$

★ **TABLE 12-3** Using the *t* Test for Paired Samples to Compare Two Methods for Quantifying Serum Glucose

Glucose Conc. (mg/dL)			Glucose Conc. (mg/dL) *(continued)*		
Method A	Method B	A–B	Method A	Method B	A–B *(continued)*
30	37	−7	79	80	−1
30	34	−4	81	88	−7
35	42	−7	84	99	−15
38	41	−3	88	98	−10
44	50	−6	89	91	−2
47	53	−6	93	99	−6
50	60	−10	96	109	−13
52	64	−12	99	110	−11
57	57	0	105	116	−11
59	60	−1	110	126	−16
61	61	0	118	128	−10
62	70	−8	126	130	−4
65	76	−11	134	145	−11
69	71	−2	150	155	−5
73	70	3	166	180	−14
74	81	−7	189	207	−18
77	88	−11	204	220	−16
				MEAN ($\bar{D}$) =	−8
				VARIANCE (s^2) =	28
				n =	34
				t-STATISTIC =	−8.816

(Equation 14 in Chapter 8, paired samples)

$$t = \frac{\bar{D}}{\sqrt{\frac{s^2}{n}}}$$

Note: These data are plotted in Figure 12-4.

A bias can be positive or negative, depending on whether the new method's mean result is greater than or less than that of the reference method.

Detecting Constant Systematic Error

The presence of interfering substances in specimens is one of the causes of constant systematic error (see Figure 11-5 in Chapter 11). An **interference experiment** is a paired comparison in which one aliquot is spiked with a selected substance that may interfere with the assay (e.g., a drug or bilirubin). The other aliquot is not spiked, although it does receive enough diluent to equalize volumes. The total constant systematic error is the value of the y-intercept, which, in the absence of interference, should be 0.

Detecting Proportional Systematic Error

A **recovery experiment** detects proportional systematic error (see Figure 11-5 in Chapter 11), and it gives the same information as does a method comparison. Therefore, if the slope calculated from a method comparison shows little or no proportional systematic error, then a recovery experiment might be unnecessary.

In a recovery experiment, the specimens are split into aliquots; the target analyte is added in known quantity to one aliquot, and diluent is added to the other (the "baseline" aliquot) to equalize the volumes. We calculate the recovery from these formulas:

$$\text{conc. recovered} = (\text{conc. in spiked aliquot}) - (\text{conc. in baseline aliquot})$$

EQUATION 9

$$\%\ \text{recovery} = \frac{\text{conc. recovered}}{\text{conc. added}} \times 100\%$$

EQUATION 10

In general, the percent recovery is acceptable when between 95% and 105%.

Ascertaining Precision

We can compare the precision of a new method with that of a reference method by means of the F test, which Chapter 8 presents in detail (see Equation 11 in Chapter 8). For the data presented in Table 12-3, the F test gives a ratio of <u>**1.143**</u>:

$$F = \frac{\text{variance}_{\text{method B}}}{\text{variance}_{\text{method A}}} = \frac{2151}{1882} = 1.143$$

For 33 degrees of freedom in the numerator and in the denominator, the critical value is hard to locate in published tables, even though they abound on the Internet. But multiples of 10 are easy to find. For 30 degrees of freedom (at a p value of 0.05), the critical value is 1.8408, whereas for 60 degrees of freedom, it is 1.5343. Therefore, the critical value for 33 degrees of freedom is between 1.5343 and 1.8408. Because the calculated value of 1.143 does not exceed the critical value, we cannot conclude that method B is more precise than method A.

DETERMINING REPORTABLE RANGE

An assay is said to be "linear" when the assayed concentration of a given analyte is directly proportional to the analyte's true concentration in the specimen being tested (or assayed count *vs.* true count, or assayed activity *vs.* true activity). After all, if an analyte's true concentration triples, the physician should rightly expect the reported result also to triple. Although in some testing systems the mathematical relationship between *assay response* and concentration is inherently nonlinear (for example, competitive-binding assays), that relationship should yield final results that satisfy the requirement for linearity between assayed concentration and true concentration.

As stated earlier, the **reportable range** represents the highest and lowest results that are accurate. Verifying or establishing the reportable range entails running several specimens of known concentrations that span the analytical range; two of those concentrations should challenge the upper and lower limits of the assay. We then evaluate the linearity of the results and identify the reportable range. Analysis of the linearity is carried out by means of the techniques explained in Chapter 8: visual inspection, linear regression, root-mean-squared error, standard error of the slope, confidence intervals, and the coefficient of determination. Other tools exist for this purpose, one example being the polynomial method. Appendix 12-1 on the website discusses the polynomial method in detail.

APPENDIX 12-1
"Polynomials and the Polynomial Method for Evaluating Nonlinearity"
www.myhealthprofessions.kit.com
PEARSON myhealthprofessionskit

Five concentrations should be tested, each one in triplicate. This is so because, if the relationship between assayed result and true result is sigmoidal, then running only four concentrations may fail to capture it. The other possible relationships—lines, hyperbolas, and parabolas—are detectable with fewer than five points. Consult Appendix 12-2 on the website for elaboration.

APPENDIX 12-2
"Capturing the Curves in Linearity Testing"
www.myhealthprofessions.kit.com
PEARSON myhealthprofessionskit

DETERMINING REFERENCE RANGES

When verifying or establishing a reference range, we should have 100–150 specimens that represent the laboratory's patient population. If the data have a normal distribution (see Figure 8-2 in Chapter 8), then the reference range runs from 2 SD below the mean up to 2 SD above the mean, an interval that includes 95% of all results (see Figure 8-3 in Chapter 8). If the data are not normally distributed, then we must employ an alternative approach to find the central 95%.

One such approach, often called "nonparametric ranking" or the "ranked percentile method," starts by ordering the data values from lowest to highest. The value that corresponds to 2.5% of the data defines the low end of the reference range, whereas the value that corresponds to 97.5% of the data defines the high end. Identifying these two values is tantamount to dropping the highest and lowest 2.5% of all the data points. An example follows.

Suppose we have 125 results with which to establish the reference range for a new assay in our laboratory. We begin by ranking the results in ascending order:

Rank	Value
1	9
2	11
3	11
4	13
5	14
6	16
.	.
.	.
.	.
120	82
121	82
122	84
123	85
124	87
125	89

The result occupying the 2.5% position is

$$2.5\% \times 125 = 3.1 \text{ (rank 3)}$$

which corresponds to a value of "11." All results below this value represent the lowest 2.5% of the data. Next, the result occupying the 97.5% position is

$$97.5\% \times 125 = 121.9 \text{ (rank 122)}$$

which corresponds to a value of "84." All results above this value represent the highest 2.5% of the data. Therefore, the reference range becomes "11–84," encompassing the central 95% of all the results.

Summary

1. *Sensitivity* is a measure of a test's ability to detect the medical condition in question in every patient who has the condition. High sensitivity is desired when the suspected medical condition is serious and treatable and when a false positive does not have harmful consequences.

$$\text{sensitivity} = \frac{TP}{TP + FN} \times 100\%$$

2. *Specificity* is a measure of a test's ability to detect only the medical condition in question. High specificity is desired when the suspected medical condition is serious but not treatable.

$$\text{specificity} = \frac{TN}{TN + FP} \times 100\%$$

3. *Efficiency* is a quantity that tells us the probability that a result, whether positive or negative, is correct. High efficiency is desired when the condition is both serious and treatable and when a false positive and false negative have equally injurious consequences.

$$\text{efficiency} = \frac{TP + TN}{TP + FP + TN + FN} \times 100\%$$

4. *Prevalence* is the frequency of the condition in the population tested at a given time.

$$\text{prevalence} = \frac{\text{persons with condition}}{\text{all people in the population}} = \frac{TP + FN}{TP + FP + TN + FN} \times 100\%$$

5. The predictive value of a positive result, or *positive predictive value (PPV)*, tells us the likelihood that a "positive" result is correct.

$$\text{positive predictive value (PPV)} = \frac{TP}{TP + FP} \times 100\%$$

6. The predictive value of a negative result, or *negative predictive value (NPV)*, gives the likelihood that a "negative" result is correct.

$$\text{negative predictive value (NPV)} = \frac{TN}{TN + FN} \times 100\%$$

7. The PPV is related to the prevalence, sensitivity, and specificity:

$$\text{PPV} = \frac{(\text{sensitivity})(\text{prevalence})}{(\text{sensitivity})(\text{prevalence}) + (1 - \text{specificity})(1 - \text{prevalence})} \times 100\%$$

8. The *referent value*, or *cutoff*, is the value above which the patient is said to have the specified medical condition and below which the patient is said not to have it.
9. Establishing a referent value is a compromise between sensitivity and specificity. False positives carry emotional and financial repercussions, and false negatives may cause a delay in life-saving treatment.
10. Quality assurance is a comprehensive program of analyzing preanalytical, analytical, and postanalytical processes for the testing of patient specimens.
11. The Clinical Laboratory Improvement Act of 1988 (CLIA 88) standardized the regulations governing all aspects of the clinical laboratory.
12. The laboratory must verify a manufacturer's performance specifications (accuracy, precision, reportable range) for any test put into use on or after April 24, 2003, if that test has been approved by the FDA and if the laboratory has not modified it.
13. The laboratory must establish performance specifications for FDA-approved tests that the laboratory has modified, for tests not subject to FDA approval, and for tests for which the manufacturer does not provide specifications. Those specifications consist of (a) accuracy, (b) precision, (c) analytical sensitivity, (d) analytical specificity, (e) reportable range, (f) reference ranges, and (g) any other characteristic required for test performance.
14. A common approach to determining accuracy is to compare, for two or three dozen specimens, the results obtained by the method under evaluation with the results obtained by an established reference method. Each specimen is divided into two aliquots, one being tested on the new method and the other on the reference method. We then plot the results for the new method against those for the reference method and examine the relationship between the two sets of results.
15. *Bias* is the difference between the average result from the new method and the average result from the reference method:

$$\text{bias} = \text{mean result from new method} - \text{mean result from reference method}$$

16. An *interference experiment* is a paired comparison in which one aliquot is spiked with a selected substance that may interfere with the assay. The other aliquot is not spiked, although it does receive enough diluent to equalize volumes. The total constant systematic error is the value of the *y*-intercept, which, in the absence of interference, should be 0.

17. In a *recovery experiment*, which detects proportional systematic error, the specimens are split into aliquots; the target analyte is added in known quantity to one aliquot, and diluent is added to the other (the "baseline" aliquot) to equalize the volumes. In general, the percent recovery is acceptable when between 95% and 105%.

$$\text{conc. recovered} = (\text{conc. in spiked aliquot}) - (\text{conc. in baseline aliquot})$$

$$\% \text{ recovery} = \frac{\text{conc. recovered}}{\text{conc. added}} \times 100\%$$

18. We can compare the precision of a new method with that of a reference method by means of the *F* test:

$$F = \frac{\text{variance}_{\text{method B}}}{\text{variance}_{\text{method A}}}$$

19. An assay is said to be "linear" when the final result for a given analyte is directly proportional to the analyte's true result for the specimen being tested.

20. The *reportable range* represents the highest and lowest results that are accurate. Verifying or establishing the reportable range entails running several specimens of known concentrations that span the analytical range; two of those concentrations should challenge the upper and lower limits of the assay.

21. When verifying or establishing a reference range, we should have 100–150 specimens that represent the laboratory's patient population. If the data have a normal distribution, then the reference range runs from 2 SD below the mean up to 2 SD above the mean. If the data are not normally distributed, then we must employ an alternative approach to find the central 95%.

22. "Nonparametric ranking" is one alternative. It starts by ordering the data values from lowest to highest. The value that corresponds to 2.5% of the data defines the low end of the reference range, whereas the value that corresponds to 97.5% of the data defines the high end.

Practice and Contextual Problems

1. (LO 1, 2, 3) Twenty-five adult patients with fever are tested for bacteremia (presence of bacteria in the blood). The following table presents leukocyte counts ($\times 10^3$ cells/mm^3) for patients who tested negative for bacteremia and for those who tested positive.

(−) Bacteremia	(+) Bacteremia
6.2	13.6
9.3	18.1
8.8	15.6
11.7	27.0
7.0	10.5
9.3	18.7
6.8	20.5
7.9	12.6
10.5	14.9
5.4	23.2
14.2	
7.8	
8.0	
10.9	
7.4	

(a) Calculate the prevalence of bacteremia in this population of patients with fever.

(b) Calculate the sensitivity and specificity when the cutoff value of the leukocyte count for diagnosing bacteremia is 10×10^3 cells/mm^3.

(c) How would raising the cutoff to 15×10^3 cells/mm^3 change the sensitivity and specificity?

(d) Calculate the positive predictive value for a cutoff of 10×10^3 cells/mm^3.

2. (LO 1) Consider a home HIV test that claims 99% sensitivity and 99% specificity. If a particular man runs the test on himself, according to directions, and the result is positive, what is the probability that he actually does have HIV? For men with demographic and clinical characteristics similar to his, HIV is present in 1 out of every 85,000 individuals.

3. (LO 1) A study was conducted to determine the usefulness of a new test for detecting human papilloma virus (HPV) in women. The data for the new test appear in the table below.

(a) Calculate the prevalence of HPV in this population as determined by the new test.

(b) Calculate the sensitivity and specificity of the new test.

(c) Calculate the positive and negative predictive values.

		Infection Status	
		Present	**Absent**
Test Result	Negative	16	280
	Positive	208	10

4. (LO 1) Suppose the prevalence of HIV is 0.3% in the population of 500,000 blood donors for your geographical area. However, among the patients at the substance-abuse clinic

in your hospital, the prevalence is 16%. The screening test for HIV has a sensitivity and specificity of 99.9%.

(a) Calculate the positive predictive value of the test for each of these two populations.

(b) If the substance-abuse clinic has 200 patients, how many of them are expected to have HIV?

(c) If there are 1132 positive results for blood donors, how many are false?

5. (LO 1) Your laboratory is evaluating two tests, *X* and *Y*, for their abilities to diagnose salmonellosis. The data appear in the two tables below.

(a) Calculate the sensitivity and specificity of each test.

(b) Which test, when its result is positive, is more reliable for diagnosing salmonellosis?

		Salmonellosis	
		Present	Absent
Result of Test *X*	Negative	0	317
	Positive	51	66

		Salmonellosis	
		Present	Absent
Result of Test *Y*	Negative	10	536
	Positive	72	4

6. (LO 1) The probability of rolling a 2, 3, 4, 5, or 6 on a single six-sided die is 83%. Suppose we officially interpret any of those five numbers as a negative result for myocardial infarction. We call this the "toss test."

(a) Calculate the specificity of the toss test.

(b) Although the toss test is patently absurd, what does it illustrate about the properties of sensitivity and specificity in general?

7. (LO 2, 3) Consider the two patient distributions appearing below, one for those without disease (pink) and the other for those with disease (blue). The orange vertical line represents the cutoff between negativity and positivity for the diagnostic test.

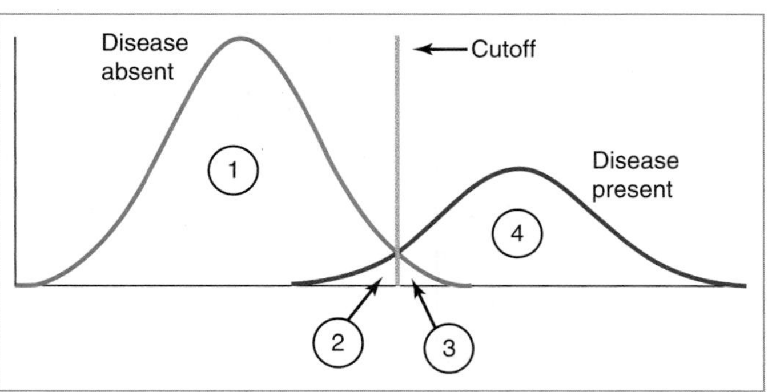

(a) Identify each of the four numbered areas by outcome (TP, FP, TN, FN).

(b) If the cutoff is shifted upward, how does the test's sensitivity change?

(c) Suppose the cutoff stands at two standard deviations above the mean for the pink curve. If the cutoff is moved to three standard deviations, how does the test's specificity change?

(d) Suppose the cutoff stands at two standard deviations below the mean for the blue curve. If the cutoff is moved to three standard deviations, how does the test's sensitivity change?

8. (LO 2, 3) Consider the two patient distributions appearing below, one for those without disease (pink) and the other for those with disease (blue).

(a) Explain whether the test is more suitable for a serious treatable disease or for a serious untreatable disease.

(b) Where should the cutoff be moved to render the test more suitable for the other kind of disease? Explain.

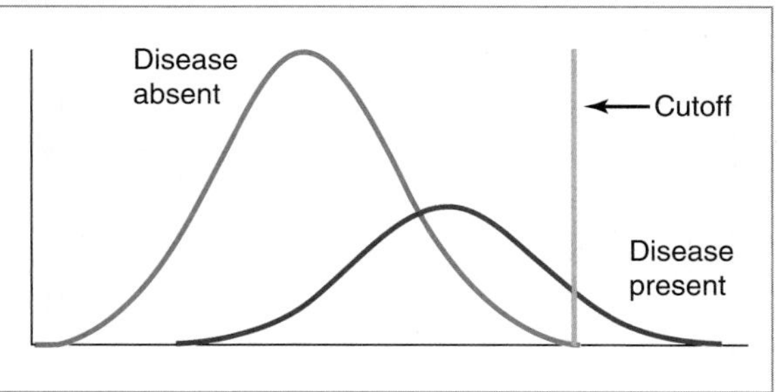

9. (LO 1, 2, 3) Suppose hormone Q is a marker for cancer when its concentration in the serum exceeds 200 ng/mL. Data on the diagnostic usefulness of hormone Q appear in the table below.

(a) What is the probability that a patient with a result < 200 ng/mL does not have cancer?

(b) What is the probability that a patient with a result > 200 ng/mL does have cancer?

(c) What is the probability that a given test result matches the diagnosis?

		Cancer	
		Present	Absent
Concentration of Hormone Q	< 200 ng/mL	59	399
	> 200 ng/mL	187	514

10. (LO 4) Solve Practice Problem 10 (a, b) in Chapter 8.

11. (LO 7) Solve Practice Problem 21 in Chapter 8.

12. (LO 7) Solve Contextual Problem 7 in Chapter 8.

13. (LO 6) A recovery experiment is performed for the validation of a new assay that quantifies chloride ion in serum.

Each test aliquot is spiked with an additional 6 mEq/L to a final volume of 150 μL, and diluent is added to each baseline aliquot to the same final volume. Calculate the average percentage of recovery. Each result in the table is the mean of triplicates.

Specimen	Conc. of Chloride (mEq/L)	
	Spiked Aliquot	Baseline Aliquot
1	107	101
2	106	99
3	110	105
4	106	100
5	102	96
6	110	104
7	106	101
8	114	108
9	105	100
10	109	104
11	103	101
12	105	98
13	113	106
14	117	110
15	105	99
16	110	103
17	106	100
18	115	111
19	115	108
20	107	102

14. (LO 4) For quantifying hemoglobin A_{1C} in whole blood, a laboratory is comparing its current analyzer with a new analyzer. Using the *t* test for paired specimens (Equation 14 in Chapter 8), determine whether the two analyzers differ significantly.

A_{1C} conc. (%)		A_{1C} conc. (%) *(continued)*	
Method A	Method B	Method A	Method B
6.2	6.1	9.0	8.6
3.9	4.5	4.6	5.0
9.8	8.9	6.0	6.2
5.0	5.1	5.4	5.2
4.7	5.2	4.7	5.0
4.8	4.7	5.2	5.2
5.9	6.1	6.6	6.9
4.0	4.4	7.9	7.8
13.2	13.8	4.9	4.2
7.1	6.9	4.2	4.3
4.5	4.2	12.2	13.0
5.2	5.0	6.0	5.9
6.1	6.5	5.1	5.1
4.9	5.0	7.6	7.4
4.8	5.0	4.6	4.4
10.7	10.3	4.8	5.0
8.3	8.8	5.0	5.0

15. (LO 9) From the following data for analyte Q, determine the reference range. The data are not normally distributed.

Rank	Value
1	0.23
2	0.23
3	0.25
4	0.26
5	0.27
6	0.29
7	0.32
.	.
.	.
.	.
157	1.33
158	1.39
159	1.42
160	1.44
161	1.49
162	1.57

PEARSON
myhealthprofessionskit™

Go to www.myhealthprofessionskit.com <http://www.myhealthprofessionskit.com/> to access the Companion Website created for this textbook. Simply select "Clinical Laboratory Science" from the choice of disciplines. Find this book and log in using your username and password to access additional practice problems, answers to the practice and contextual problems, additional information, and more.

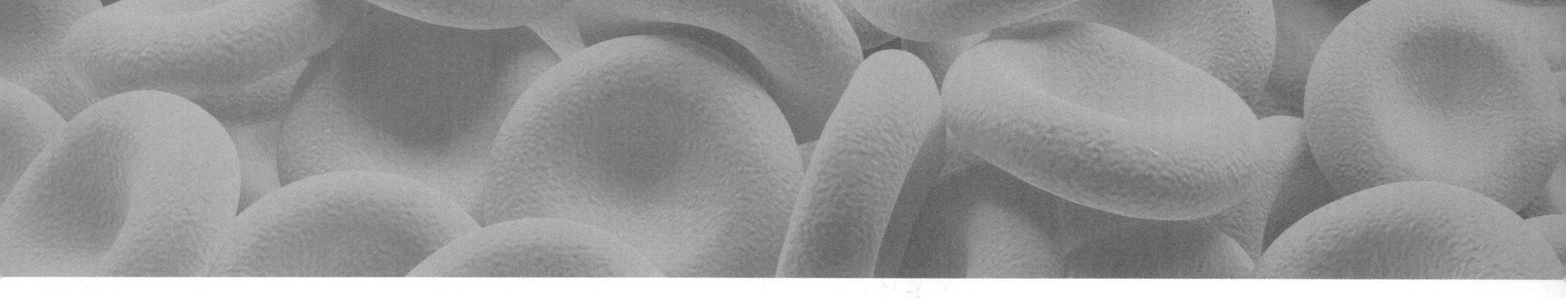

Frequently Asked Questions and Common Misunderstandings

Are the units "milliliter" and "cubic centimeter" interchangeable?
Are the constants K_M and K_S the same?
In calculating the standard deviation (SD), which denominator is better: n or $n-1$?
Is the coefficient of variation (CV) useable with positive and negative data values?
Is the standard deviation (SD) better than the mean absolute deviation (MAD)?
When is the p value misleading?
How is the p value misinterpreted?
How is the null hypothesis (H_0) misleading?
What do the terms "micron," "lambda," and "gamma" mean?
Can pH be negative?
When applied to acids and bases, are "strength" and "concentration" synonymous?
Why does the pH scale run from 1 to 14?
Why is "mcg," instead of "μg," sometimes used to abbreviate "microgram"?
Is there an easy way to rationalize the equations for Celsius–Fahrenheit conversions?
Why do only some equilibrium constants appear with units?
What are the criteria for choosing a measure of central tendency?

ARE THE UNITS "MILLILITER" AND "CUBIC CENTIMETER" INTERCHANGEABLE?

For almost all practical circumstances in a clinical setting, laboratories included, the answer to this question is "yes." In exacting scientific work, however, there is possibly a fine difference between these two units that may matter. The details follow.

In 1791, during the French Revolution, the National Assembly of France accepted a proposal from a commission of savants to define various units of measure. The unit of volume, eventually becoming known as the "liter," was defined as the volume of a cube with each side being one-tenth of a meter in length, that is, a volume of 1 cubic decimeter (dm^3).

The unit of mass, eventually called the "kilogram," was defined as the mass of one liter of distilled water at the temperature of melting ice. This followed naturally from the existing definition of "gram" as the mass of one cubic centimeter of water at that same temperature. Soon afterwards, however, it was argued that the temperature used should be the one at which the density of water is greatest (4°C). At that slightly higher temperature, it was discovered that one liter of water had an actual mass of 0.9999707 kg; that is, 1 kilogram actually occupied 1000.029—not 1000 exactly—cubic centimeters. Therefore, 1 milliliter equaled 1.000029 cm^3.

In 1901, the third meeting of the General Conference on Weights and Measures (*Conférence Général des Poids et Mesures* [CGPM]) decided officially to maintain the liter as the equivalent of 1000.029 cm^3 (the volume of 1 kilogram of pure water at maximum density and standard atmospheric pressure). In 1964, the 12th meeting of the CGPM abrogated that definition, declaring the term "liter" to be a special name for the cubic decimeter. This action reestablished the liter as a true volume by divorcing it from the kilogram. Nowadays, consequently, nearly all concerned parties treat the milliliter as being exactly equal to one cubic centimeter, although the tiny difference between them may affect measurements with certain existing volumetric ware, and only out at the fifth decimal place.

References

1. *Décret relatif aux poids et aux mesures*, Art. 5, 18 germinal an 3 (7 avril 1795).
2. Stott, V. (1929). The milliliter. *Nature*, 124, 622–623.
3. International Committee of Weights and Measures (1902). *Nature*, 65, 538.
4. General Conference on Weights and Measures, Bureau International des Poids et Mesures. Retrieved July 1, 2011, from http://www.bipm.org/en/convention/cgpm/.

ARE THE CONSTANTS K_M AND K_S THE SAME?

No, they are not the same. However, they sometimes can be treated as being equal when dissociation of the Michaelis complex (ES $\rightarrow$ E + S) is much faster than conversion of substrate to product (ES $\rightarrow$ E + P), that is, when $k_{-1} \gg k_2$.

IN CALCULATING THE STANDARD DEVIATION (SD), WHICH DENOMINATOR IS BETTER: *n* OR *n*–1?

The denominator $n-1$ is better. The alternative, n, is acceptable when its value is so high that it returns the same SD as does $n-1$.

IS THE COEFFICIENT OF VARIATION (CV) USEABLE WITH POSITIVE AND NEGATIVE DATA VALUES?

The CV makes sense only when every data value is positive. When both positive and negative values are present, one of three problems arises:

a. the mean is zero, in which case the CV cannot be computed;

b. the mean is less than zero, in which case the CV is negative (and meaningless); or

c. the mean is close to zero, in which case the CV can be misleading, even preposterous.

Consider an example of scenario **c**. Assume the following eight data values:

$$-7, -5, -3, -1, 1, 3, 5, 8$$

The mean of these values is 0.125 and the standard deviation is 5.11; therefore, the CV is 4089%. This means that the standard deviation is 40.89 times larger than the mean, implying that the data are spread very much farther apart than they really are. In this case, the CV is useless.

IS THE STANDARD DEVIATION (SD) BETTER THAN THE MEAN ABSOLUTE DEVIATION (MAD)?

The answer to this question depends on the person asked and on the information needed from a given analysis.

The MAD is the average absolute difference between the mean and the data values:

$$\text{MAD} = \frac{\sum_{i=1}^{n} |x_i - \overline{x}|}{n}$$

The SD, or *s*, is the square-root of the average *squared* difference between the mean and the data values:

$$SD = s = \sqrt{\frac{\sum_{i=1}^{n}(x_i - \bar{x})^2}{n - 1}}$$

Reasons to Prefer the SD over the MAD

1. The notation for absolute value is difficult to use in algebra and calculus. In the early 20th century, this property set the course for modern statistics, with the result that using the SD became traditional. Furthermore, its usefulness became compelling as statisticians discovered they could express the proportion of a normal distribution lying within a certain multiple of the SD.
2. Consider an experiment in which a large, normally distributed population is sampled repeatedly, and the SD and MAD are calculated for each sampling. The result is a set of SDs and a set of MADs. Under ideal conditions (absence of error in the observations), the standard deviation of the MAD values is greater than the standard deviation of the SD values.[1] This means that the SD is more consistent than the MAD at estimating the standard deviation (σ) of the whole population.
3. By squaring the differences between the mean and the data values, the SD captures whatever greater variation may be present in the data, whereas the MAD may not. For example, consider these two data sets: (*a*) 10, 10, 15, 20, 20 and (*b*) 13, 7, 15, 23, 17. Even though set *b* has more variation than set *a*, the MAD for each data set is 4. The SD, however, reflects the difference; it is 5.0 for set *a* and 5.8 for set *b*.

Reasons to Prefer the MAD over the SD

1. The MAD is less sensitive to outliers. The SD exaggerates larger deviations by squaring them; taking the square root of the sum of the squares does not fully offset the bias.
2. Under nonideal conditions, that is, where there are "naturally occurring deviations from the ideal model" as one would encounter in a scientific experiment, the MAD is more consistent than the SD at estimating the standard deviation (σ) of the whole population.[2] This is the opposite of what happens under ideal conditions (bullet #2 above, under "Reasons to prefer the SD over the MAD"). Thus, the MAD may be superior in real-world experiments, where vicissitudes are present in measurements and observations.
3. The MAD may be more appropriate than the SD for non-normal distributions,[1] which may be more common than is generally believed. Distributions that *seem* normal (*i.e.*, that are approximately normal) may not actually *be* normal, even in the clinical laboratory. There is a tendency to reject extreme values as outliers because they so greatly influence the SD, even though those values may be legitimate and may offer important information about the underlying phenomena at work.
4. The MAD is more intuitive than the SD. The average distance of the data values from their mean is more straightforward to interpret than is the square root of the average squared distance from that same mean.

References

1. Stigler, S. M. (1973). Studies in the history of probability and statistics. XXXII: Laplace, Fisher and the discovery of the concept of sufficiency. *Biometrika*, 60, 439–445.
2. Huber, P. J. (2004). *Robust statistics*. Hoboken, NJ: Wiley.

WHEN IS THE *p* VALUE MISLEADING?

The *p* value can be misleading whenever the sample size is too small or too large. If the sample size is too small, statistical significance may fail to appear, even if the effect is large. However, if the sample size is too large, even very small effects can show statistical significance.

HOW IS THE *p* VALUE MISINTERPRETED?

Researchers sometimes use the p value to answer the wrong question. The p value is the probability of obtaining the results that were actually observed if the null hypothesis (H_0) is true. The null hypothesis states that the two groups come from the same overall population, that is, that there is no real difference between the two groups. The question that the p value properly answers is the following.

a. What is the probability of observing a large difference between the means (D) if the two groups, control and experimental, are the same (H_0)? In short, what is the probability of D, given H_0?

However, the question that researchers often—and wrongly—try to answer with the p value is the reverse of **a:**

b. What is the probability that the two groups, control and experimental, are the same (H_0) if there is a large difference between their means (D)? In short, what is the probability of H_0, given D?

Here is a simple analogy. Consider question **c** and its reverse, question **d**.

c. What is the probability of a man's feet being purple (P) if he has been stomping red grapes (G)? In short, what is the probability of P, given G?

d. What is the probability that a man has been stomping red grapes (G) if his feet are purple (P)? In short, what is the probability of G, given P?

The probability in **c** is very high, perhaps 0.98, but the probability in **d** is lower, depending on the man's circumstances. Clearly, the two questions are not equivalent and they should not be treated as though they were.

The Correct and Incorrect Conclusions

Suppose we observe a large difference between the means for our control and experimental groups, with $p = 0.05$. If the null hypothesis is true, then it is *correct* to conclude that the large difference we saw, or a larger one, would occur five out of every 100 times we ran the experiment. Another way to say this is that, if the null hypothesis (H_0) is true, there is only a 5% probability of observing such a large difference between the means (D). With this conclusion, we have answered question **a**, for which the p value is appropriate.

It is *incorrect* to conclude that the null hypothesis (H_0) has a 5% probability of being true because there was such a large difference between the means (D). This conclusion would be an effort to answer question **b**, for which the p value is inappropriate. And it is this question that some researchers mistakenly answer with the p value.

Using the grape-stomping analogy, we *correctly* conclude that 98 out of every 100 men have purple feet (P) if all the men have been stomping red grapes (G). In other words, if the men have indeed been stomping red grapes (G), then there is a 98% probability of finding one with purple feet (P). This answers question **c**. However, we *incorrectly* conclude that a man has a 98% probability of having been stomping red grapes (G) if his feet are purple (P). This would be a mistaken effort to answer question **d**.

HOW IS THE NULL HYPOTHESIS (H_0) MISLEADING?

Strictly speaking, the assumption that H_0 is true is often, if not always, wrong. In other words, we do not know that there is no difference between the means of two groups. On the contrary, there probably *is* a difference. For example, if we are establishing reference ranges for analyte **Q** in the two sexes, we measure its concentration in randomly selected men and women. If we see no statistically significant difference between the means of the two groups, then we conclude that H_0 cannot be rejected.

However, if we measured the concentration of **Q** for every person in each sex (an impossible task), then there would almost certainly be a difference between the two means. Even if we failed to see such a difference at a precision of 0.1 mg/dL, it would appear as our precision increased, say to 0.0001 mg/dL. The only question would be that of the size, or clinical meaningfulness, of the difference. This is the reason that many researchers now report effect size in addition to, or instead of, the p value. For an explanation of effect size, see Advanced Topic II, "Effect Size."

WHAT DO THE TERMS "MICRON," "LAMBDA," AND "GAMMA" MEAN?

These terms come from older versions of the metric system, and are no longer acceptable in formal scientific or technical communications. However, some laboratorians still use them informally because of convenience or habit; so, it is reasonable to be familiar with them.

Micron = micrometer (μm)
Lambda = microliter (μL)
Gamma = microgram (μg)

CAN *p*H BE NEGATIVE?

Theoretically, yes, but a negative *p*H has little meaning. At a concentration of H^+ of 1 mol/L, the *p*H is 0. Therefore, as the concentration of H^+ rises above 1 mol/L, the *p*H becomes negative. The familiar equation

$$pH = -\log[H^+]$$

is valid only for dilute acids and bases, because *p*H is actually a function of activity rather than concentration (see Advanced Topic IV, "Activity as Opposed to Concentration"):

$$pH = -\log a_{H^+}$$

At high $[H^+]$ (or high $[OH^-]$), activity differs enough from concentration that *p*H readings are unreliable. At very high concentrations, such as those of concentrated acids and bases, the difference is so large that specific gravity must be used to express the amount present per unit volume.

WHEN APPLIED TO ACIDS AND BASES, ARE "STRENGTH" AND "CONCENTRATION" SYNONYMOUS?

No. The *strength* of an acid or base is its tendency to lose or accept a hydrogen ion, respectively. By contrast, the *concentration* of an acid or base is its amount in solution (per unit volume or weight), regardless of strength. For example, acetic acid (CH_3CO_2H) is a weak acid whether its concentration in a given solution is high or low. But even a weak acid, such as acetic, can be dangerous if its concentration is high.

WHY DOES THE *p*H SCALE RUN FROM 1 TO 14?

The *p*H scale runs from 1 to 14 because of the ion product of water (see Advanced Topic III, "Ion Product of Water"). In an aqueous solution, the concentrations of H^+ and OH^- always adjust themselves to keep their product equal to 1.0×10^{-14}:

$$[H^+][OH^-] = 1.0 \times 10^{-14}$$

Taking the negative logarithm of each side gives

$$-\log([H^+][OH^-]) = -\log(1.0 \times 10^{-14})$$

$$-\log[H^+] + -\log[OH^-] = 14$$

$$pH + pOH = 14$$

Just as the product of the $[H^+]$ and $[OH^-]$ is always 10^{-14}, the sum of the *p*H and the *p*OH is always 14. Therefore, the *p*H scale of 1 to 14 is convenient for the acids and bases usually encountered in clinical and research laboratories, because their concentrations fall between 10^{-1} M (*p*H 1) and 10^{-14} M (*p*H 14). And whenever the concentration lies outside that range (i.e., whenever the *p*H is less than 1 or greater than 14), its value is unreliable anyway (see Advanced Topic IV, "Activity as Opposed to Concentration").

Consider an example of K_W in operation. If NaOH is added to water to a concentration of 0.01 M, then the final concentration of OH^- in the solution is 0.01 M plus the starting concentration of OH^-, which was 1.0×10^{-7} M:

$$[OH^-]_{final} = 0.01\ \text{M} + 1.0 \times 10^{-7}\ \text{M} = 0.0100001\ \text{M}$$

However, the starting amount is so small relative to the added amount that the final concentration is, for all practical purposes, the same as 0.01 M:

$$[OH^-]_{final} = 0.01\ \text{M}$$

In response to this increase in the concentration of OH^-, the concentration of H^+ falls from 1.0×10^{-7} M down to 1.0×10^{-12} M, in order to satisfy K_W:

$$K_W = [H^+][OH^-] = (1.0 \times 10^{-12}\ \text{M})(0.01\ \text{M}) = 1.0 \times 10^{-14}\ \text{M}^2$$

This adjusted H^+ concentration corresponds to a *p*H of 12.

WHY IS "mcg," INSTEAD OF "μg," SOMETIMES USED TO ABBREVIATE "MICROGRAM"?

The proper symbol for the prefix "micro" is the Greek letter *micron*, or "μ." Some clinics and hospitals, however, prefer the abbreviation "mc" because the handwritten letter "μ" can be mistaken for "M" or "m." In those clinical settings, therefore, "mcg" refers to a microgram (and "mcL" to a microliter). In formal scientific contexts, however, the abbreviation "mcg" refers to a millicentigram, which actually equals 10 micrograms:

$$1\ \text{mcg} = 1 \times 0.001 \times 0.01\ \text{g} = 0.00001\ \text{g} = 10 \times 10^{-6}\ \text{g} = 10\ \mu\text{g}$$

IS THERE AN EASY WAY TO RATIONALIZE THE EQUATIONS FOR CELSIUS–FAHRENHEIT CONVERSIONS?

To remember the equations more easily, memorize the ratio 180/100, or 9/5. From the freezing point to the boiling point, there are 180 degrees on the Fahrenheit scale (32° ⟶ 212°) and 100 on the Celsius scale (0° ⟶ 100°):

100°C — 212°F

Δ = 100 C° — Δ = 180 F°

0°C — 32°F

Therefore, there are 9 Fahrenheit degrees for every 5 Celsius degrees:

$$\frac{180\ \text{F}^\circ}{100\ \text{C}^\circ} = \frac{9\ \text{F}^\circ}{5\ \text{C}^\circ}$$

This means that the slope of the line relating Fahrenheit (*y*) to Celsius (*x*) is 9/5, or 1.8 (see the figure on the next page). Notice that the *y*-intercept, where water freezes, is 32°F. What all this means is that every Fahrenheit temperature is 32 greater than 9/5 times the Celsius temperature. Therefore, to convert from Celsius (the *x*-value) to Fahrenheit (the *y*-value), just multiply by the ratio 9/5 (or 1.8) and then add 32:

$$^\circ\text{F} = \left(^\circ\text{C} \times \frac{9}{5}\right) + 32^\circ$$

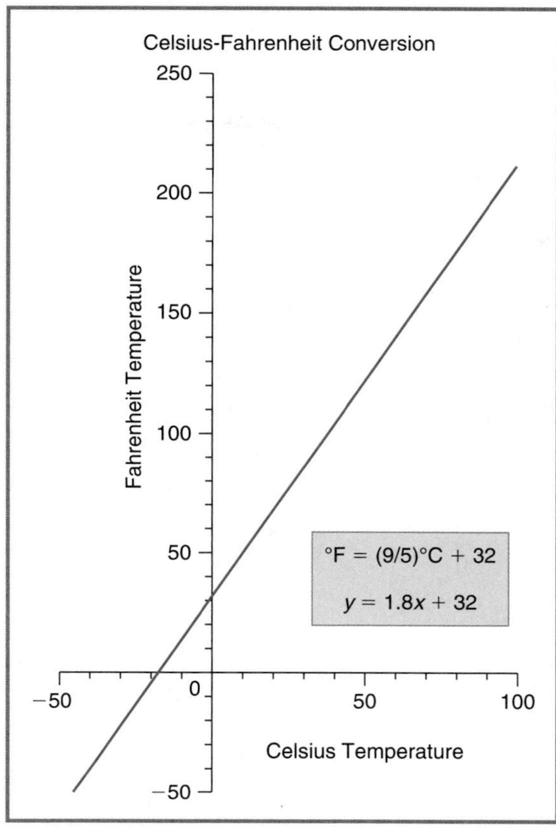

To convert in the opposite direction, carry out the arithmetic in reverse: first, subtract 32 from the Fahrenheit temperature, and then divide by 9/5 (which is the same as multiplying by 5/9):

$$°C = \frac{5}{9}(°F - 32°)$$

WHY DO ONLY SOME EQUILIBRIUM CONSTANTS APPEAR WITH UNITS?

Strictly speaking, equilibrium constants do *not* have units; they are dimensionless. However, it is often helpful to keep the units because they serve as a check on the calculations. Consider, for example, this reaction in aqueous solution:

$$A(aq) + 2B(aq) \rightleftharpoons 2C(aq)$$

The familiar equilibrium constant is

$$K_{eq} = \frac{[C]^2}{[A]^1[B]^2}$$

Because each concentration is "M," the unit on K_{eq} has to be "M^{-1}":

$$K_{eq} = \frac{M^2}{M \cdot M^2} = \frac{1}{M} = M^{-1}$$

Therefore, if our calculation produces a unit of, say, "M^{2}" or "M^{-3}," then we know the computation went wrong somewhere and we can look for the error.

But for the general reaction

$$aA(aq) + bB(aq) \rightleftharpoons cC(aq)$$

the rigorous equation for K_{eq} is

$$K_{eq} = \frac{\left(\frac{[C]}{1\ \text{M}}\right)^c}{\left(\frac{[A]}{1\ \text{M}}\right)^a\left(\frac{[B]}{1\ \text{M}}\right)^b}$$

when the solution is dilute with respect to all three solutes. The actual molar concentration of each is divided by its standard-state concentration, which is 1 M. Therefore, all the units in the equation cancel and K_{eq} is dimensionless. For a detailed explanation of equilibrium constants, including the reason for canceling the units, see Advanced Topic I, "Equilibrium Constants."

WHAT ARE THE CRITERIA FOR CHOOSING A MEASURE OF CENTRAL TENDENCY?

The purpose of reporting the central tendency is to typify the data, that is, to give a value that is typical or representative of the results. The best measure of central tendency depends on the nature of the data.

For Continuous Variables

Continuous variables have equally spaced divisions and can take any value between the minimum and maximum of the range. For example, consider a glass cylinder graduated from 5 mL to 25 mL. The difference between 6 mL and 8 mL is exactly the same as the difference between 22 mL and 24 mL. Furthermore, the measured volume can take any value between 5 mL and 25 mL.

a. If the distribution is normal, that is, if the data are symmetrical, then the best measure of central tendency is *the mean*.

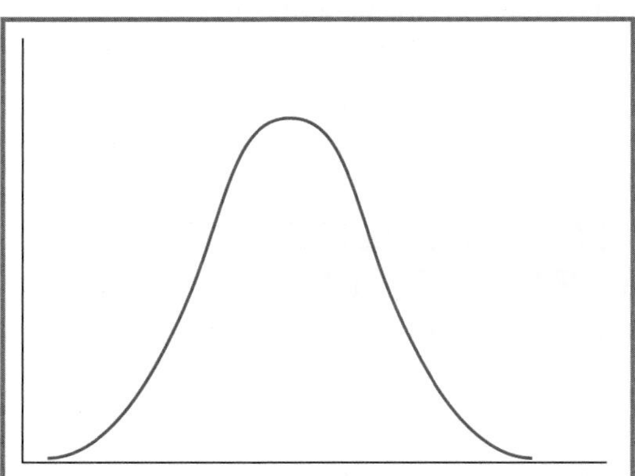

b. If the distribution is skewed, then the best measure of central tendency is *the median*. Outliers affect the median less than they do the mean.

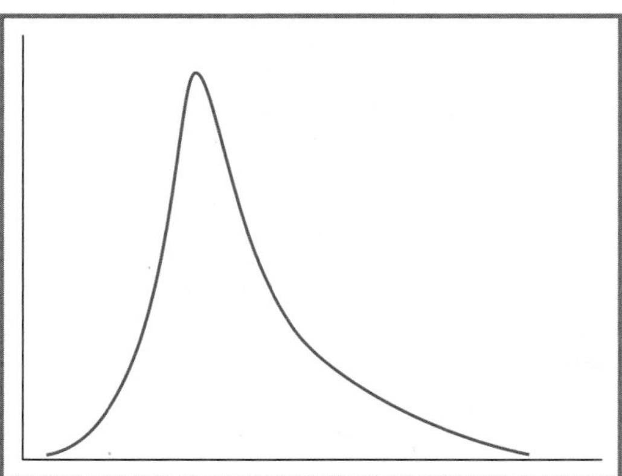

c. If the distribution is polymodal, that is, if the data have more than one peak, then there may be two populations, each having its own central tendency. In such a case, reporting one measure of central tendency for the entire data set might be misleading.

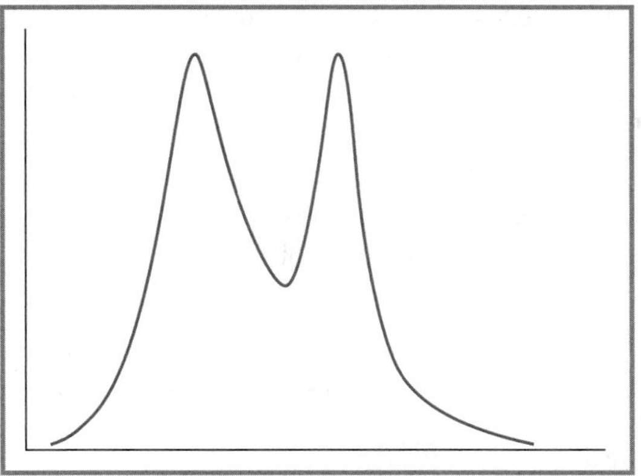

For Ordinal Variables

The measure of central tendency for ordinal variables is *the median* or *the mode*. Ordinal variables consist of categories in a logical order, but the quantitative relationships among those categories are unknown. For example, consider an employee-satisfaction survey that offers five responses to each statement it makes:

1 = strongly disagree
2 = disagree
3 = neither agree nor disagree
4 = agree
5 = strongly agree

The numbers serve only to rank the responses—not to quantify them. In other words, this scale does *not* mean that someone who responds "5" agrees 1.25 times more strongly than someone who responds "4." Similarly, it does not mean that a person who responds "1" agrees half as much as a person who responds "2."

For another example, consider a subjective scale from 1 to 5 that a particular clinic asks patients to use for ranking their physical pain:

1 = mild
2 = moderate
3 = distressing
4 = intense
5 = unbearable

These numbers, "1" through "5," represent categories. The following figure depicts some hypothetical results for this pain scale from 27 patients. The median of these data is "4."

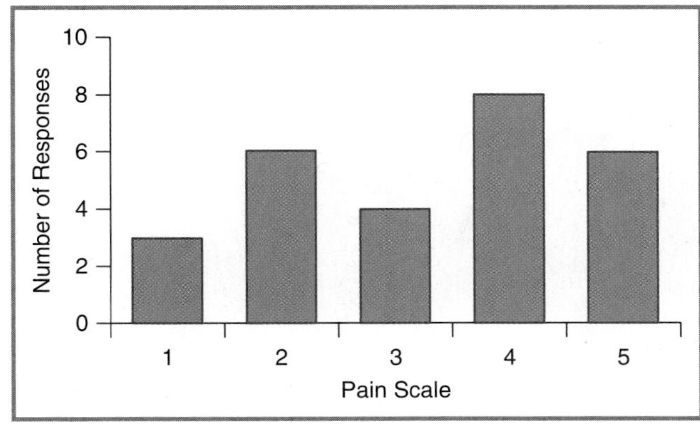

It is impossible to conclude that level-4 pain is twice as severe as level-2 pain. Likewise, these data do not imply that a patient who reports "1" feels only 20% as much pain as a patient who reports "5." Once again, the numbers serve only to rank the responses.

For ordinal data, the mean is inappropriate as a measure of central tendency because it incorrectly assumes that the numbers assigned to the categories have quantitative relationships. Neither the median nor the mode, however, makes this false assumption. The median is merely the value with the same number of responses above it as below it, and the mode is just the value with the most responses.

For Nominal Variables

The measure of central tendency for nominal (non-numerical) variables is *the mode.* For example, the following graph shows the frequency of side effects observed for a certain drug in a clinical trial. The mode for these data is "nausea."

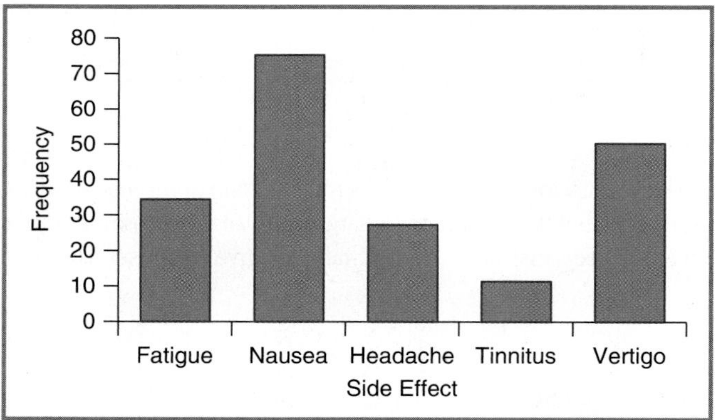

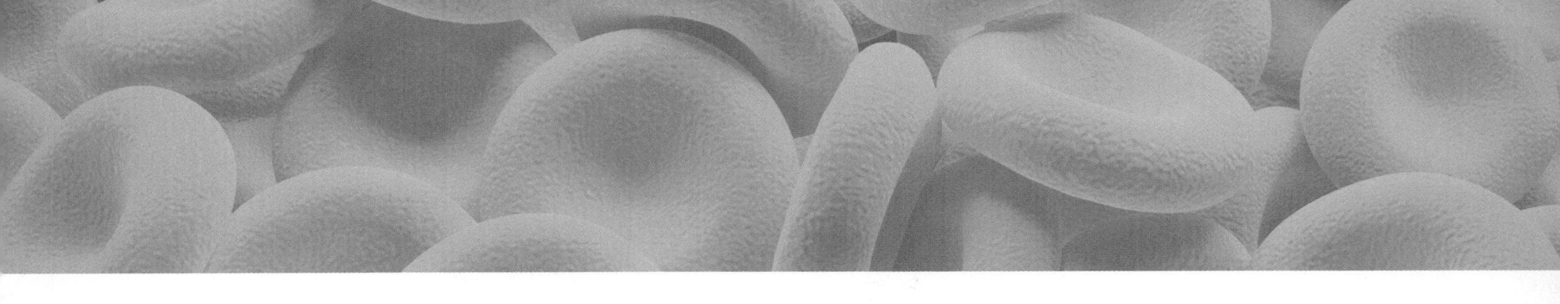

Answer Key

Chapter 1

Practice Problems

1. (a) −3 (b) 3 (c) −2 (d) −18.7 (e) 0.259 (f) 12.097 (g) 125 (h) −2.32 (i) 2 (j) −0.00122 (k) 10,031 (l) 90

2. (a) −7 (b) −90 (c) 80 (d) 33 (e) −21.3 (f) −366 (g) 330 (h) −0.0098 (i) 1650 (j) 0.45 (k) −250,000 (l) −100

3. (a) 1.978 (b) 7.5 (c) 0.164 (d) 2 (e) −0.4 (f) 2500 (g) −58.6 (h) −0.0055 (i) 400 (j) −0.5 (k) 519 (l) 2.81

4. (a) $\frac{3}{20}$ (b) $8\frac{4}{7}$ (c) $\frac{3}{8}$ (d) $\frac{2}{35}$ (e) $2\frac{1}{4}$ (f) $\frac{1}{3}$ (g) $3\frac{1}{3}$ (h) $2\frac{1}{3}$ (i) $\frac{9}{20}$ (j) $\frac{3}{32}$ (k) 1 (l) 5000

5. (a) $1\frac{3}{10}$ (b) $\frac{5}{12}$ (c) $3\frac{13}{24}$ (d) $\frac{1}{10}$ (e) $2\frac{1}{4}$ (f) $\frac{4}{39}$ (g) $12\frac{1}{2}$ (h) $\frac{41}{56}$ (i) $\frac{9}{10}$

6. (a) 0.67 (b) 0.8 (c) 0.875 (d) 0.4 (e) 0.25 (f) 0.25

7.

Percentage	Decimal Number	Fraction
12	0.12	$\frac{12}{100}$ or $\frac{3}{25}$
4	0.04	$\frac{4}{100}$ or $\frac{1}{25}$
75	0.75	$\frac{3}{4}$
91	0.91	$\frac{91}{100}$
0.55	0.0055	$\frac{0.55}{100}$ or $\frac{0.11}{20}$
33	0.33	$\frac{1}{3}$

8. (a) 38 (b) 0.07056 (c) 0.616 (d) 66 (e) 3 (f) 0.005742

9. (a) $x = 9.5$ (b) $x = 32.2$ (c) $x = 3$ (d) $x = 10$ (e) $x = 4$ (f) $x = 0.28$

10. (a) $x = 138$ (b) $x = 70$ (c) $x = 161.8$ (d) $x = 30$ (e) $x = 0.294$ (f) $x = 48$

Contextual Problems

1. (a) LDL cholesterol = 190 mg/dL − 36 mg/dL − (288 mg/dL ÷ 5) = 96 mg/dL
(b) 175 mg/dL

(c) Algebraically rearrange the formula to isolate the total concentration of cholesterol:

$$\text{LDL} = \text{total} - \text{HDL} - \frac{\text{triglycerides}}{5}$$

$$\text{LDL} + \text{HDL} + \frac{\text{triglycerides}}{5} = \text{total}$$

$$101 \text{ mg/dL} + 46 \text{ mg/dL} + \frac{150 \text{ mg/dL}}{5} = 177 \text{ mg/dL}$$

(d) Algebraically rearrange the formula to isolate the concentration of triglycerides:

$$(\text{LDL} - \text{total} + \text{HDL}) \times (-5) = \text{triglycerides}$$

$$(129 \text{ mg/dL} - 208 \text{ mg/dL} + 59 \text{ mg/dL}) \times (-5) = 100 \text{ mg/dL}$$

2. The 23 patient specimens necessitate 23 × 0.10, or 2.3, volumes of stock reagent *A*. Therefore,

$$\frac{3 \text{ volumes of } B}{0.5 \text{ volumes of } A} = \frac{x}{2.3 \text{ volumes of } A}$$

Cross-multiplying gives

$$x = 13.8 \text{ volumes of } B$$

3. (a) Group 4 is 1/2 of 1/3 of the 624 specimens. Thus, it comprises 104 specimens:

$$\frac{1}{2} \times \frac{1}{3} = \frac{1}{6}$$

$$\frac{1}{6} \times 624 = 104$$

One-fourth of these specimens equals 26. Therefore, if 26 of them have become unusable, then 78 good specimens remain in the group.

(b) Group 2 is 1/3 of the 624 specimens, or 208. Three-eighths of that group consists of 78 specimens:

$$\frac{3}{8} \times 208 = 78$$

(c) Group 1 is 1/3 of the 624 specimens, or 208. Of these, 25% represents 52 specimens:

$$25\% \text{ of } 208 = 0.25 \times 208 = 52$$

4. (a) No. The hemoglobin value should be

$$14.4 = 4.8 \times 3$$

and the hematocrit should be

$$41 = 13.6 \times 3$$

(b) Yes. The hemoglobin value is 5.1 × 3, and the hematocrit is 15.3 × 3, as both those numbers should be.

(c) Because the hemoglobin value should be the RBC count × 3, then the RBC count should be the hemoglobin value divided by 3:

$$\text{RBC count} = \frac{\text{hemoglobin value}}{3}$$

Thus, because the hemoglobin value is 14.0, the RBC count should be 14.0 ÷ 3, or 4.7.

5. Yes. The concentration is 3.9 g/dL:

$$56\% \text{ of } 7.0 \text{ g/dL} = 0.56 \times 7.0 \text{ g/dL} = 3.9 \text{ g/dL}$$

6. Yes. The expected range for CSF glucose in this patient runs from 60% of 81 mg/dL up to 75% of 81 mg/dL:

$$60\% \text{ of } 81 \text{ mg/dL} = 0.60 \times 81 \text{ mg/dL} = 49 \text{ mg/dL}$$

$$75\% \text{ of } 81 \text{ mg/dL} = 0.75 \times 81 \text{ mg/dL} = 61 \text{ mg/dL}$$

7. Let the unknown variable, x, be the glucose concentration at the time of collection.

$$\text{Glucose concentration at time of collection} = x$$

$$\text{Change in glucose concentration during standing for 1 hour} = 0.07x$$

$$x - 0.07x = 61 \text{ mg/dL}$$

$$(1 - 0.07)x = 61 \text{ mg/dL}$$

$$0.93x = 61 \text{ mg/dL}$$

$$x = \frac{61 \text{ mg/dL}}{0.93}$$

$$x = 65.6 \text{ mg/dL (approximately 66 mg/dL)}$$

8. (a) Yes, there is enough acetonitrile left for today's run. Your colleague used 1/3 of the 1/2 that he took from your bottle. Thus, he used 1/6 of the original amount of acetonitrile:

$$\frac{1}{3} \times \frac{1}{2} = \frac{1}{6}$$

This means that 5/6 of the original amount remains between your half and the remainder that your colleague returns to you. Five-sixths is greater than 3/4—the minimum for today's run. This inequality is easier to see when the fractions are expressed as decimal numbers:

$$\frac{5}{6} = 0.83 \quad \text{is greater than} \quad \frac{3}{4} = 0.75$$

(b) Not quite. Between your half and the 1/5 he returns to you, you have only 7/10, or 70%, of the original amount, slightly less than the 75% (3/4) needed.

$$\frac{1}{2} + \frac{1}{5} = \frac{5}{10} + \frac{2}{10} = \frac{7}{10} = 0.7 = 70\%$$

(c) Let the unknown variable, x, be the amount consumed in period 1.

$$\text{Number of liters consumed in period 1} = x$$

$$\text{Change in number of liters consumed} = 0.30x$$

$$x + 0.30x = 4.6 \text{ L}$$

$$(1 + 0.30)x = 4.6 \text{ L}$$

$$1.30x = 4.6 \text{ L}$$

$$x = \frac{4.6 \text{ L}}{1.30}$$

$$x = 3.5 \text{ L (rounded off from 3.538 L)}$$

9. (a) $\frac{400 \text{ mL methanol}}{90 \text{ mL water}} = \frac{320 \text{ mL methanol}}{x}$

$$(400 \text{ mL methanol})x = (90 \text{ mL water})(320 \text{ mL methanol})$$

$$x = 72 \text{ mL water}$$

(b) Yes. The two ratios are equal:

$$\frac{400 \text{ mL methanol}}{90 \text{ mL water}} = \frac{600 \text{ mL methanol}}{135 \text{ mL water}}$$

$$4.44 \text{ mL methanol/mL water} = 4.44 \text{ mL methanol/mL water}$$

(c) Doubling the ratio of methanol to water raises it from 4.44 to 8.88. Therefore, the volume of water you should mix with 500 mL of methanol is

$$\frac{8.88 \text{ mL methanol}}{\text{mL water}} = \frac{500 \text{ mL methanol}}{x}$$

$$(8.88 \text{ mL methanol})x = (\text{mL water})(500 \text{ mL methanol})$$

$$x = 56.3 \text{ mL water}$$

Chapter 2

Practice Problems

1. (a) $10^{4.8234} = 66{,}590$ (b) $10^{7.4771} = 30{,}000{,}000$ (c) $10^{2.3149} = 206.5$ (d) $2^4 = 16$ (e) $5^6 = 15{,}625$ (f) $3^{10} = 59{,}049$ (g) $10^{0.903} = 8$ (h) $10^{-0.0969} = 0.8$ (i) $10^{-2.64} = 0.0023$

2. (a) $\log_6 (67.193) = 2.3$ (b) $\log (0.537) = -0.27$ (c) $\log (1{,}000{,}000) = 6$ (d) $\log_2 (16{,}384) = 14$ (e) $\log (0.0001) = -4$ (f) $\log_{5.1} (26.01) = 2$ (g) $\log (2137.96) = 3.33$ (h) $\log (0.00251) = -2.6$ (i) $\log_{4.9} (2.90) = 0.67$

3. (a) 2.48 (b) 4.04 (c) 5 (d) 2.303 (e) 7 (f) 6.50 (g) 4.99 (h) 631,000,000 (i) 1.39 (j) 128 (k) 0.956 (l) 0.631 (m) −1.35 (n) −0.357 (o) 5.01×10^{-8}

4. (a) 6.55×10^{-4} (b) 9.03×10^6 (c) 1.012×10^5 (d) 4×10^2 (e) 1.65×10^{-1} (f) 3.7×10^{12} (g) 9.2×10^{-7} (h) 3.775×10^3 (i) 1.602×10^4

5. (a) 1,900,000 (b) 0.0004722 (c) 0.0090 (d) 551,000 (e) 6,080,000,000 (f) −26,000 (g) 74,553,000 (h) −0.00883 (i) 205

6. (b) The appropriate rule is

$$b^m/b^n = b^{(m-n)}$$

The value 4 is $2^{(m-n)}$, which must equal 2^2. Therefore,

$$m - n = 2$$

For example, $m = 6$ and $n = 4$.

(c) The product rule for exponents is appropriate:

$$\log x + \log y = \log xy$$

The value 5 is $\log xy$, which means that

$$10^5 = xy = 100{,}000$$

For example, $x = 100$ and $y = 1000$.

(d) The appropriate rule is

$$(b^n c^n) = (bc)^n$$

The value 2500 is $(10 \times 5)^n$, or 50^n. Therefore, n = 2.

(e) The appropriate rule is

$$n \log x = \log x^n$$

Thus, $-12.5581 = n \log x$, where $n = 6.2$. Therefore,

$$\log x = (-12.5581) \div (6.2) = -2.0255$$

$$x = \text{antilog}\,(-2.0255) = 0.00943$$

7. (a) 6.08955 (b) −5.0773 (c) −1.96 (d) −2.699209 (e) −3.469 (f) 9.986782

8. (a) 0.1083 (b) 80,000 (c) 4599 (d) 120 (e) 7.71×10^{-6} (f) 3.689×10^{10}

9. By a factor of 10^4, or 10,000:

$$\frac{10^8}{10^4} = 10^4$$

10. The answer is *b* because

$$2 \times (3.8 \times 10^4) = 7.6 \times 10^4 = 0.76 \times 10^5$$

11. The answer is *a*, *b*, and *c*. All three of these numbers are the same; each is 1/10 of 9.7×10^{-5}:

$$\frac{9.7 \times 10^{-5}}{10} = 9.7 \times 10^{-6}$$

12. The answer is *a* and *b*. They are equal, and each gives 10^{-2} when multiplied by 1000:

$$0.00001 \times 1000 = 0.01 = 10^{-2}$$

13. Increasing the logarithm by 1 increases the argument by a factor of 10. For example, if $y = 1000$,

$$\begin{aligned} \log x &= 1 + \log(1000) \\ &= 1 + 3 \\ &= 4 \end{aligned}$$

Therefore,

$$\begin{aligned} x &= \text{antilog}\,(4) \\ &= 10{,}000 \end{aligned}$$

This means that *x* is 10 times greater than *y*:

$$x = 10y$$

14. The number *r* is 1000 times smaller than *q*. Decreasing the logarithm by 3 decreases the argument by a factor of 10^3, or 1000. For example, if $q = 100{,}000$,

$$\begin{aligned} \log(100{,}000) - 3 &= \log r \\ 5 - 3 &= \log r \\ 2 &= \log r \end{aligned}$$

Therefore,

$$\begin{aligned} r &= \text{antilog}\,(2) \\ &= 100 \end{aligned}$$

15. The number c is the largest. The first equation shows that

$$\log a - \log b = 2$$
$$\log(a/b) = 2$$
$$a/b = 10^2$$
$$a/b = 100$$
$$a = 100b$$

and the second equation shows that

$$\log b + 3 = \log c$$
$$3 = \log c - \log b$$
$$3 = \log(c/b)$$
$$10^3 = c/b$$
$$1000 = c/b$$
$$1000b = c$$

Therefore, a is 100 times greater than b, but c is 1000 times greater than b. The order is $c > a > b$.

16. (a) $(2.4 \times 10^{-5})(4.6 \times 10^3) = (2.4 \times 4.6)(10^{-5} \times 10^3) = (2.4 \times 4.6) \times 10^{(-5+3)} = 11 \times 10^{-2} = 0.11$

(b) $(7.08 \times 10^6)(0.113) = (7.08 \times 0.113) \times 10^6 = 0.800 \times 10^6 = 8.00 \times 10^5$

(c) $(3.55/3.8) \times 10^{-7} = 0.93 \times 10^{-7} = 9.3 \times 10^{-8}$

(d) $(3.0/-3.0)(10^5/10^5) = -1.0 \times 1 = -1.0$

(e) $(-4.04 \times 3.66)(10^8 \times 10^{-8}) = -14.8 \times 10^0 = -14.8$

(f) $(144/6.67) \times (1/10^3) = 21.6 \times 10^{-3} = 2.16 \times 10^{-2}$

17.

	log a	log b	b / a
(a)	2	5	1000
(b)	2	4	100
(c)	4	6	100
(d)	4	5	10
(e)	−1	2	1000
(f)	−8	−3	100,000
(g)	2.17	3.17	10
(h)	4.9	6.9	100
(i)	−3.5	3.5	10,000,000

Sample calculations:

(a)

$$\log b - \log a = \log(b/a)$$
$$5 - 2 = \log(b/a)$$
$$3 = \log(b/a)$$
$$\text{antilog } 3 = b/a$$
$$10^3 = b/a$$
$$1000 = b/a$$

(f)

$$\log b - \log a = \log(b/a)$$
$$\log b = \log(b/a) + \log a$$
$$= \log(100{,}000) + (-8)$$
$$= 5 - 8$$
$$= -3$$

18. (a) True.

$$\log x = \log y$$
$$\text{antilog}(\log x) = \text{antilog}(\log y)$$
$$x = y$$

(b) True.

$$\log x = 2 \log y$$
$$\text{antilog}(\log x) = \text{antilog}(2 \log y)$$
$$10^{(\log x)} = 10^{(2 \log y)}$$
$$x = (10^{\log y})^2 \qquad \text{(Power Rule)}$$
$$x = y^2$$

Prove by setting the value of y at, say, 10,000

$$x = y^2$$
$$x = (10{,}000)^2$$
$$x = (10^4)^2$$
$$x = 10^8$$

Therefore,

$$\log(10^8) = 2 \log(10^4)$$
$$8 = 2(4)$$
$$8 = 8$$

(c) True.

$$\log(10{,}000) = 4 \quad \text{and} \quad \log(100{,}000) = 5$$

Because 28,446 lies between 10,000 and 100,000, its logarithm lies between 4 and 5.

(d) True.

$$\log(1{,}000{,}000) = 6 \quad \text{and} \quad \log(10{,}000{,}000) = 7$$

Because 6.39 lies between 6 and 7, its argument lies between 1,000,000 and 10,000,000.

(e) False.

$$\log x = -4$$
$$\text{antilog}(\log x) = \text{antilog}(-4)$$
$$10^{(\log x)} = 10^{-4}$$
$$x = 10^{-4}$$
$$x = 0.0001$$

Therefore, $x < y$ because $0.0001 < 0.00025$.

(f) True.

$$\log x = -7.3$$
$$\text{antilog}(\log x) = \text{antilog}(-7.3)$$
$$10^{(\log x)} = 10^{-7.3}$$
$$x = 10^{-7.3}$$

Therefore, because $10^{-7.3}$ is greater than 10^{-8}, x is *greater* than y.

(g) True.

$$y = 10x$$
$$\log y = \log (10x)$$
$$\log y = \log 10 + \log x \qquad \text{(Product Rule)}$$
$$\log y = 1 + \log x$$
$$\log y = \log x + 1$$

Therefore, log y is larger than log x by 1. Prove this by setting the value of x at, say, 10,000

$$y = 10x$$
$$y = 10(10{,}000)$$
$$y = 100{,}000$$

Then, substitute:

$$\log y = 1 + \log x$$
$$\log (100{,}000) = 1 + \log (10{,}000)$$
$$\log (10^5) = 1 + \log (10^4)$$
$$5 = 1 + 4$$
$$5 = 5$$

(h) True.

$$x = (1/1000)y$$
$$x = 0.001y$$
$$x = (10^{-3})y$$
$$\log x = \log [(10^{-3})y]$$
$$\log x = \log 10^{-3} + \log y \qquad \text{(Product Rule)}$$
$$\log x = (-3) + \log y$$
$$\log x = \log y - 3$$

Therefore, log x is less than log y by 3. Prove this by setting the value of y at, say, 1,000,000:

$$x = (10^{-3})y$$
$$x = (10^{-3})(1{,}000{,}000)$$
$$x = (10^{-3})(10^6)$$
$$x = 10^{(-3+6)} \qquad \text{(Product Rule)}$$
$$x = 10^3$$

Then, substitute:

$$\log x = \log y - 3$$
$$\log (10^3) = \log (10^6) - 3$$
$$3 = 6 - 3$$
$$3 = 3$$

Contextual Problems

1. **W:** Yes, they achieved it. A 1-log drop from the previous viral load of 13,200,000 would be 1,320,000. The present load, however, is 1,200,000, representing more than a 1-logarithm drop.

X: Yes, they achieved it. A 1-log drop from the previous viral load of 2.4 million would be 240,000. The present load, however, is 230,000, representing more than a 1-logarithm drop.

Y: No, they did not achieve it. A 1-log drop from the previous viral load of 990,000 would be 99,000. The present load, however, is 120,000, representing less than a 1-logarithm drop.

Z: Yes, they achieved it. A 1-log drop from the previous viral load of 1.9×10^6 would be 1.9×10^5. The present load, however, is 1.8×10^5, representing more than a 1-logarithm drop.

2. **N:** 1 log. One way to approach this problem is to calculate the ratio of the present load to the previous load:

$$\frac{380{,}000}{4{,}400{,}000} = 0.086$$

What this means is that the present load is slightly less than 1/10 of the previous load; that is, the load has fallen by a factor of somewhat more than 10, or more than 1 logarithm. Another approach to this question is to take the ratio of the previous load to the present load, which is just the reciprocal of the ratio above.

$$\frac{4{,}400{,}000}{380{,}000} = 11.6$$

What this means is that the previous load was more than 10 times higher than the present load. Therefore, the load has indeed fallen by a factor of slightly more than 10, or more than 1 logarithm.

O: 2 logs. The ratio of the present load to the previous load is

$$\frac{75{,}000}{9.6 \times 10^6} = 0.008$$

The present load, therefore, is less than 1/100 (0.01) of the previous load, that is, the load has fallen by a factor of more than 100, or more than 2 logarithms. Alternatively, the ratio of the previous load to the present load is 128, meaning that the previous load was more than 100 times, or 2 logarithms, greater than the present load.

P: 2 logs. The ratio of the present load to the previous load is 0.01.

Q: 3 logs. The ratio of the present load to the previous load is 0.0005.

3. (a) There are at least two advantages: (1) logarithms are easier to write and read than are counts, and (2) logarithms make it easier to discern at a glance whether the present result differs from the previous result by a factor of 10.

(b) The count is the antilog of 6.933, which is $10^{6.933}$, or 8,570,000 counts/mL.

(c) The log of 18,450,000 is 7.266.

(d) To calculate the factor by which the load decreased, convert each logarithm into "counts/mL" and then take the ratio. Before treatment, the log was 7.223, which corresponds to a viral load of $10^{7.223}$, or 16,700,000. After treatment, it was 4.187, which corresponds to a viral load of $10^{4.187}$, or 15,400. The ratio of "before treatment" to "after treatment" is

$$\frac{\text{load before treatment}}{\text{load after treatment}} = \frac{16{,}700{,}000}{15{,}400} = 1080$$

Therefore, the viral load decreased by a factor of 1080, which is more than 3 orders of magnitude, or more than 3 logarithms. This accords with the difference between the two logarithms themselves: $7.223 - 4.187 = 3.036$.

4. (a) 2,300,000 copies/mL

$$884{,}000 \text{ IU/mL} \left(\frac{2.6 \text{ copies/mL}}{1 \text{ IU/mL}}\right) = 2{,}300{,}000 \text{ copies/mL}$$

(b) 9,700,000 IU/mL

$$1.45 \times 10^7 \text{ copies/mL} \left(\frac{1 \text{ IU/mL}}{1.5 \text{ copies/mL}}\right) = 9{,}700{,}000 \text{ IU/mL}$$

(c) 1,420,000 IU/mL

(d) The answer is 539,000 IU/mL. First, calculate the copies/mL from the logarithm, which is 6.223: $10^{6.223} = 1{,}670{,}000$ copies/mL. Next, convert this value into "IU/mL":

$$1{,}670{,}000 \text{ copies/mL} \left(\frac{1 \text{ IU/mL}}{3.1 \text{ copies/mL}}\right) = 539{,}000 \text{ IU/mL}$$

(e) The answer is 6.511. First, at 2.7 copies per IU, 1.2 million IU/mL equals 3,240,000 copies/mL. The logarithm of that number is 6.511.

5. Laboratory 2 found the highest amount of viral RNA. First, convert all three results into a common unit, say, "copies/mL." Thus, Laboratory 1's result is the antilog of 7.548, which is $10^{7.548}$, or 35,300,000 copies/mL. Laboratory 3's result is equivalent to 31,900,000 copies/mL:

$$1.45 \times 10^7 \text{ copies/mL} \left(\frac{1 \text{ IU/mL}}{2.2 \text{ copies/mL}}\right) = 31{,}900{,}000 \text{ IU/mL}$$

6. (a) No. The reduction would have been 1000-fold or greater only if the difference between the two logarithms had been at least 3.

(b) Patient B. The difference between the two logarithms is 2.0, corresponding to 10^2, or 100.

(c) 97%. The logarithms 2.64 and 1.17 correspond to cell numbers of 440 and 15, respectively. Thus, the difference is 425, which is 97% of 440.

7. (a) 0.61 (b) 29% (c) 0.66 ($1 - 0.34 = 0.66$) (d) 0.086 ($A = -\log[1 - 0.18]$) (e) 0.301 ($A = -\log[0.5]$) (f) 0.022 ($A = -\log[0.95]$)

8. (a)

Concentration (mIU/mL)	A_{450}	Log of Concentration	Log(A_{450})
2.50	0.042	0.398	−1.38
5.00	0.081	0.699	−1.09
20.0	0.319	1.301	−0.496
50.0	0.773	1.699	−0.112
100.	1.459	2.000	0.1641
200.	2.586	2.301	0.4126

(b)

(1)

(2)

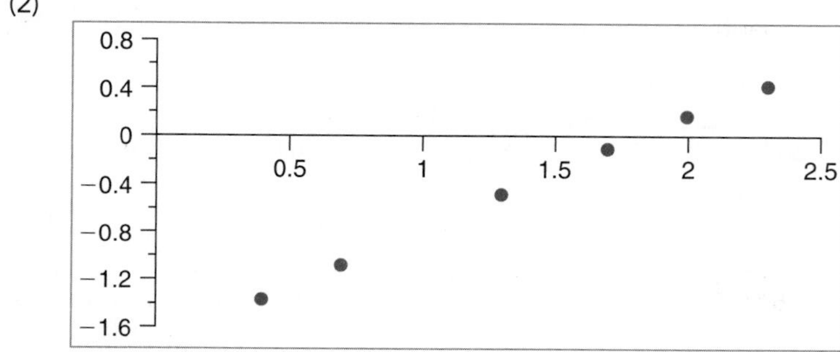

(3)

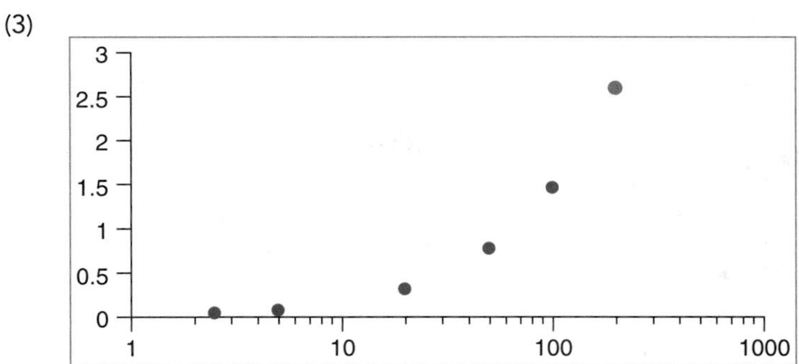

(4)

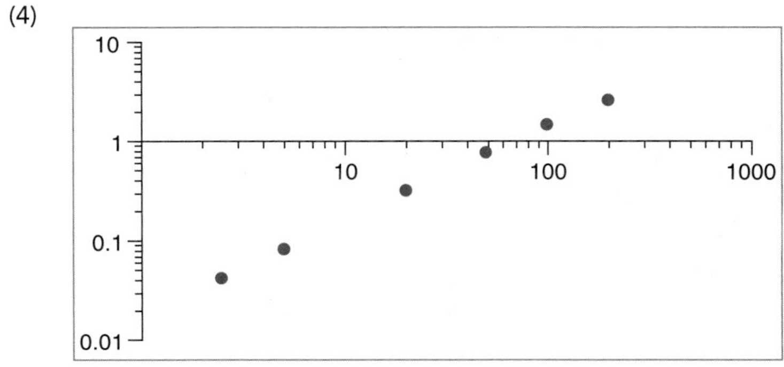

(c) The spacing among the data points is more uniform, allowing for a more accurate visual interpretation, especially at low concentrations.

(d) The plot is linear, allowing for an easier visual interpretation, especially at low concentrations.

(e) Data are plotted directly, without the need for converting to logarithms.

9. (a)

Concentration (mIU/mL)	A_{450}	Log of Concentration	Log(A_{450})
12.0	0.019	1.079	−1.72
32.0	0.056	1.505	−1.25
97.0	0.171	1.987	−0.767
249	0.448	2.396	−0.349
495	0.814	2.695	−0.0894
890.	1.507	2.949	0.1781

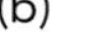
(b)

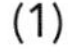
(1)

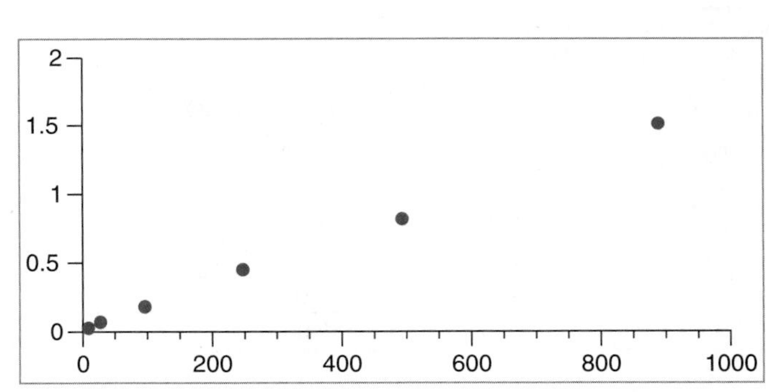

(2)

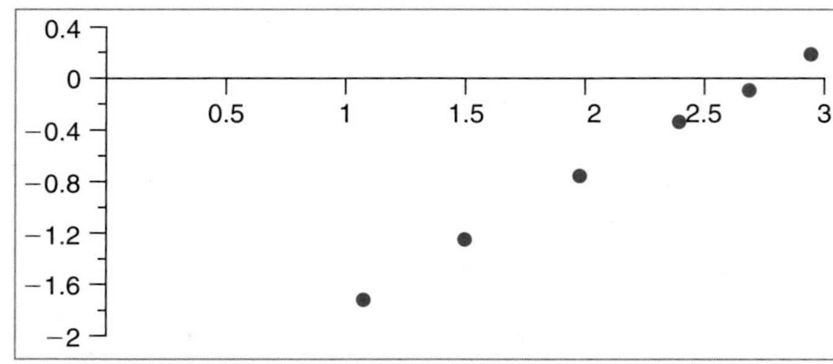

(3)

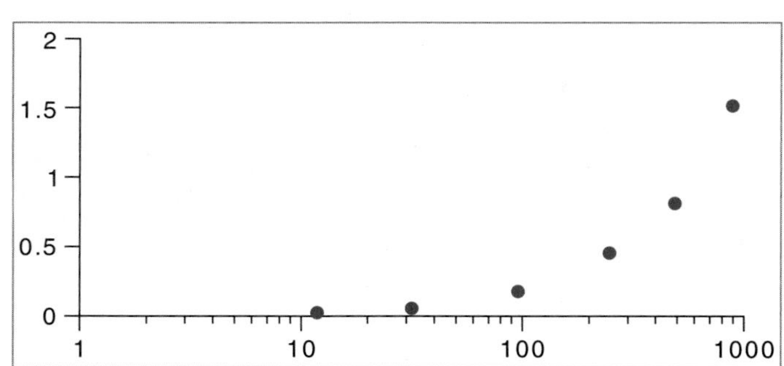

(4)

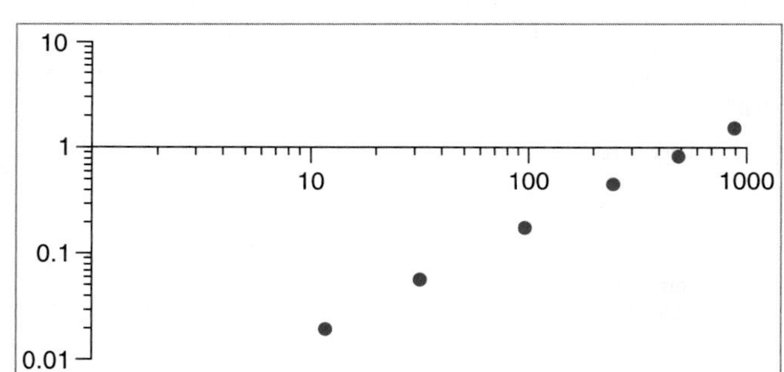

(c) The spacing among the data points is more uniform, allowing for a more accurate visual interpretation, especially at low concentrations.

(d) The plot is linear, allowing for an easier visual interpretation, especially at low concentrations.

(e) Data are plotted directly, without the need for converting to logarithms.

10. (a)

Concentration of Endogenous Vitamin D (ng/mL)	% of Added Radiolabeled Vitamin D Bound to Antibody (%Bound)	Log of Concentration	Log (%Bound)
0.500	96.00	−0.301	1.9822
5.00	82.36	0.699	1.9157
12.0	61.57	1.079	1.7894
20.0	44.25	1.301	1.6459
40.0	28.05	1.602	1.4479
100.	16.68	2.000	1.2222

(b)

(1)

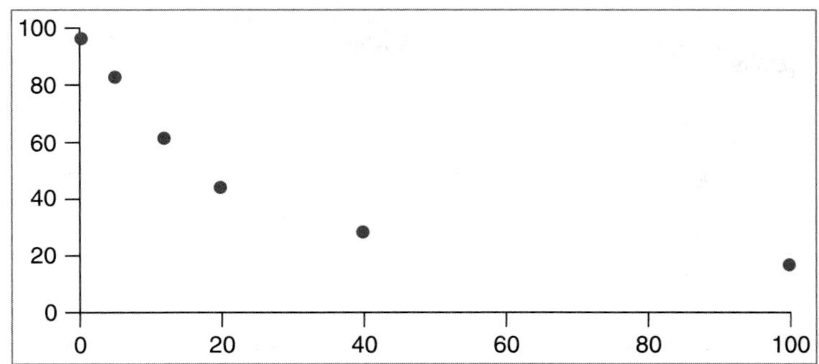

(2)

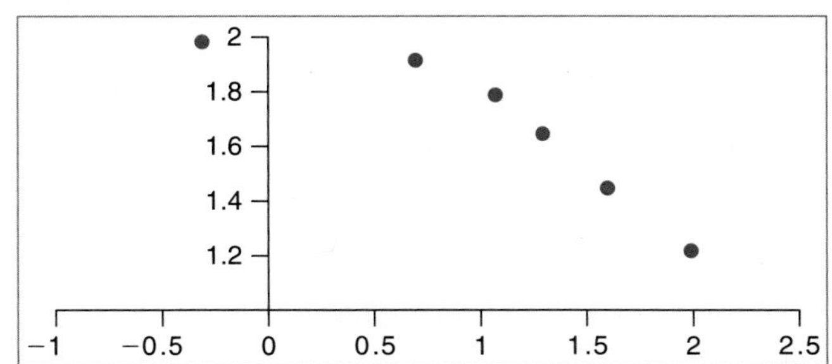

(3)

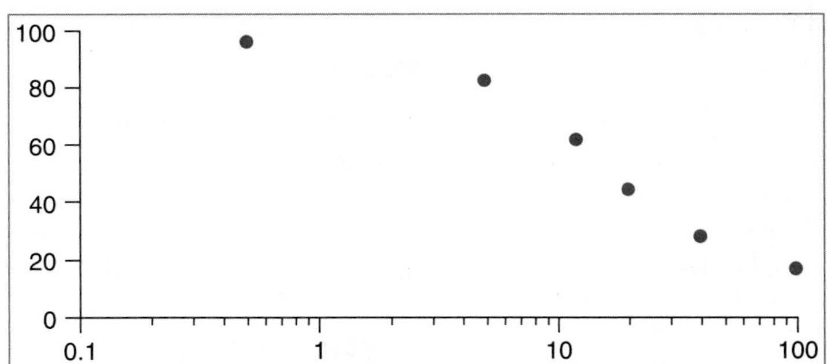

(c) The "0" value corresponds to a vitamin D concentration of 1 ng/mL. This is so because $10^0 = 1$. The "1" value corresponds to 10 ng/mL because $10^1 = 10$. The "1.8" value corresponds to 63 ng/mL because antilog (1.8) = 63.

(d) It is easier to see the change in the *y* value as the concentration changes in the middle and high ranges.

(e) It is easier the see the change in the *y* value as the concentration changes in the low range.

(f) The logarithm is negative at concentrations less than 1, complicating interpretation of the graph.

11. (a)

Tube	Chemical Substance	Result for Protein Q (pg/mL)	Relative Result for Protein Q
1	none	3.4	1.0
2	caffeine	3.5	1.0
3	vancomycin	6.7	2.0
4	acetaminophen	4.0	1.2
5	lead	1.7	0.50

(b) Vancomycin multiplies the result by 2, and lead divides it by 2.

(c) Tube 1: log 1.0 = 0. Tube 3: log 2.0 = 0.301. Tube 5: log 0.50 = −0.301.

(d) The logarithms for vancomycin and lead are equal and opposite, showing that they affect the result by the same factor but in opposite directions.

Chapter 3

Practice Problems

1. (a) 42.8 (b) 0.2 (c) 106.0 (d) 9.0 (e) 0.8 (f) 50.1 (g) 2866.0 (h) 17.1 (i) 7.0 (j) 33.6 (k) 0.7 (l) 91.2

2. (a) 13,410 (b) 20 (c) 510 (d) 70 (e) 380 (f) 4600 (g) 1010 (h) 220 (i) 50 (j) 9.07×10^3 (k) 2.286×10^4 (l) 600

3. (a) 3 (b) 28 (c) 103 (d) 100 (e) 18,405 (f) 4 (g) 55 (h) 600 (i) 1003 (j) 8 (k) 9091 (l) 14

4. (a) 4.134 (b) 0.932 (c) 12.002 (d) 8×10^{-3} (e) 20.009 (f) 20.010 (g) 7.2×10^{-2} (h) 0.203 (i) 61.774 (j) 15.001 (k) 2.491 (l) 185.237

5. (a) 5.02 (b) 199.76 (c) 0.69 (d) 2×10^{-2} (e) 2.51 (f) 35.38 (g) 0.03 (h) 1.00 (i) 40.53 (j) 0.02 (k) 9.08 (l) 58.11

6. (a) 4 (b) 1 (c) 3 (d) 5 (e) 4 (f) 3 (g) 6 (h) 3 (i) 2 (j) 3 (k) 7 (l) 1 (m) 3 (n) 2 (o) 3 (p) 5 (q) 6 (r) 4 (s) 2 (t) 2

7. (a) 3 (b) 4 (c) 2 (d) 5 (e) 4 (f) 5 (g) 2 (h) 5 (i) 1 (j) 4 (k) 1 (l) 5

8. (a) −3.437 (b) 5.0282 (c) 3.85 (d) −2.00842 (e) 6.3010 (f) −8.39728 (g) 13.70 (h) −7.76195 (i) 5.8 (j) 2.8866 (k) −11.1 (l) 4.47714

9. We report measurements such that only the last digit is uncertain.

(a) <u>0.088</u> (calculated value = 0.08794) The digit in the second decimal place, an "8," is the same in all five measurements. But the digit in the third decimal place is the first one to vary. Therefore, the average may have no more than three decimal places.

(b) <u>2.6</u> (calculated value = 2.630) The first uncertain digit in the five measurements occupies the first decimal place. Therefore, the final answer must terminate there.

(c) <u>60</u> (calculated value = 60.2) The first uncertain digit in the six measurements is in the tens place. Therefore, we should round the final answer to the nearest 10. Note the absence of a decimal point in the final answer, telling us that the zero is not significant.

(d) <u>1.24</u> (calculated value = 1.238) The first uncertain digit in the six measurements is in the second decimal place. Therefore, the final answer may include both decimal places.

(e) <u>7.6×10^4</u> (calculated value = 7.61×10^4) The first uncertain digit in the five measurements is in the first decimal place. Therefore, the final answer must terminate there.

10. (a) 4 (b) 3 (c) 5 (d) 5 (e) 4 (f) 2

11. (a) 3 (b) 4 (c) 3 (d) 4 (e) 1 (f) 5

12. (a) Rounding to even numbers would not change the average. The two values of "13.5" would be rounded *up* under either rounding rule.

(b) Rounding to even numbers would change the average. The value "137.5" would be rounded *up* under either rule. The values "136.5" and "134.5", however, would be rounded *up* under the standard rule but *down* under the even-number rule.

(c) Rounding to even numbers would change the average. The value "43.5" would be rounded *up* under either rule. The values "46.5" and "42.5," however, would be rounded *up* under the standard rule but *down* under the even-number rule.

(d) Rounding to even numbers would not change the average. The value "1.5" would be rounded *up* under either rounding rule.

13. (a) $\frac{0.005}{4.667} = 0.001 = 0.1\%$ (b) 0.7% (c) 3%

14. (a) $\frac{0.005}{0.48} = 0.01 = 1\%$ (b) 2% (c) 0.3%

(d) 1.7% (Note decimal point in measurement.) (e) 0.1% (f) 2.5% (g) 17% (h) 0.7%

15. (a) STEP 1: 19.2 + 8.66 = 27.86, rounded to 27.9

STEP 2: 27.9 × 1.3 = 36.27, rounded to **36**

(b) 12.2 (c) 0.007511

(d) STEP 1: 7.9 × 1.44 = 11.376, rounded to 11

STEP 2: 13.62 − 11 = 2.62, rounded to **3**

(e) 11.083 (f) 5815 (g) 134 (h) 1.1 (i) 400,000 (j) 0.0038

16. (a) 39 (b) 25 (c) 20. (d) 89 (e) 61 (f) 8 (g) 32 (h) 104 (i) 2 (j) 50. (k) 30. (l) 122 (m) 1 (n) 77 (o) 10. (p) 100.

17. (a) 39 Same value, same implied range, NO bias.

(b) 26 Implied range: 25.5–26.5. Implied range in #16: 24.5–25.5. Bias = 1.

(c) 20. (same) (d) 90 (bias = 1) (e) 61 (same) (f) 8 (same) (g) 32 (same)

(h) 104 (same) (i) 2 (same) (j) 50. (same) (k) 30. (same) (l) 123 (bias = 1)

(m) 2 (bias = 1) (n) 77 (same) (o) 10. (same) (p) 100. (same)

18.

Row	Mass of an Object (g)	Implied Range (g)	Implied Relative Uncertainty
1	480	475–485	2.1%
2	480.	479.5–480.5	0.21%
3	480.0	479.95–480.05	0.021%
4	48	47.5–48.5	2.1%

What the completed table confirms is the rule that *trailing zeros are significant only if a decimal point is present in the number.*

The zero in "480" in row 1 is not significant. Removing that zero to give "48" (row 4) fails to change the implied relative uncertainty. In other words, that particular zero gives no information about precision in the measurement, confirming its status as a nonsignificant figure.

By contrast, the zero in "480." in row 2 *is* significant. Removing that zero *does* change the implied relative uncertainty, meaning that the zero does indeed give information about precision.

This observation confirms the zero's status as a significant figure. One can draw the same conclusion from the removal of both zeros from "480.0" in row 3.

Contextual Problems

1. (a) The value implies astonishing precision. The manufacturer is saying that the average life expectancy of its lamp falls between 2118.55 hours (2118 hours, 33 minutes) and 2118.65 hours (2118 hours, 39 minutes). Thus, the manufacturer claims to know how long, on average, its lamp lasts, plus or minus only 3 minutes. In the absence of supporting data, this assertion is unjustifiable.

(b) No. The value of 2100 hours implies a range of 2050–2150 hours. Because the competitor's lamp life of 2060 hours falls within that range, we cannot conclude that manufacturer *A*'s lamp lasts longer.

(c) The lower value (9.66 μg/mL) has three significant figures, whereas the higher value (102.17 μg/mL) has four. This implies that the precision of your method increases with the concentration.

(d) No. The ratio of 6.1 mg/dL to 2.2 mg/dL should have no more than two significant figures. Therefore, it would be proper to say that the concentration rose **2.8**-fold.

2. We should round the value to "**9.0** pg/mL." The implied relative uncertainty in "9.0" is the same as the relative uncertainty in the original value.

Value (pg/mL)	Absolute Uncertainty (pg/mL)	Relative Uncertainty
8.94	0.05	0.6%
9	0.5	6%
9.0	0.05	0.6%

3. (a) The best value is **5.5 ng/mL**. The reasoning follows.

(i) The unrounded average is 5.539 ng/mL, which implies more precision than is present in the original values.

(ii) Rounding the average to 5.54 is unreasonable because it places the true average between 5.535 and 5.545, a range that is unjustifiably small because it implies certainty in the first two digits, even though there are no certain digits in the raw data.

(iii) Rounding the average to "6" is risky because only 3 of the 10 concentrations are higher than that value and because it has much less precision than the data have.

(iv) Reporting "5.5" is a good compromise between a value ("6") that may be too high and that has too little precision and a value ("5.54") that carries too much precision.

(b) The best value is **5.6 ng/mL**. The reasoning follows.

After rounding to one decimal place, the values are these (in the same order as above):

4.5 5.0 3.5 6.8 7.7 9.2 4.9 5.7 3.3 4.9 (ng/mL)

(i) The unrounded average of these values is 5.55 ng/mL, but that suggests the range for the true average to be 5.545 to 5.555. As in part *a* above, this is unjustifiably small because it implies certainty in the first two digits, even though there are no certain digits in the data.

(ii) Also as in part *a*, rounding the average to "6" is risky because only 3 of the 10 concentrations are higher than that value and because it has a high implied relative uncertainty (8%).

(iii) The value "5.6," however, is a good compromise between a value ("6") that may be too high and that has too little precision and a value ("5.55") that carries too much precision.

(c) The bias is **0.1 ng/mL**. The average of 5.5 in part *a* implies a range for the true average of 5.45 to 5.55, whereas the average of 5.6 in part *b* implies a range of 5.55 to 5.65. Thus, the range shifted up by 0.1.

(d) The best value is **6 ng/mL**. After rounding by the researcher, the values are these (in the same order as above):

5 5 4 7 8 9 5 6 3 5 (ng/mL)

(i) The average of these whole numbers is 5.7 ng/mL. Each whole-number value has an uncertainty of 0.5, which gives an implied relative uncertainty ranging from a high of 17% for the "3" down to 6% for the "9."

(ii) The value of "5.7" has an implied relative uncertainty of 0.9%, which represents too much precision for the values as written.

4. The unrounded average is "4,728,333." Because the average in this case may not have more than four significant figures, we immediately round it to "4,728,000." Each count carries an uncertainty of 500 and an implied relative uncertainty of 0.01%. Reporting the average as "4,728,000" is risky for at least two reasons:

(a) It implies that the "7" and "2" are known with confidence and that only the "8" is an estimate.

(b) It puts the true average between 4,727,500 and 4,728,500, which implies too much certainty, given that the first "7" and the "2" are each questionable.

Listed in the table below, there are three other rounding options: the nearest million, nearest 100,000, and nearest 10,000.

Average After Rounding (RBCs/μL)	Absolute Uncertainty (RBCs/μL)	Implied Relative Uncertainty	Strengths	Weaknesses
5,000,000	500,000	10%		1. Lies outside range of actual counts. 2. Relative uncertainty is 1000 times higher than that of actual counts. 3. Changes the certain digit "4" to the uncertain "5."
4,700,000	50,000	1%	1. Retains the certain digit "4." 2. Lies near center of actual counts.	1. Retains the uncertain digit "7." 2. Relative uncertainty is 100 times higher than that of actual counts.
4,730,000	5000	0.1%	1. Retains the certain digit "4." 2. Lies near center of actual counts. 3. Of all three rounding possibilities, implied relative uncertainty is closest to that of actual counts.	1. Has two uncertain digits: "7" and "3." 2. Relative uncertainty is 10 times higher than that of actual counts.

Chapter 4

Practice Problems

1. (a) $3.1\ \text{mL} \times \dfrac{\text{L}}{1000\ \text{mL}} \times \dfrac{1 \times 10^6\ \mu\text{L}}{\text{L}} = 3100\ \mu\text{L}$

(b) $420\ \text{ng} \times \dfrac{\text{g}}{1 \times 10^9\ \text{ng}} \times \dfrac{1000\ \text{mg}}{\text{g}} = 4.2 \times 10^{-4}\ \text{mL}$ (c) 2 μL (d) 780 ng

(e) 0.85 L (f) 1.445 g (g) 36.4 mL (h) 0.013 ng (i) 0.620 μmol (j) 0.097 mmol (k) 400 mL (l) 0.073 mg (m) 0.400 mL (n) 250 pg (o) 0.0609 mol (p) 6.2 dL (q) 705,000 pmol (r) 2000 pg

2. (a) 74.55 g/mol (b) 17.04 g/mol (c) 212.10 g/mol
(d) (2 × 22.99 g/mol) + 32.07 g/mol = 78.05 g/mol (e) 95.21 g

3. (a) $3.50\ \text{g} \times \dfrac{\text{mol}}{58.44\ \text{g}} = 0.0599\ \text{mol}$ (b) 0.137 (c) 0.012 (d) 10.8 (e) 0.00314

4. (a) 98.6°F (b) 179.6°F (c) 284°F (d) −4°F (e) 39.2°F

5. (a) 22.2°C (b) 110°C (c) −21.7°C (d) 7.2°C (e) −12.2°C

6. (a) 273.15 K (b) 373.15 K (c) 0 K

7. (a) $53\ \text{km} \times \dfrac{\text{mi}}{1.61\ \text{km}} = 32.9\ \text{mi}$ (b) 14.2 cm (c) 58.2 kg (d) 70.4 oz

(e) $31\ \text{ft} \times \dfrac{\text{mi}}{5280\ \text{ft}} \times \dfrac{1.61\ \text{km}}{\text{mi}} \times \dfrac{1000\ \text{m}}{\text{km}} = 9.5\ \text{m}$ (f) 3.2 km (g) 2.3 gal

(h) 47.2 mL (i) 5.8 L

Contextual Problems

1. First, convert one of the units into the other:

$$1 \text{ mL} \times \frac{1 \text{ L}}{1000 \text{ mL}} \times \frac{1 \times 10^{15} \text{ fL}}{1 \text{ L}} = 1 \times 10^{12} \text{ fL}$$

Next, we take the ratio of the 1-mL volume to the 90-fL volume:

$$\frac{1 \times 10^{12} \text{ fL}}{90 \text{ fL}} = 1.1 \times 10^{10}$$

Thus, we conclude that 1.1×10^{10} (11 billion) red blood cells could theoretically occupy a volume of 1 mL.

2. First, convert one of the units into the other:

$$250 \text{ mL} \times \frac{\text{L}}{1000 \text{ mL}} = 0.250 \text{ L}$$

Next, set up an equation of ratios:

$$\frac{30 \text{ mL concentrate}}{0.250 \text{ L solution}} = \frac{x}{1 \text{ L solution}}$$

$$(30 \text{ mL concentrate})(1 \text{ L solution}) = (0.250 \text{ L solution})x$$

$$120 \text{ mL concentrate} = x$$

3. $450 \text{ mg} \times \frac{\text{g}}{1000 \text{ mg}} = 0.450 \text{ g}$

4. $0.080 \text{ mL} \times \frac{\text{L}}{1000 \text{ mL}} \times \frac{1 \times 10^{6} \text{ µL}}{\text{L}} = 80 \text{ µL}$

This step can be shorter because 1 µL = 0.001 mL. Therefore, just multiply the number of milliliters by 1000 to give the number of microliters:

$$0.080 \text{ mL} \times 1000 \text{ µL/mL} = 80 \text{ µL}$$

5. (a) Here are four approaches to this problem.

APPROACH 1
Straightforward dimensional analysis.

$$\frac{628 \text{ pg}}{\text{mL}} \times \frac{\text{g}}{1 \times 10^{12} \text{ pg}} \times \frac{1 \times 10^{9} \text{ ng}}{\text{g}} \times \frac{1000 \text{ mL}}{\text{L}} = \frac{628 \text{ ng}}{\text{L}}$$

APPROACH 2
Use the relationship that 1 ng = 1000 pg.

$$\frac{628 \text{ pg}}{\text{mL}} \times \frac{\text{ng}}{1000 \text{ pg}} \times \frac{1000 \text{ mL}}{\text{L}} = \frac{628 \text{ ng}}{\text{L}}$$

APPROACH 3
Two-step reasoning.

Step 1.

$$\frac{628\ \text{pg}}{\text{mL}} \times \frac{\text{ng}}{1000\ \text{pg}} = \frac{0.628\ \text{ng}}{\text{mL}}$$

Step 2. Every mL contains 0.628 ng. Thus, 1 L, which is 1000 mL, contains 1000 times as much, or 628 ng. The concentration is **628 ng/L**.

APPROACH 4
The ratio method.

$$\frac{1 \times 10^{12}\ \text{pg}}{\text{g}} = \frac{628\ \text{pg}}{x} \qquad x = 6.28 \times 10^{-10}\ \text{g}$$

$$\frac{\text{g}}{1 \times 10^{9}\ \text{ng}} = \frac{6.28 \times 10^{-10}\ \text{g}}{x} \qquad x = 0.628\ \text{ng}$$

Because 1 L = 1000 mL,

$$\frac{0.628\ \text{ng}}{\text{mL}} = \frac{x}{1000\ \text{mL}} \qquad x = 628\ \text{ng}$$

Therefore, there are **628 ng in every liter.**

(b) 19.8 pmol/mL (c) 17.4 mg/mL (d) 49 μmol/dL

Chapter 5
Practice Problems

1. In each case, calculate the number of grams present in 100 mL of solution. Given that 100 mL is the same as 0.1 L, we may solve problem ***a*** this way:

$$\left(\frac{400\ \text{g}}{1\ \text{L}}\right)\left(\frac{0.1\ \text{L}}{100\ \text{mL}}\right) = 40\ \text{g}/100\ \text{mL} = 40\%\ (\text{w/v})$$

And because 100 mL = 1 dL, we might also solve the problem this way:

$$\left(\frac{400\ \text{g}}{1\ \text{L}}\right)\left(\frac{0.1\ \text{L}}{\text{dL}}\right) = 40\ \text{g/dL} = 40\%\ (\text{w/v})$$

(b) 12% (w/v) (c) 0.9% (w/v) (d) 0.5% (w/v) (e) 0.08% (w/v) (f) 6.16% (w/v)

2. (a) The total solution mass is 800 g + 9.2 g = 809.2 g. Therefore, the concentration is the mass of the solute divided by the total solution mass:

$$\frac{9.2\ \text{g}}{809.2\ \text{g}} \times 100\% = 1.1\%\ (\text{w/w})$$

(b) 9% (w/w) (c) 0.8% (w/w)

3. The concentration is the volume of alcohol divided by the total solution volume:

$$\frac{50\ \text{mL}}{150\ \text{mL}} \times 100\% = 33\%\ (\text{v/v})$$

4. (a) $4.0\text{ g}\left(\frac{\text{mol}}{56.1\text{ g}}\right)\left(\frac{1}{1\text{ L}}\right) = 0.071\text{ M}$ (b) $60.0\text{ g}\left(\frac{\text{mol}}{58.5\text{ g}}\right)\left(\frac{1}{0.400\text{ L}}\right) = 2.56\text{ M}$

(c) 9.0×10^{-4} M (d) 0.014 M (e) 0.10 M (f) 2.37×10^{-3} M

5. (a) 1 mol KCl = 1 Eq KCl. Therefore,

$$14.9\text{ g}\left(\frac{\text{mol}}{74.6\text{ g}}\right)\left(\frac{1}{0.200\text{ L}}\right) = 1.0\,N$$

(b) 4 *N* (c) 2.0 *N*

6. Sample calculation, first row in the table. A 1.0 M solution of $MgCl_2$ is the same as 0.10 moles per 100 mL:

$$\frac{1.0\text{ mol}}{\text{L}} = \frac{0.10\text{ mol}}{100\text{ mL}}$$

Therefore, it is necessary to convert "0.10 moles" into "grams" (formula mass of $MgCl_2$ is 95.21 g/mol):

$$\frac{95.21\text{ g}}{1.0\text{ mol}} = \frac{x}{0.10\text{ mol}} \qquad x = 9.5\text{ g (in 100 mL)}$$

Thus,

$$\frac{9.5\text{ g}}{100\text{ mL}} \times 100\% = 9.5\%\text{ (w/v)}$$

Sample calculation, second row in the table. At 2.6% (w/v), the solution has 2.6 g of $MgCl_2$ in every 100 mL.

$$2.6\%\text{ (w/v)} = \frac{2.6\text{ g}}{100\text{ mL}}$$

Therefore, it is necessary to convert "2.6 grams" into "moles":

$$\frac{95.21\text{ g}}{1\text{ mol}} = \frac{2.6\text{ g}}{x} \qquad x = 0.027\text{ mol (in 100 mL, or 0.1 L)}$$

The number of moles in 1 liter, then, is

$$\frac{0.027\text{ mol}}{0.1\text{ L}} = 0.27\text{ mol/L} = 0.27\text{ M}$$

Molarity	% (w/v)
1.0	9.5
0.27	2.6
3.4×10^{-4}	0.0032
3.06	29.1
0.0025	0.024

7. See problem 6 for sample calculations (formula mass of NaCl is 58.44 g/mol).

Molarity	% (w/v)
2.0	12
0.15	0.90
1.7×10^{-3}	0.0099
2.74	16.0
0.082	0.48

8. See problem 6 for sample calculations (formula mass of glucose is 180.16 g/mol).

Molarity	% (w/v)
0.80	14
0.28	5.0
9.6×10^{-4}	0.017
0.046	0.83
0.066	1.2

Contextual Problems

1. A result of 2.3 mmol/L is within range. Dimensional analysis converts mmol/L to mg/dL:

$$2.3\text{ mmol}\left(\frac{1\text{ mol}}{1000\text{ mmol}}\right)\left(\frac{40.08\text{ g}}{\text{mol}}\right)\left(\frac{1000\text{ mg}}{\text{g}}\right)\left(\frac{1}{10\text{ dL}}\right) = 9.2\text{ mg/dL}$$

The ratio method gives the same result:

$$\frac{1000\text{ mmol}}{1\text{ mol}} = \frac{2.3\text{ mmol}}{x} \qquad x = 0.0023\text{ mol}$$

$$\frac{1\text{ mol}}{40.08\text{ g}} = \frac{0.0023\text{ mol}}{x} \qquad x = 0.092\text{ g}$$

$$\frac{1\text{ g}}{1000\text{ mg}} = \frac{0.092\text{ g}}{x} \qquad x = 92\text{ mg}$$ ← The mass present in 1 L (in 10 dL)

$$\frac{92\text{ mg}}{10\text{ dL}} = \mathbf{9.2\text{ mg/dL}}$$ ← The final concentration in the new units

A result of 4.8 mEq/L is also within range. Remember that because 1 mole of Ca^{2+} can theoretically replace 2 hydrogen ions, it is the same as 2 equivalents:

$$1\text{ mol Ca}^{2+} = 2\text{ Eq Ca}^{2+}$$

Likewise, 1 millimole is the same as 2 milliequivalents:

$$1\text{ mmol Ca}^{2+} = 2\text{ mEq Ca}^{2+}$$

Therefore, 4.8 mEq/L equals 2.4 mmol/L, which falls in the reference range:

$$4.8\text{ mEq Ca}^{2+}\left(\frac{1\text{ mmol Ca}^{2+}}{2\text{ mEq Ca}^{2+}}\right) = 2.4\text{ mmol} \quad \text{(the amount in every liter)}$$

By the ratio method:

$$\frac{2\text{ mEq Ca}^{2+}}{1\text{ mmol Ca}^{2+}} = \frac{4.8\text{ mEq Ca}^{2+}}{x} \qquad x = 2.4\text{ mmol Ca}^{2+} \quad \text{(the amount in every liter)}$$

2. A result of 2.6 mEq/L is not within range. Dimensional analysis converts mEq/L to mg/dL:

$$2.6\text{ mEq}\left(\frac{0.5\text{ mmol}}{1\text{ mEq}}\right)\left(\frac{\text{mol}}{1000\text{ mmol}}\right)\left(\frac{24.305\text{ g}}{\text{mol}}\right)\left(\frac{1000\text{ mg}}{\text{g}}\right)\left(\frac{1}{10\text{ dL}}\right) = 3.2\text{ mg/dL}$$

A result of 0.8 mmol/L is within range:

$$0.8\text{ mmol}\left(\frac{\text{mol}}{1000\text{ mmol}}\right)\left(\frac{24.305\text{ g}}{\text{mol}}\right)\left(\frac{1000\text{ mg}}{\text{g}}\right)\left(\frac{1}{10\text{ dL}}\right) = 1.9\text{ mg/dL}$$

3. To go from *p*H to [H⁺], rearrange Equation 4 to give

$$10^{-pH} = [H^+]$$

Thus, we can solve the first row of the table using this equation:

$$10^{-3.90} = [H^+]$$

$$1.26 \times 10^{-4}\text{M} = [H^+]$$

Going from $[H^+]$ to *p*H requires direct substitution into Equation 4. The second row of the table gives

$$pH = -\log(1.91 \times 10^{-6})$$

$$pH = 5.72$$

*p*H	$[H^+]$ (M)
3.90	1.3×10^{-4}
5.72	1.9×10^{-6}
7.05	8.9×10^{-8}
9.640	2.29×10^{-10}
11.38	4.2×10^{-12}
13.060	8.71×10^{-14}

4. To go from *p*H to $[H^+]$ in "mol/L," use the same equations as in problem 3 above. But to convert from mol/L to mmol/L, multiply by 1000; to convert from mmol/L to mol/L, divide by 1000. Thus, the first row of the table gives $[H^+]$ = 0.00245 M, which is equal to 2.45 mM.

In the second row, $[H^+]$ = 0.0200 mM, which is the same as 2.00×10^5 M. The corresponding *p*H is 4.70.

*p*H	$[H^+]$ (mM)
2.616	2.42
4.699	0.0200
7.00	1.0×10^{-4}
10.149	7.10×10^{-8}
12.27	5.4×10^{-10}
14.000	1.00×10^{-11}

5. The total mass is 721 g (0.721 kg). A 2.00 *m* solution contains 2 moles (360 g, 0.360 kg) of glucose for every kilogram of water present. Thus,

$$1\text{ kg water} + 0.360\text{ kg glucose} = 1.360\text{ kg of solution}$$

Glucose accounts for 26.5% of the solution's mass:

$$\frac{0.360\text{ kg of glucose}}{1.360\text{ kg of solution}} \times 100\% = 26.5\%$$

The total mass of glucose, then, is 26.5% of 2720 g, or 721 g (0.721 kg):

$$0.265 \times 2720\text{ g} = 721\text{ g}$$

6.

Analyte	Your Result	Result in Requested Units
creatinine (112.3 g/mol)	6.4 mg/L	57 μM
folic acid (441.6 g/mol)	14 ng/mL	32 nmol/L
phenobarbital (230.8 g/mol)	15 μg/mL	65 μM
lead	4.2 μM	870 μg/L
phosphorus	1.62 mM	50.2 mg/L
iron	22.9 μmol/L	1280 μg/L
glucose	160 mg/dL	8.9 mmol/L
uric acid (168.1 g/mol)	77 mg/L	458 μM

Sample calculation, first row in the table.

$$\left(\frac{6.4\text{ mg}}{\text{L}}\right)\left(\frac{\text{g}}{1000\text{ mg}}\right)\left(\frac{\text{mol}}{112.3\text{ g}}\right)\left(\frac{10^6\ \mu\text{mol}}{\text{mol}}\right) = 57\ \mu\text{mol/L} = 57\ \mu\text{M}$$

By the ratio method:

$$\left(\frac{1000\text{ mg}}{1\text{ g}}\right) = \left(\frac{6.4\text{ mg}}{x}\right) \qquad x = 0.0064\text{ g}$$

$$\left(\frac{112.3\text{ g}}{1\text{ mol}}\right) = \left(\frac{0.0064\text{ g}}{x}\right) \qquad x = 5.7 \times 10^{-5}\text{ mol}$$

$$\left(\frac{1\text{ mol}}{1 \times 10^6\ \mu\text{mol}}\right) = \left(\frac{5.7 \times 10^{-5}\text{ mol}}{x}\right) \qquad x = 57\ \mu\text{mol}$$

$$\frac{57\ \mu\text{mol}}{1\text{ L}} = 57\ \mu\text{mol/L} = 57\ \mu\text{M}$$

7. Yes. The concentration is 0.62% (w/v).

$$\left(\frac{0.083\text{ mol}}{\text{L}}\right)\left(\frac{74.44\text{ g}}{\text{mol}}\right)\left(\frac{1\text{ L}}{10\text{ dL}}\right) = 0.62\text{ g/dL} = 0.62\text{ g/100 mL} = 0.62\%\text{ (w/v)}$$

By the ratio method:

$$\left(\frac{1\text{ mol}}{74.44\text{ g}}\right) = \left(\frac{0.083\text{ mol}}{x}\right) \qquad x = 6.2\text{ g} \quad \text{(in 1 liter, or 1000 mL)}$$

$$\frac{6.2\text{ g}}{1\text{ L}} = \frac{6.2\text{ g}}{1000\text{ mL}} = 0.0062\text{ g/mL}$$

$$\left(\frac{0.0062\text{ g}}{1\text{ mL}}\right) = \left(\frac{x}{100\text{ mL}}\right) \qquad x = 0.62\text{ g/100 mL} = 0.62\text{ g/dL} = 0.62\%\text{ (w/v)}$$

8. Calculate the factor that converts "mg/dL" to "mmol/L":

$$\left(\frac{1\text{ mg}}{\text{dL}}\right)\left(\frac{\text{g}}{1000\text{ mg}}\right)\left(\frac{\text{mol}}{40.08\text{ g}}\right)\left(\frac{1000\text{ mmol}}{\text{mol}}\right)\left(\frac{10\text{ dL}}{\text{L}}\right) = 0.2495\text{ mmol/L}$$

Your supervisor is correct.

By the ratio method:

$$\left(\frac{1000\text{ mg}}{1\text{ g}}\right) = \left(\frac{1\text{ mg}}{x}\right) \qquad x = 0.001\text{ g (in 1 dL)}$$

$$\left(\frac{40.08\text{ g}}{1\text{ mol}}\right) = \left(\frac{0.001\text{ g}}{x}\right) \qquad x = 2.495 \times 10^{-5}\text{ mol (in 1 dL)}$$

$$\left(\frac{1\text{ mol}}{1000\text{ mmol}}\right) = \left(\frac{2.495 \times 10^{-5}\text{ mol}}{x}\right) \qquad x = 0.02495\text{ mmol (in 1 dL, or 0.1 L)}$$

$$\left(\frac{0.02495\text{ mmol}}{1\text{ dL}}\right) = \left(\frac{0.02495\text{ mmol}}{0.1\text{ L}}\right) = 0.2495\text{ mmol/L}$$

9. In order to answer this question, the result of 9.2 mmol/L must be converted to "mg/dL."

$$\left(\frac{9.2\text{ mmol}}{\text{L}}\right)\left(\frac{1\text{ mol}}{1000\text{ mmol}}\right)\left(\frac{62\text{ g}}{\text{mol}}\right)\left(\frac{1000\text{ mg}}{1\text{ g}}\right)\left(\frac{\text{L}}{10\text{ dL}}\right) = 57\text{ mg/dL}$$

Because the concentration is greater than 50 mg/dL, the patient is indeed a candidate for hemodialysis.

By the ratio method:

$$\left(\frac{1000\text{ mmol}}{1\text{ mol}}\right) = \left(\frac{9.2\text{ mmol}}{x}\right) \qquad x = 0.0092\text{ mol (in 1 L)}$$

$$\left(\frac{1\text{ mol}}{62\text{ g}}\right) = \left(\frac{0.0092\text{ mol}}{x}\right) \qquad x = 0.57\text{ g (in 1 L)}$$

$$\left(\frac{1\text{ g}}{1000\text{ mg}}\right) = \left(\frac{0.57\text{ g}}{x}\right) \qquad x = 570\text{ mg (in 1 L, or in 10 dL)}$$

$$\left(\frac{570\text{ mg}}{1\text{ L}}\right) = \left(\frac{570\text{ mg}}{10\text{ dL}}\right) = 57\text{ mg/dL}$$

10. The answer is 2.8 mL. The target solution will contain 1 equivalent weight in every liter. For sulfuric acid (98.08 g/mol), an equivalent weight is half a mole, or 49.04 g. Thus, 100 mL of the dilute acid contains

$$100\text{ mL}\left(\frac{\text{L}}{1000\text{ mL}}\right)\left(\frac{49.04\text{ g}}{\text{L}}\right) = 4.90\text{ g}$$

The volume of concentrated acid that corresponds to this mass of 4.90 g is

$$0.97 \times \left(\frac{1.84\text{ g}}{\text{mL}}\right) = 1.78\text{ g}$$

Thus, each mL of the concentrated acid contains 1.78 g of H_2SO_4. The volume needed for dilution, then, is

$$4.90\text{ g} \times \left(\frac{\text{mL}}{1.78\text{ g}}\right) = 2.8\text{ mL}$$

Chapter 6

Practice and Contextual Problems

1. (a) 5 (b) 4 (c) 3 (1st), 10 (2nd), 30 (final) (d) 30 (e) 40 (f) 4
(g) 10 (1st), 5 (2nd), 50 (final) (h) 1001 (i) 50 (j) 201
(k) 7.5 (1st), 10 (2nd), 75 (final) (l) 7.7 (m) 1.8 (n) 1.5

2. (a) 0.18 (b) 30 (c) 3 (d) 80 (e) 0.45 (f) 5 (g) 20 (h) 0.30 (i) 8

3.

	Tube A			Tube *B*			Tube C			
	Volume of Serum (mL)	**Volume of Diluent (mL)**	**Tube Dilution**	**Volume from Tube *A* (mL)**	**Volume of Diluent (mL)**	**Tube Dilution**	**Volume from Tube *B* (mL)**	**Volume of Diluent (mL)**	**Tube Dilution**	**Sample Dilution**
a	0.20	1.80	1:10	0.20	1.80	1:10	0.20	1.80	1:10	1:1000
b	0.50	4.50	1:10	0.10	0.90	1:10	0.05	0.100	1:3	1:300
c	0.10	0.40	1:5	0.05	0.45	1:10	0.10	4.90	1:50	1:2500
d	0.10	4.90	1:50	0.10	4.90	1:50	0.10	0.30	1:4	1:10,000
e	0.01	0.24	1:25	0.01	0.09	1:10	0.01	0.02	1:3	1:750
f	0.02	0.98	1:50	0.02	0.78	1:40	0.02	0.04	1:3	1:6000
g	0.01	0.50	1:51	0.01	0.50	1:51	0.01	0.10	1:11	1:28,611
h	0.40	3.60	1:10	0.02	0.58	1:30	0.02	0.58	1:30	1:9000
i	0.025	0.475	1:20	0.025	0.475	1:20	0.025	0.725	1:30	1:12,000

4. (a) Add the 10 µL to 490 µL of diluent.
(b) Add the 20 µL to 100 µL of diluent.
(c) Add the 15 µL to 435 µL of diluent.
(d) In each step, dilute 50 µL with 450 µL of diluent.
(e) In each step, dilute 10 µL with 190 µL of diluent.
(f) In each step, dilute 1.0 mL with diluent up to 5.0 mL.
(g) In each step, dilute 0.20 mL with 1.80 mL of diluent.

5. (a) Choose a convenient initial volume, say, 100 µL. The final volume, then, must be three times greater, or 300 µL. Therefore, mix 200 µL of diluent and 100 µL of sample. Any combination of volumes is acceptable if it meets the restrictions specified above and if the ratio of initial volume to final volume is 1:3.

(b) Because the dilution factor is 20, the initial volume must be 50 µL or less in order to keep the final volume at 1.0 mL or less. Therefore, add 50 µL of patient sample to 950 µL of diluent. Any combination of volumes is acceptable if it meets the restrictions specified above and if the ratio of initial volume to final volume is 1:20.

(c) Because the dilution factor is 100, a simple dilution is impossible. With the available pipets, there is no initial volume that can be diluted 100-fold in one step to a final volume of 1.0 mL or less. Therefore, a serial dilution is necessary. For example, two sequential 1:10 dilutions would succeed, such as adding 50 µL of sample to 450 µL of diluent. A 1:20 followed by a 1:5 would achieve the same goal, first by adding 20 µL of sample to 380 µL of diluent and then by mixing 100 µL of the resulting dilution into 400 µL of diluent. Another option is a 1:25 followed by a 1:4; done by adding 20 µL of specimen to 480 µL of diluent and then transferring 100 µL of the resulting dilution into 300 µL of diluent.

(d) With a dilution factor of 201, a simple dilution is impossible. With the available pipets, there is no initial volume that can be diluted 201-fold in one step to a final volume of 1.0 mL or less. Therefore, a serial dilution is necessary. For example, a 20.1-fold dilution followed by a 10-fold dilution would succeed. To do this, add 20 µL of specimen to 382 µL of diluent for the 20.1-fold dilution. Then, add 20 µL of the first dilution to 180 µL of diluent, giving the 10-fold dilution. Other combinations are possible. For example, execute a 40.2-fold and then a 5-fold dilution by adding 20 µL of specimen to 784 µL of diluent and then transferring 50 µL of the first dilution into 200 µL of diluent.

6. (a) 250 ng/dL. If the raw result for the second run had been 50 ng/dL, the corre[illegible] concentration would be 250 ng/dL. But, because the raw result is > 50[illegible] concentration must be > 250.

(b) 31 ng/dL. Simply multiply the raw result by the dilution factor of 5.

(c) 500 ng/dL. The overall dilution factor is 10 (5×2). If the third raw result had been 50 ng/dL, the corrected concentration would be 500 ng/dL. But, because the result is > 50, the real concentration must be > 500.

(d) 920 ng/dL. The sample dilution is 20-fold (5×4). Because the raw result of 46 ng/dL falls within the range of reliability, simply multiply it by the dilution factor of 20.

7. It is too low by 25%. The technologist should have multiplied the result by 4. Thus, the corrected concentration is only 3/4 of the real value or 1/4 less than it should be.

8. It is too low by 4%. The dilution is actually 26-fold.

9. (a) 92 cells/mL. Use the serial-dilution equation,

$$D_{\text{sample}} = (D_{\text{tube}})^N$$

where D_{tube} (the tube dilution) $=$ 1:10 (1.0 mL $+$ 9.0 mL) and N (the number of the tube in the sequence) equals 3. The sample dilution for tube **3** is 1/1000; divide the starting concentration (92,300 cells/mL) by 1000.

(b) 1.9×10^6 cells/mL. The sample dilution in tube **4** is 1:10,000. Therefore, multiply the concentration in tube **4** (190 cells/mL) by 10,000.

(c) The target concentration is 50 cells per 0.10 mL, or 500 cells/mL. This represents a sample dilution of about 1000-fold, which corresponds to tube **3**.

(d) The tube dilution in the series changes from 1:10 to 1:11 because 1.0 mL of specimen is added to 10.0 mL, giving a total volume of 11.0 mL. Therefore, the sample dilution (D_{sample}) in tube **4** is 1:14,600.

10. Solve the serial-dilution equation for N.

$$D_{\text{sample}} = (D_{\text{tube}})^N$$

$$\frac{1}{243} = \left(\frac{1}{3}\right)^N$$

$$\log\left(\frac{1}{243}\right) = N\log\left(\frac{1}{3}\right)$$

$$5 = N$$

Therefore the sample has been diluted 243-fold in the fifth tube.

11. (a) The raw result is "275 mg/dL," but it represents a 1:5 dilution because the technologist diluted 200 µL of the sample with diluent to a total volume of 1000 µL. Therefore, he must multiply the result by 5 to give the corrected concentration for the patient sample: 1375 mg/dL.

(b) The 1:2 dilution gave a raw result of 688 mg/dL, which yields a corrected result of 1376 mg/dL. Because this is effectively the same as the corrected result for the 1:5 dilution (1375 mg/dL), the value of 688 may have been reliable.

12. Rearrange the dilution equation to isolate V_{final}:

$$V_{\text{final}}C_{\text{final}} = V_{\text{initial}}C_{\text{initial}}$$

$$V_{\text{final}} = \frac{V_{\text{initial}}C_{\text{initial}}}{C_{\text{final}}}$$

[illegible]e known values into the equation in order to give the target value, V_{final}:

$$V_{\text{final}} = \frac{(9.8\ \text{mL})(86\ \text{mg/dL})}{1500\ \text{mg/dL}} = 0.56\ \text{mL}$$

[illegible]he final volume is 0.42–0.56 mL.

13. The result for the straight serum (>12.0) is greater than the result for the 1:3 dilution after correction (9.0). The corrected result should have given a number higher than 12.

14. There are two corrections to make on the raw concentration of 1946 nM BCE.

1. From the total BCE, subtract the contribution of sample *B* in the mixture of samples *A* and *B*.
2. Correct the concentration of BCE in diluted sample *A* for the dilution.

There are several approaches to solving these problems. Two of them follow.

APPROACH 1

Consider the fact that the total number of moles of BCE from sample *A* is the sum of the number of moles from samples *A* and *B*:

$$\text{Total moles BCE in mixture} = \text{moles BCE from } A + \text{moles BCE from } B$$

To simplify the calculation, assume the mixture of *A* and *B* to have a final volume of 1.00 mL (1.00×10^{-3} L). Therefore, 0.20×10^{-3} L of *A* was diluted with 0.80×10^{-3} L of *B*. The total number of nanomoles of BCE in the mixture is 1.95 (1.00×10^{-3} L $\times$ 1946 nmol/L), and the number of nanomoles of BCE from sample *B* is 0.26 (0.80×10^{-3} L $\times$ 331 nmol/L). Substitute these values into the above equation:

$$1.95 \text{ nmol BCE in mixture} = \text{nmol BCE from } A + 0.26 \text{ nmol BCE from } B$$

Therefore,

$$1.95 \text{ nmol BCE in mixture} - 0.26 \text{ nmol BCE from } B = \text{nmol BCE from } A$$

$$1.69 = \text{nmol BCE from } A$$

What this means is that there are 1.68 nmol of BCE in 0.20×10^{-3} L, giving a concentration of 8400 nM for undiluted sample *A*.

APPROACH 2

Envision five test tubes, each containing 0.20 mL of sample *B*. If the contents of all five of the tubes are mixed, the concentration of the mixture is still 331 nM. Now, if a test tube containing 0.20 mL of *A* is substituted for one of the tubes containing *B*, then the final mixture is only 80% *B*; this means that the mixture's BCE concentration coming from sample *B* is not 331 nM but 80% of 331 nM, or 265 nM. Therefore:

$$\text{BCE concentration in mixture} = \text{conc. coming from } A + (80\% \text{ of conc. coming from } B)$$

$$1946 \text{ nM} = \text{conc. coming from } A + 265 \text{ nM}$$

$$1946 \text{ nM} - 265 \text{ nM} = \text{conc. coming from } A$$

$$1681 \text{ nM} = \text{conc. coming from } A$$

Correcting this concentration for the 1:5 dilution gives 8405 nM.

15. (a) Because the sample on circle 1 is straight (undiluted), its dilution is considered 1:1. Here is a summary of the other four serial dilutions.

Circle	Starting Dilution	Dilution Relative to Preceding Circle	Sample Dilution
2	1:1	1:2	1:2
3	1:2	1:2	1:4
4	1:4	1:2	1:8
5	1:8	1:2	1:16

(b) Sample is diluted 1:16 at the start of this procedure (100 μL is added to 1500 μL, for a total volume of 1600 μL); this 1:16 dilution is what goes onto circle 1. Here is a summary of all five dilutions.

Circle	Starting Dilution	Dilution Relative to Preceding Circle	Sample Dilution
1	—	—	1:16
2	1:16	1:2	1:32
3	1:32	1:2	1:64
4	1:64	1:2	1:128
5	1:128	1:2	1:256

(c) Sample is diluted 1:4 at the start of this procedure (e.g., 100 μL + 300 μL of normal saline solution). Then, use a pipet to put 75 μL of diluent onto each of circles 2–5. Next, dispense 75 μL of the diluted sample onto circle 1 and 25 μL onto circle 2. Of the mixture on circle 2, transfer 25 μL to circle 3, and repeat this dilution procedure through the fifth circle. From the fifth circle, remove and discard 25 μL, equalizing the volumes on all five circles. Here is a summary of all five dilutions.

Circle	Starting Dilution	Dilution Relative to Preceding Circle	Sample Dilution
1	—	—	1:4
2	1:4	1:4	1:16
3	1:16	1:4	1:64
4	1:64	1:4	1:256
5	1:256	1:4	1:1024

Chapter 7

Practice Problems

1. (a) yes (b) yes (c) no (d) yes

2.

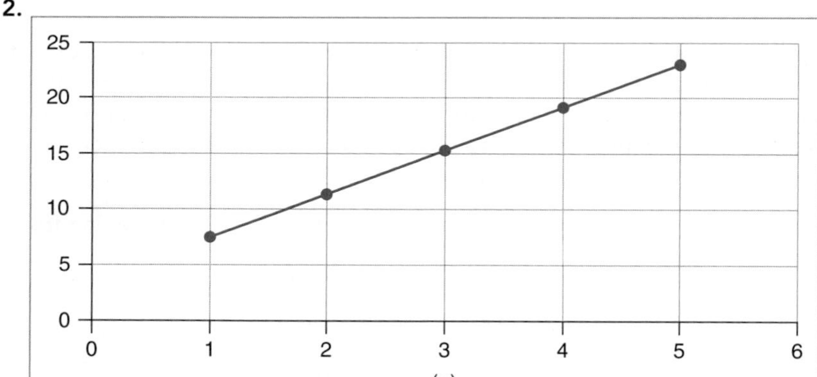

(a)

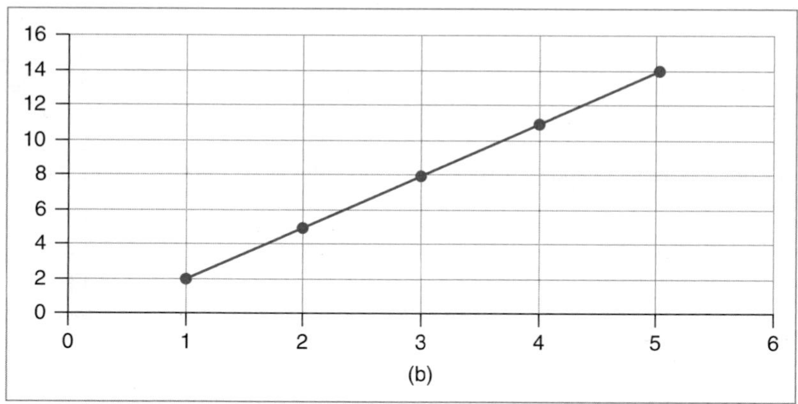

(b)

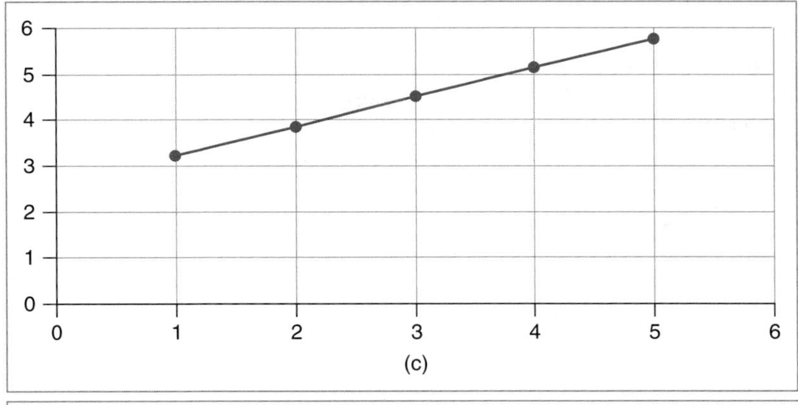
6
5
4
3
2
1
0
0 1 2 3 4 5 6
(c)

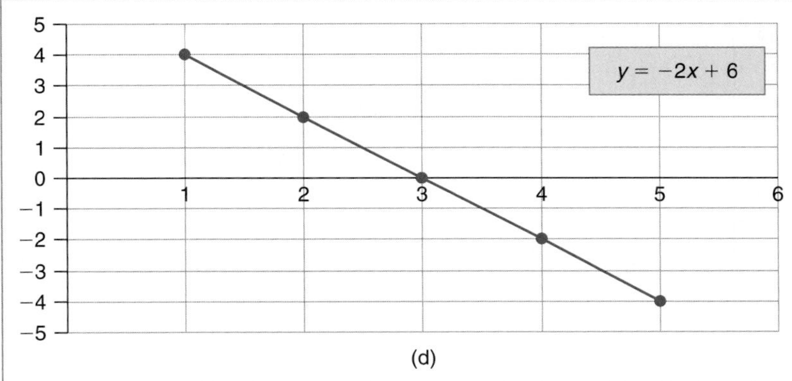
$y = -2x + 6$
5
4
3
2
1
0
−1
−2
−3
−4
−5
1 2 3 4 5 6
(d)

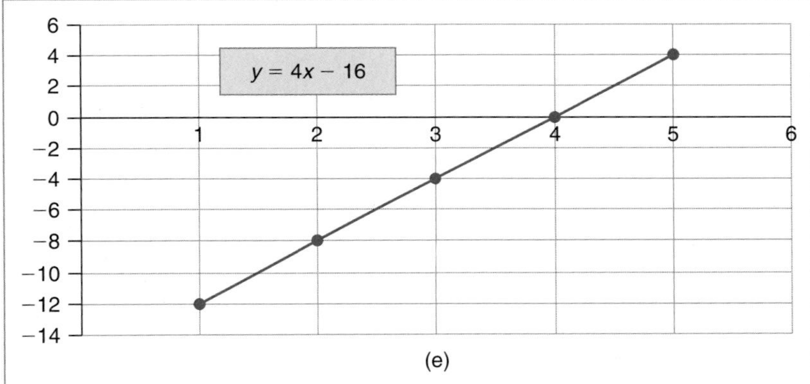
$y = 4x - 16$
6
4
2
0
−2
−4
−6
−8
−10
−12
−14
1 2 3 4 5 6
(e)

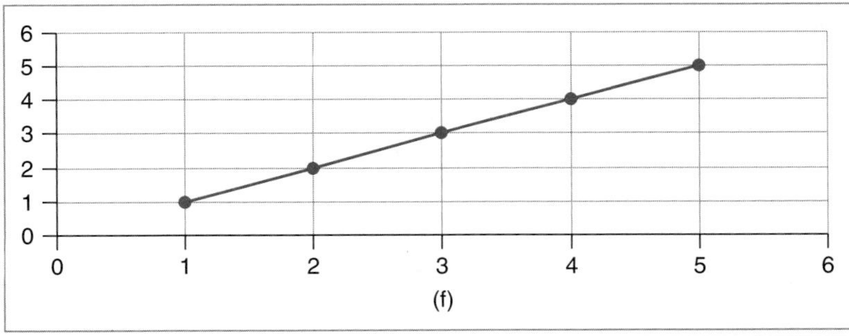
6
5
4
3
2
1
0
0 1 2 3 4 5 6
(f)

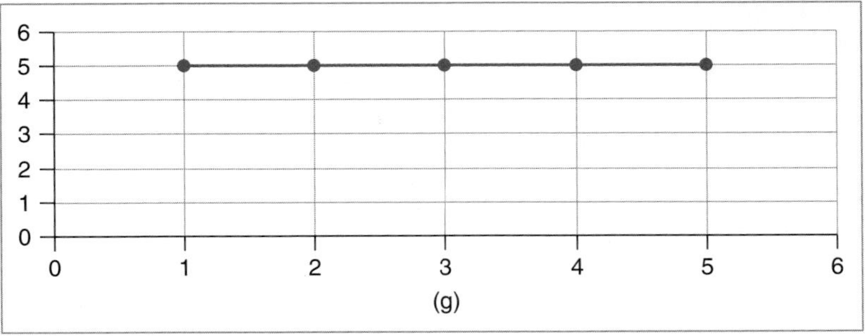
6
5
4
3
2
1
0
0 1 2 3 4 5 6
(g)

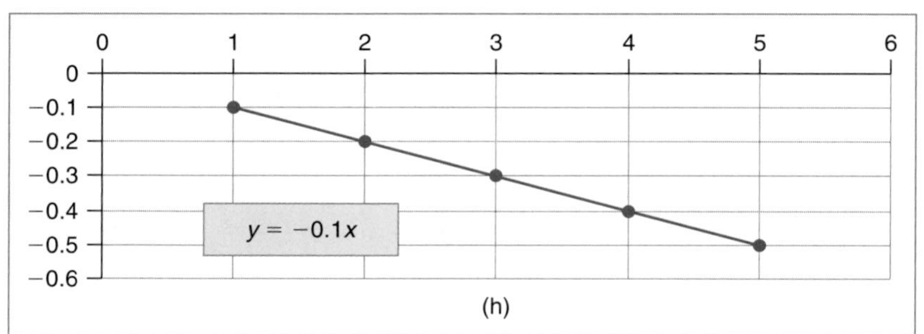
y = −0.1x
(h)

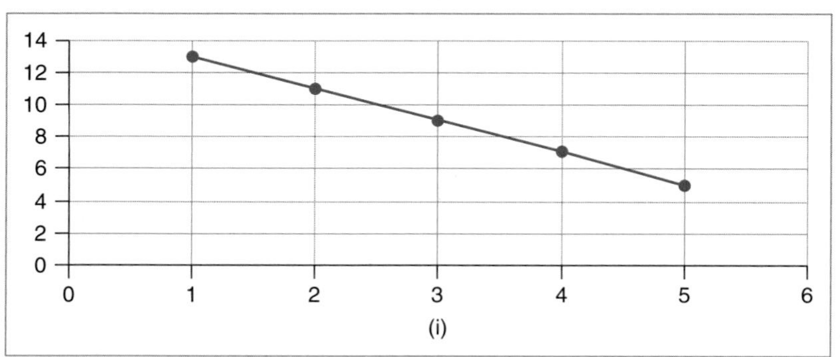
(i)

3.

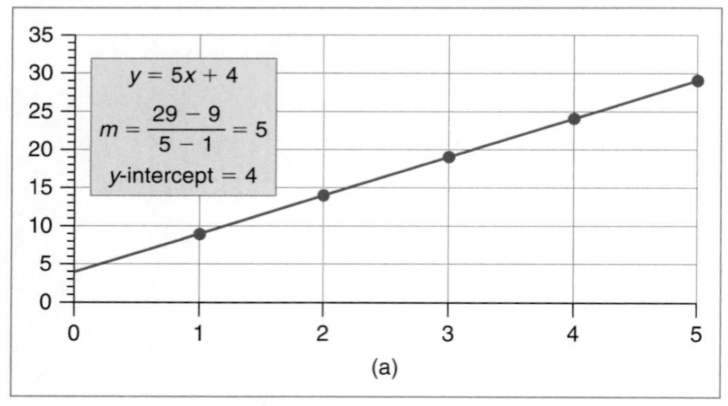
y = 5x + 4
m = (29 − 9)/(5 − 1) = 5
y-intercept = 4
(a)

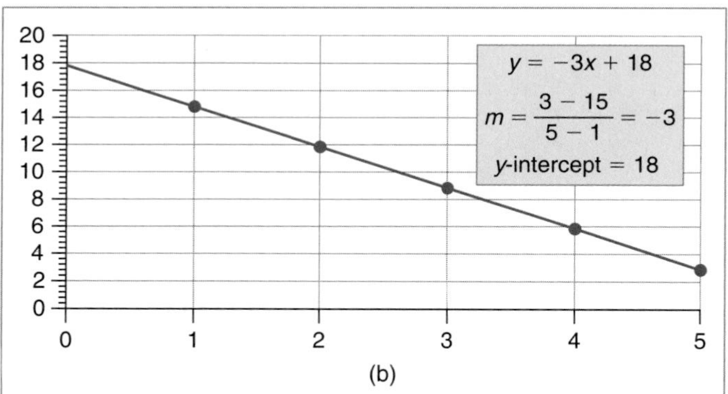
y = −3x + 18
m = (3 − 15)/(5 − 1) = −3
y-intercept = 18
(b)

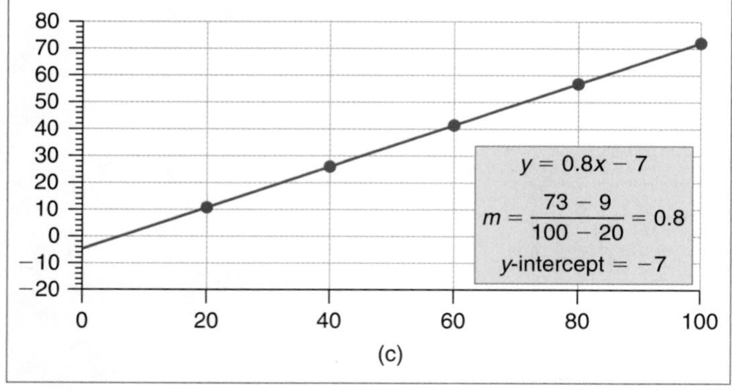
y = 0.8x − 7
m = (73 − 9)/(100 − 20) = 0.8
y-intercept = −7
(c)

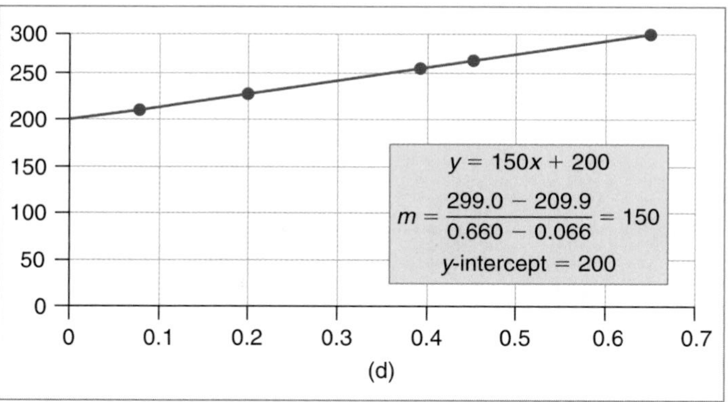
y = 150x + 200
m = (299.0 − 209.9)/(0.660 − 0.066) = 150
y-intercept = 200
(d)

4. (a) $m = \dfrac{110\text{ nmol} - 30\text{ nmol}}{50\text{ s} - 10\text{ s}} = 2\text{ nmol/s}$

(b) $m = \dfrac{5\ \mu\text{mol} - 21\ \mu\text{mol}}{10\text{ s} - 2\text{ s}} = -2\ \mu\text{mol/s}$

(c) $m = \dfrac{30\text{ mmol} - 10\text{ mmol}}{2.5\text{ min} - 0.5\text{ min}} = 10\text{ mmol/min}$

(d) $m = \dfrac{6.5\ \mu\text{g} - 1.3\ \mu\text{g}}{13.0\text{ min} - 2.6\text{ min}} = 0.5\ \mu\text{g/min}$

5.

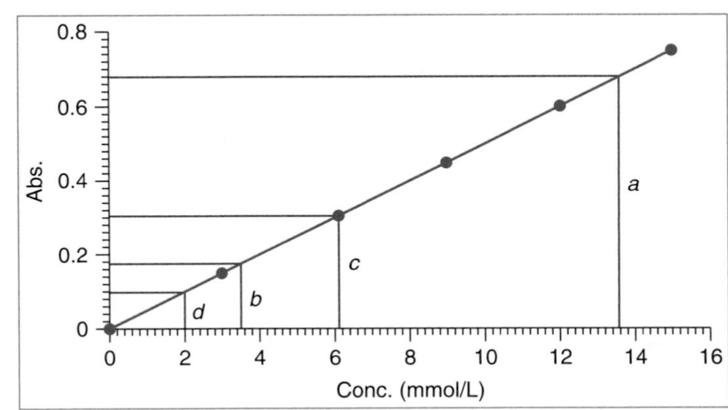

(a) 13.6 mmol/L (b) 3.5 mmol/L (c) 6.1 mmol/L (d) 1.9 mmol/L

6.

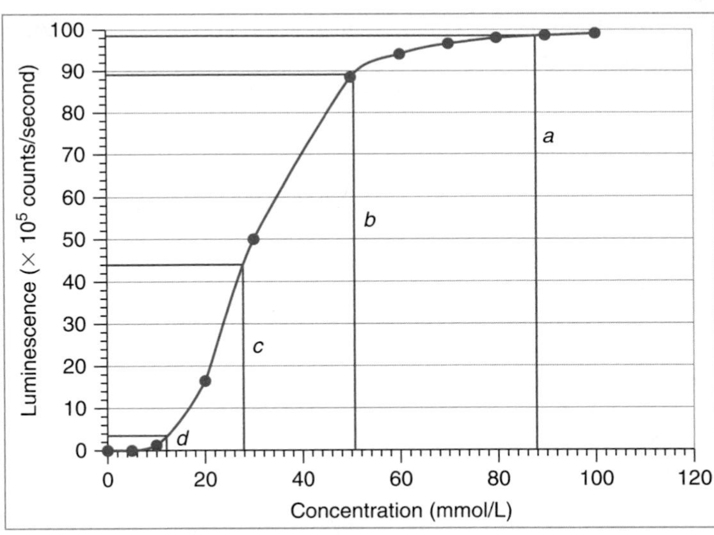

(a) 88 mmol/L (b) 51 mmol/L (c) 28 mmol/L (d) 12 mmol/L

7. Interpolation *a* is the most prone to error. In the region where the horizontal line from the *y*-axis touches the curve, the two are nearly parallel. Therefore, visually locating the point of intersection is more questionable than it is for any of the other interpolations.

8. (*A*) $y = x$ (*B*) $y = 5$ (*C*) $y = -x + 10$ (*D*) $x = 6$ (*E*) $y = 0.2x + 5$
(*F*) $y = -0.2x + 5$ (*G*) $y = 0.7x + 4$ (*H*) $y = -0.7x + 7$ (*I*) $y = 0.7x + 1$
(*J*) $y = -0.7x + 9$

9. (a) True. The graph shows that the slope of **C** is less than the slope of **A**. Therefore, if the equation for **A** is $y = 2x + 5$, then its slope is 2, and the slope of **C** must be < 2.

(b) True. The graph shows that **B** and **C** have the same *y*-intercept. Therefore, if the equation for **C** is $y = x + 10$, then the *y*-intercept of each line is 10.

(c) True. The graph shows that

- line **A** rises about twice as fast as line **C** (the slope of **A** is about two times the slope of **C**), and
- the *y*-intercept of **A** is about twice that of **C**.

Line	Equation	Slope	*y*-Intercept	Comment
A	$y = 4x + 12$	4	12	Both the slope and *y*-intercept of line **A** are twice as large as they are for line **C**.
C	$y = 2x + 6$	2	6	

(d) False. The slope (−3) is negative, but each of the three lines moves upward.

(e) False. The *y*-intercept (−7) is negative, but each of the three lines crosses the *y*-axis above "0."

10. (a) $y = 1/x^2$ (b) $y = 3 \log x$ (c) $y = x^2 + 2$ (d) $y = x^3/(x^3 + 10)$ (e) $y = 1/x$ (f) $y = \log x$ (g) $y = e^x$ (h) $y = 2x^2 + 3x + 20$ (i) $y = x/(x + 10)$

Contextual Problems

1. (a) A luminescence of 700,000 RLU corresponds to a concentration of 0.61 ng/mL. The other two interpolations are 1,900,000 RLU → 0.020 ng/mL and 200,000 RLU → 4.6 ng/mL.

(b) This problem necessitates reading the graph at the seven data points and replotting them on arithmetic axes. A comparison of the two graphs reveals a difference in the reliability of interpolation at high concentrations. Consider, for example, a luminescence of 200,000 RLU. It is much harder to discern where the interpolation line touches the curve, which is nearly horizontal in this range.

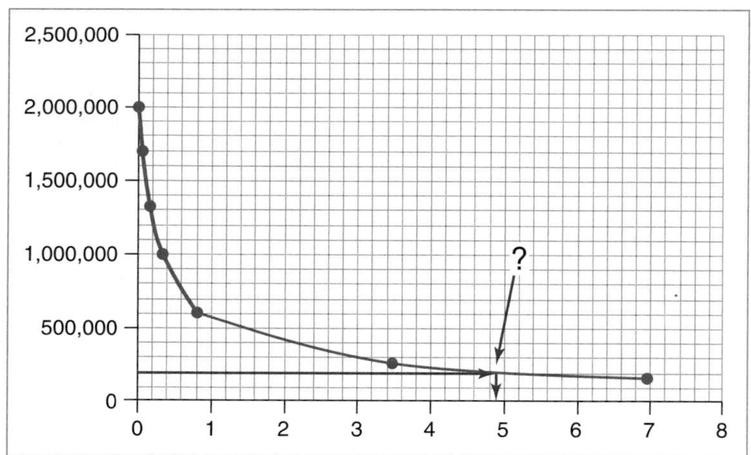

2. (a) Slope = 278; *y*-intercept = 41,582.

(b) New slope = 299. New *y*-intercept = 44,131. The acceptability range of the existing slope is 278 ± 27.8, or 250.2–305.8. The acceptability range of the existing *y*-intercept is 41,582 ± 10%, or 37,424–45,740. Both the new slope and *y*-intercept fall within their acceptability ranges. Therefore, the existing standard curve is still valid.

(c) The new line from scenario *A* is slightly closer to the existing standard curve. To reach this conclusion, there are at least two approaches.

APPROACH 1

On a single graph, accurately plot the existing standard curve (from part *a*), along with the two new curves from scenarios *A* and *B*. By visual inspection, the new line from scenario *A* is closer to the existing standard curve at a concentration of 120 μmol/L and above.

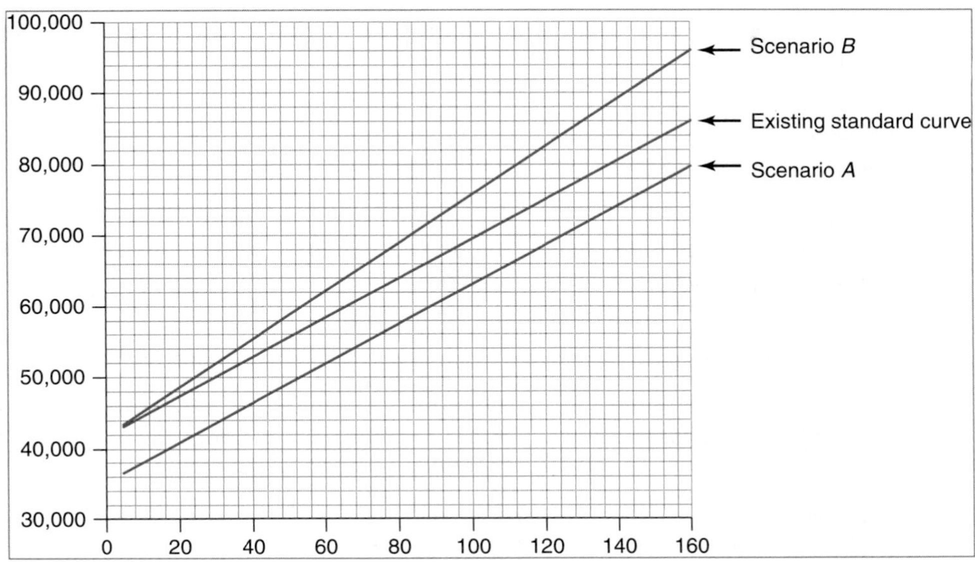

APPROACH 2

Find the equations of all three lines in question (existing standard curve, scenario *A*, scenario *B*). Then, for each line, calculate the value of *y* (counts per second) at a concentration of 120 μmol/L and above. Finally, compare the two new lines for distance from the existing standard curve at 120 μmol/L and above.

	Equation	Value of *y* at $x = 120$ μmol/L	Difference from Existing Standard Curve at $x = 120$ μmol/L
Existing standard curve	$y = 278x + 41{,}582$	74,942	—
New line from scenario *A*	$y = 278x + 35{,}193$	68,553	$74{,}942 - 68{,}553 = 6389$
New line from scenario *B*	$y = 340x + 41{,}582$	82,382	$82{,}382 - 74{,}942 = 7440$

As the graph shows, at concentrations above 120 μmol/L, the new line from scenario *B* diverges even more from the existing standard curve because of its greater slope. The new line from scenario *A*, however, has the same slope as the existing standard curve; at all concentrations, therefore, it lies at the same distance from the existing curve.

Chapter 8

Practice Problems

1. (1) mean = 150 median = 150

(2) mean = 450 median = 150

(3) mean = 135 median = 150

The median resists outliers, whether high or low, but the mean is strongly affected by them.

2. (1) mean = 2.5 median = 2.5 mode = 2.6

(2) mean = 108 median = 107 mode = 106

(3) mean = 43.5 median = 44.1 mode = 44.8

3. (a) 5.5 ± 2.0 (b) 92.2 ± 4.2 (c) 0.033 ± 0.007 (d) $1.00 \times 10^6 \pm 4.5 \times 10^4$ (e) 2277 ± 1177

4. (a) mean = 5, median = 5, balanced

The beam is balanced on the mean. If the median equals the mean, then the beam is balanced on the median. If the median is greater than the mean, then there is more weight to the median's left, causing the beam to tip leftward. If the median is less than the mean, then there is more weight to the median's right, causing the beam to tip rightward.

(b) mean = 6.6, median = 7, tips to left

(c) mean = 113.8, median = 108, tips to right

(d) mean = 0.67, median = 0.655, tips to right

(e) mean = 1.4×10^5, median = 1.2×10^5, tips to right

5. The number of standard deviations can be calculated by determining the ratio of the individual deviation to the standard deviation:

$$(\text{data value} - \text{mean}) \div \text{SD}$$

(a) 1 SD (b) 1.2 SD (c) −1 SD (d) 1.7 SD (e) 2.8 SD (f) −2.1 SD

6. Ninety-five percent. The range of 30 to 70 extends from two standard deviations below the mean to two standard deviations above the mean. For a normal distribution, 95% of the data lie between −2 and +2 standard deviations of the mean.

7. Pipet *A* is the most accurate because its mean is closest to the nominal volume of 200 μL. Pipet *C* is the most precise because its coefficient of variation is the smallest at 0.8%.

8. (a) $y = 2.05x + 4.93$, $r = 0.99$ (b) $y = -19.67x + 45.17$, $r = -0.99$
(c) $y = 0.03x - 0.18$, $r = 0.99$ (d) $y = 14{,}674x + 151$, $r = 0.97$
(e) $y = 0.976x - 15.19$, $r = 1.0$ (0.9996) (f) $y = -34x + 404$, $r = -0.96$

9. To predict *x*, substitute the specified value of *y* into the regression equation found in problem 1 and solve for *x*.

(a) 8.6 (b) 0.56 (c) 59.3 (d) 0.47 (e) 357 (f) 10.4

10. (a) Slope = 0.94, *y*-intercept = 0.28 mmol/L, $r^2 = 0.9935$.

To find the result for method *Q* when the result for method *P* is 5.5, use the regression equation $y = 0.94x + 0.28$. Therefore,

$$y = 0.94(5.5) + 0.28 = 5.45$$

Likewise, when *P* is 2.5, *Q* is 2.63.

(b) Slope = 1.05, *y*-intercept = −0.27 mmol/L, $r^2 = 0.9935$.

To find the result for method *P* when the result for method *Q* is 5.5, use the regression equation $y = 1.05x - 0.27$. Therefore,

$$y = 1.05(5.5) - 0.27 = 5.51$$

Likewise, when *Q* is 2.5, *P* is 2.36.

(c) To one decimal place, the two regression lines give the same result for the dependent variable (5.5 mmol/L) when the independent variable is 5.5 mmol/L. However, they give different results (2.6 and 2.4 mmol/L) when the independent variable is 2.5 mmol/L. This happens because the difference in slope has its smallest effect near the center of the range and its greatest effect near the ends of the range.

11. (a) Slope = 0.028 AU per mg/dL, *y*-intercept = −0.0029AU, $r^2 = 0.9941$.

The regression equation is $y = 0.028x - 0.0029$. To predict the concentration when the absorbance is 0.300, rearrange the equation to give $x = (y + 0.0029) \div 0.028$. Thus, when $y = 0.300$, $x = 10.8$ mg/dL. When $y = 0.547$, $x = 19.6$ mg/dL.

(b) Slope = 35.09 mg/dL per AU, *y*-intercept = 0.17 mg/dL, $r^2 = 0.9941$.

The regression equation is $y = 35.09x + 0.17$. To predict the concentration when the absorbance is 0.300, substitute the value directly into the equation. Thus, when $x = 0.300$, $y = 10.7$ mg/dL. When $x = 0.547$, $y = 19.4$ mg/dL.

(c) Yes. Generally, standard curves are more suitable for interpolation when the independent variable predicts the dependent variable. In this case, however, the results of the two regression equations are so close that the difference may be negligible.

12. The assay for analyte *A* shows stronger agreement. Although analyte *B* gave the higher correlation, the slope of the line is such that the *y* value is more than 2.6 times the *x* value. By contrast, analyte *A* yields *x* and *y* values much closer to equality.

13. (a) The equation is $CI = m \pm (t \times S_m)$. The *t* value corresponds to 30 degrees of freedom because there are 32 data points and to a *p* value of 0.01 because the desired confidence interval should enclose 99% of the data. Thus, substitution into the equation gives $CI = (-8.23) \pm (2.75 \times 0.041)$, which means that the 99% confidence interval for the slope extends from −8.34 to −8.12.

(b) It says that every increase of 1 μg/dL in the concentration of *V* causes a decrease in the measured concentration of *M* between 8.12 and 8.34 μg/dL.

(c) The equation is $CI = b \pm (t \times S_b)$. The *t* value corresponds to 30 degrees of freedom because there are 32 data points and to a *p* value of 0.10 because the desired confidence interval should enclose 90% of the data. Thus, substitution into the equation gives $CI = 66.52 \pm (1.70 \times 2.92)$, which means that the 90% confidence interval for the intercept extends from 61.56 to 71.48 μg/dL.

14. (a) and (b)

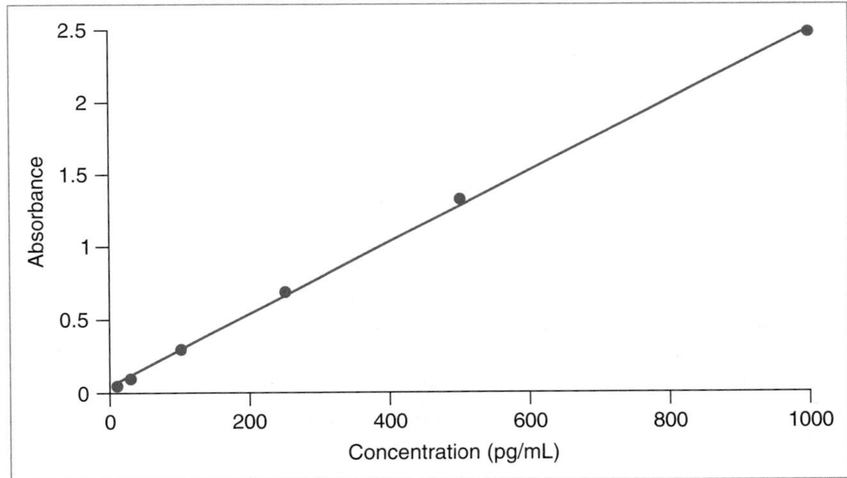

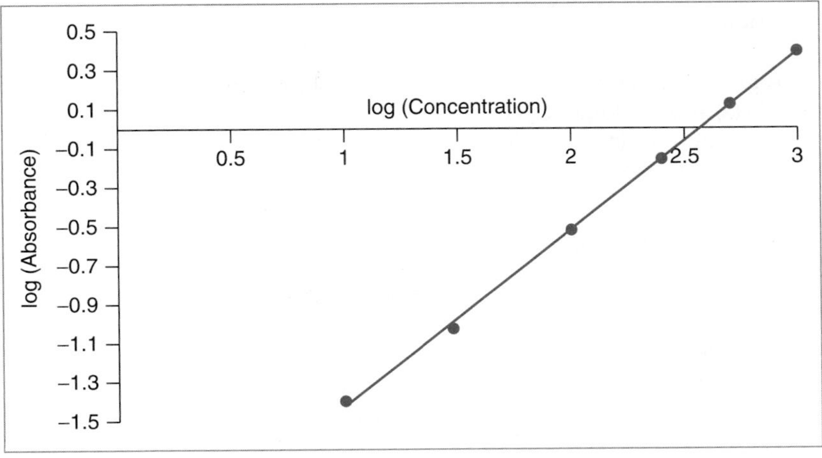

(c) The log-log plot is superior because it spaces the data points more evenly, thereby reducing uncertainty in the regression line. Moreover, it renders the linearity easier to see in the first test for goodness-of-fit. The regression equation is

$$\log y = 0.910(\log x) - 2.34$$

An absorbance of 0.844 predicts a concentration of 309 pg/mL. The y value is 0.844, the logarithm of which is −0.07366; this gives a value for log x of 2.49, making the x value 309. Likewise, an absorbance of 0.107 predicts a concentration of 32.0 pg/mL.

15. (a) $y = 0.078x - 0.060$, $r = 0.987$

(b) Solve the regression equation for x at each specified absorbance, which is the y value.

y (absorbance)	x (concentration)
0.130	2.4
0.330	5.0
0.530	7.6

(c)

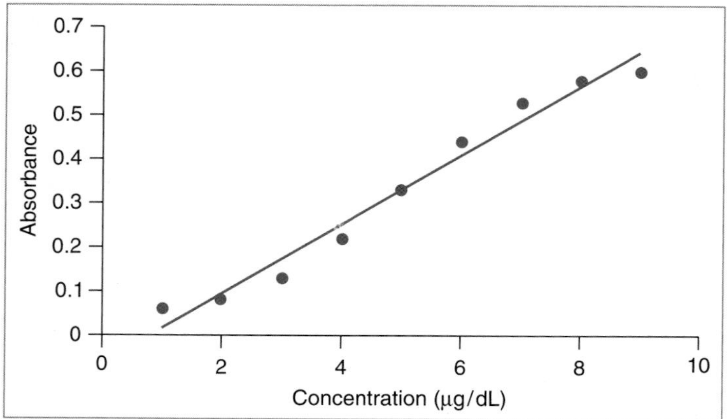

(d) The regression line is arguably unsuitable as a standard curve because, as the plot reveals, the data points are not linear. In fact, they describe a sigmoidal curve. The consequence of this misfitting appears in the table in part *b* above, which shows that, at an absorbance of 0.130, the line predicts a concentration of 2.4, although the true concentration is 3.0. The difference, 0.6, is 20% of the true value.

At an absorbance of 0.530, the line predicts a concentration of 7.6, as opposed to the true value of 7.0; the difference, 0.6, is about 9% of the true concentration. At an absorbance of 0.330, the line predicts the true concentration. In fact, the line is close to the points in only three parts of the curve, that is, where the concentration is about 2, 5, or 8.

16. The equation describes a straight line, in which elapsed time (t) is the independent variable (x) and the logarithm of cell number at time t (c_t) is the dependent variable (y). (Alternatively, the difference [$\log c_t - \log c_i$] can be treated as y, but the final result is the same.) The slope of the line is $0.301/d$. Thus, finding the slope by linear regression leads to the value of d.

The regression equation is

$$y = 0.0166x + 1.38$$

It follows that

$$\text{slope} = \frac{0.301}{d} = 0.0166\ \text{min}^{-1}$$

Therefore, the doubling time (d) is 18.1 min. A plot of the data with the regression line appears below.

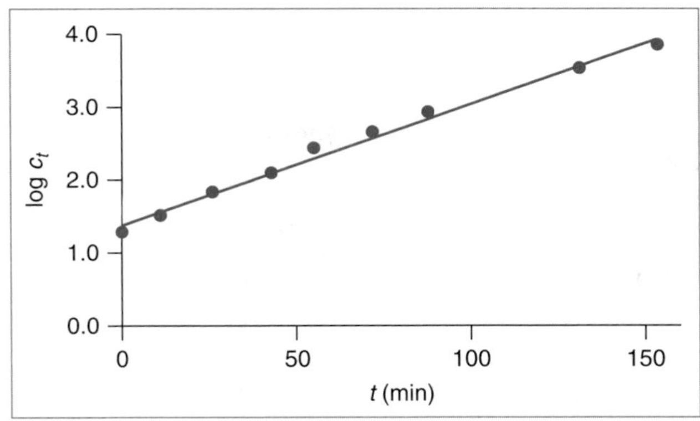

17. (a) 0.997 (b) 0.071 (c) −0.541 (d) 0.914 (e) −0.980

18. To determine significance, compare the calculated *t* value with the critical value, for $n_1 + n_2 - 2$ degrees of freedom. For (**a**), there are 8 degrees of freedom, and the corresponding critical value is 2.306. Because the calculated *t* statistic is less than the critical value, there is no significant difference between the means.

(b) significant (c) not significant (d) not significant
(e) significant

19. There are 11 degrees of freedom:

$$d.f. = n_1 + n_2 - 2 = 6 + 7 - 2 = 11$$

At a *p* value of 0.05, the critical value of the *t* value is 2.201. Because the calculated *t* value exceeds the critical value, there is a significant difference between the means at this level of certainty. At a *p* value of 0.01, however, the calculated value is less than the critical value (3.106); thus, the difference between the means is not significant at this level of certainty.

20. Yes. A preliminary *F* test shows the two variances to be similar:

$$F = \frac{14.78}{13.34} = 1.108$$

At $p = 0.05$, with 20 degrees of freedom in the numerator and 20 in the denominator, the critical value is 2.124. Because the calculated *F* value is less, the variances are considered equal. Student's *t* test requires the two variances to be similar.

21.

	Instrument #1		Instrument #2			Is Difference Significant?
	Variance	*n*	Variance	*n*	*F*	(yes/no)
(a)	0.0446	21	0.0793	21	1.778	no
(b)	8.094	8	10.772	11	1.331	no
(c)	46.812	11	23.004	11	2.035	no
(d)	0.3755	61	0.6122	61	1.630	yes
(e)	32.881	21	15.112	21	2.176	yes

SAMPLE CALCULATION (for comparison **a**):

$$F = \frac{0.0793}{0.0446} = 1.778$$

For 20 degrees of freedom in the numerator and 20 in the denominator, and $p = 0.05$, the critical value is 2.124. Because the calculated *F* value is smaller, the difference between the two variances is not statistically significant.

Critical values for the other comparisons:

(b) 3.637 (not sig.) (c) 2.978 (not sig.) (d) 1.534 (sig.) (e) 2.124 (sig.)

22.

		Response Variable			TOTAL
		X	Y	Z	
Explanatory Variable	A	12 (13.6)	26 (31.8)	83 (75.6)	121
	B	18 (16.1)	34 (37.5)	91 (89.4)	143
	C	15 (15.3)	45 (35.7)	76 (85)	136
	TOTAL	45	105	250	400

Expected counts are in parentheses.

The null hypothesis is that there is no difference between the observed counts and the expected counts.

SAMPLE CALCULATION (for category **X**): The expected frequency of category **X** is 45/400, or 0.1125. Therefore, when the explanatory variable is **A**, the expected count for category **X** is 0.1125 × 121 or 13.6. The other expected counts are calculated similarly.

To calculate the χ^2 statistic, it is helpful to set up a table.

Observed	Expected	Observed – Expected	(Observed − Expected)^2	$\frac{(\text{Observed} - \text{Expected})^2}{\text{Expected}}$
12	13.6	−1.6	2.56	0.188
18	16.1	1.9	3.61	0.224
15	15.3	−0.3	0.09	0.006
26	31.8	−5.8	33.64	1.058
34	37.5	−3.5	12.25	0.327
45	35.7	9.3	86.49	2.423
83	75.6	7.4	54.76	0.724
91	89.4	1.6	2.56	0.029
76	85	−9	81	0.953
			SUM (= χ^2)	5.931

The number of degrees of freedom is

$$d.f. = (\text{number of rows in contingency table} - 1) \times (\text{number of columns in contingency table} - 1)$$

$$d.f. = (3 - 1)(3 - 1) = 4$$

At $p = 0.05$ and 4 degrees of freedom, the critical value of χ^2 is 9.488. Because the calculated value of χ^2 is smaller, the observed results do not differ significantly from the expected results. In other words, we do not reject the null hypothesis.

23. The null hypothesis is that there is no difference between the observed counts and expected counts.

(a) $\chi^2 = 211.915$, $d.f. = 2$. Calculated χ^2 exceeds critical value (9.210) at $p = 0.01$. Thus, we reject the null hypothesis.

(b) $\chi^2 = 1.696$, $d.f. = 4$. Calculated χ^2 is less than critical value (7.779) even at $p = 0.10$. Thus, we do not reject the null hypothesis.

(c) $\chi^2 = 378.132$, $d.f. = 3$. Calculated χ^2 exceeds critical value (11.345) at $p = 0.01$. Thus, we reject the null hypothesis.

24. To determine significance, compare the calculated t value to the critical value, for $n_1 + n_2 - 2$ degrees of freedom. For **a**, there are 100 degrees of freedom, and the corresponding critical value is 2.626. Because the calculated t value is less than the critical value, there is no significant difference between the means.

(b) not significant (c) significant (d) significant (e) not significant

25. (a) True (b) True

(c) False. There is no relationship between the size of p and the size of the difference between the two means. A difference of 50 between two means can be significant at $p = 0.05$, while a difference of 500 can be significant at $p = 0.01$.

26. This statement is true.

27. The statement is true. In the table of critical values, with 10 degrees of freedom, the t value of 2.046 falls between the p values of 0.10 and 0.05.

28. The statement is true. In the table of critical values, with 7 degrees of freedom, the t value of 2.880 falls between the p values of 0.05 and 0.01.

Contextual Problems

1. $\bar{x} = \dfrac{\sum_{i=1}^{n} x_i}{n}$

By the equation above, the mean is 54.2 ng/dL.

$$\text{standard deviation} = s = \sqrt{\frac{\sum_{i=1}^{n}(x_i - \bar{x})^2}{n - 1}}$$

By the equation above, the sample standard deviation is 7.52 ng/dL. The value of 40.4 ng/dL lies at −13.8 ng/dL from the mean, which is the same as −1.8s:

$$\frac{-13.8 \text{ ng/dL}}{7.52 \text{ ng/dL}} = -1.8$$

Therefore, your result of 40.4 does fall within 2s, and you may begin running patient samples and releasing results.

2. (a) No, the error is not negligible. Adding only 1.90 mL to the bottle containing the dehydrated material increases the resulting troponin-T concentration by a factor of 1.05, bringing it up to 3.09 ng/mL. This value, however, lies at 5 standard deviations above the mean of 2.94, well outside the limits of acceptability. This error will cause a delay in running patient samples and releasing the results.

(b) Yes, it will be affected appreciably. The resulting concentration is 2.87 ng/mL, which is 2.3 standard deviations below the mean of 2.94 ng/mL. This error will cause a delay in running patient samples and releasing the results.

3. (a) If the two pipets were correctly calibrated, the curve would show an approximately normal distribution. In this case, however, the curve is bimodal; one peak occurs at 100 ng/dL, corresponding to the correct volume of 50.0 μL, whereas the other peak occurs at about 110 ng/dL, corresponding to the incorrect volume of 55.0 μL. The two peaks are distinct because each pipet has its own standard deviation of 1.0 μL. What this means is that, for the correctly calibrated pipet, 99% of the results fall between about 94 and 106 ng/dL, a range extending from three standard deviations below the mean pipet volume to three above the mean pipet volume. Likewise, for the miscalibrated pipet, 99% of the results fall between about 104 and 116 ng/dL. (This explanation, of course, ignores other sources of error in the assay procedure.)

(b) Each peak would be narrower, and the separation between them would be deeper.

(c) The peak at about 110 ng/dL, corresponding to the miscalibrated pipet, would have been shorter because of a smaller number of data points arising from it. In other words, the frequency of values between about 104 and 116 ng/dL would have been lower.

4. The answer is "16." By the 68-95-99.7 Rule, one standard deviation under the mean, which is 5760, contains 34% of the data. Therefore, a total of 32% (100% − [2 × 34%]) of the data lie above and below one standard deviation, which means that 16% of the data lie below one standard deviation.

5. Despite having a standard deviation between the other two, analyzer *A* has the smallest coefficient of variation, at 4.1%. Therefore, it has the greatest precision.

6.

	Mean (μg/dL)	Standard Deviation (μg/dL)	Coefficient of Variation (%)
Day-to-Day	20	1.6	8
Within-Run	22	0.8	4

The within-run precision is greater. This is so because the day-to-day data include more errors (that is, there are more opportunities for errors to occur from one day to the next and affect the results).

7. The *F* test is appropriate for this problem. The variances, however, must first be calculated by squaring their respective standard deviations.

$$F = \frac{32.49}{22.09} = 1.471$$

Because $n = 16$ for each data set, the number of degrees of freedom is 15 for the numerator and for the denominator. The critical value at $p = 0.05$ is 2.4035. Because the observed *F* value is less than this, the observed difference between the precisions of methods 1 and 2 is statistically nonsignificant.

8. A preliminary *F* test reveals statistical equivalence between the variances:

$$F = \frac{0.08990}{0.03584} = 2.508$$

This *F* value is less than the critical value (2.9782) at $p = 0.05$ for 10 degrees of freedom in the numerator and the denominator. Therefore, Student's *t* test is an appropriate choice. The calculated *p* value is 0.0127, which falls between 0.01 and 0.02, making the difference between the mean concentrations significant at a *p* value of 0.02.

9. A paired *t* test is appropriate because each result from laboratory 1 is matched to a result from laboratory 2.

	Concentration of Hemoglobin (g/dL)		
Specimen	**Laboratory 1**	**Laboratory 2**	**1–2**
1	14.1	14.6	−0.5
2	16.8	16.9	−0.1
3	14.9	15.8	−0.9
4	15.5	15.9	−0.4
5	13.9	14.4	−0.5
6	16.7	17.0	−0.3
7	17.0	17.6	−0.6
8	15.6	16.2	−0.6
9	16.1	16.3	−0.2
10	17.6	18.0	−0.4
		MEAN	−0.45
		VARIANCE	0.05167

The *t* value is −6.26:

$$t = \frac{-0.45}{\sqrt{\frac{0.05167}{10}}} = -6.26$$

At a p value of 0.01 (99% confidence level), and with 9 degrees of freedom, the calculated t value of -6.26 is more negative than the critical value of -3.250. Therefore, the difference between the two instruments is statistically significant.

10. Because one variable is the technologist and the other is the cell type, both variables are categorical. Thus, the χ^2 test is appropriate.

		Count from Manual Differential			TOTAL
		Neutrophils	Lymphocytes	Monocytes	
Technologist	#1 (new)	64 (61)	30 (32.3)	6 (6.7)	100
	#2	60 (61)	33 (32.3)	7 (6.7)	100
	#3	59 (61)	34 (32.3)	7 (6.7)	100
	TOTAL	183	97	20	300

The null hypothesis is that there is no relationship between who the technologist is and the count from the manual differential.

SAMPLE CALCULATION:

For neutrophils, the expected frequency is 183/300, or 0.61. Therefore, the expected neutrophil count for technologist #1 is 0.61×100, or 61.

The χ^2 statistic is 0.598.

The number of degrees of freedom is

$$d.f. = (\text{number of rows} - 1)(\text{number of columns} - 1)$$

$$d.f. = (3 - 1)(3 - 1) = 4$$

For a p of 0.05 at 4 degrees of freedom, the critical value of χ^2 is 9.488. Thus, the observed counts do not differ significantly from the expected counts, and we do not reject the null hypothesis.

11. A paired t test is appropriate because each result from the current instrument is matched to a result from the new one.

	Urine Osmolality (mOsm/kg)		
Specimen	Current Instrument	New Instrument	Current – New
1	446	450	−4
2	307	299	8
3	661	648	13
4	537	555	−18
5	498	494	4
6	410	431	−21
7	372	401	−29
8	526	540	−14
9	462	450	12
10	602	619	−17
		MEAN	−6.6
		VARIANCE	229.38

The t value is -1.378:

$$t = \frac{-6.6}{\sqrt{\dfrac{229.38}{10}}} = -1.378$$

At a p value of 0.05, and with 9 degrees of freedom, the calculated t value of -1.378 is less negative than (is greater than) the critical value of -2.262. Therefore, the difference between the two instruments is statistically nonsignificant.

12. Because one variable is categorical and the other numerical, a t test is called for. A preliminary F test reveals statistical nonequivalence between the variances:

$$F = \frac{5.408}{1.223} = 4.422$$

This F value is greater than the critical value (3.522) at $p = 0.01$ for 15 degrees of freedom in the numerator and in the denominator. Therefore, the t test for unequal variances is the appropriate choice.

The t value is 6.708. There are 21 degrees of freedom (calculated by statistics software in a spreadsheet program). At $p = 0.01$, the calculated t value of 6.708 exceeds the critical value of 2.831. Therefore, there is a significant difference between the means of the two data sets.

CHAPTER 9

Practice and Contextual Problems

1. Beer's law is suitable for each case.

(a) $c = 6.35 \times 10^{-5}$ (b) $c = 6.84 \times 10^{-5}$ (c) $\epsilon = 660$ (d) $l = 0.5$
(e) $c = 3.41 \times 10^{-5}$ (f) $A = 0.400$ (g) $\epsilon = 1676$ (h) $c = 2.63 \times 10^{-4}$

2. (a) The concentration of #2 is two times that of #1 because the absorbance of #2 is two times that of #1. This conclusion is sound because the absorbance values of #1 and #2 are both in the linear range of the standard curve, where Beer's law is valid.

Lowest concentration of linear range	1.0×10^{-5} M
Highest concentration of linear range	6.8×10^{-5} M
Concentration of #1	1.8×10^{-5} M
Concentration of #2	3.6×10^{-5} M

(b) No. The absorbance of #3, despite being four times that of #1, is outside the linear range, where Beer's law is invalid. The highest absorbance value of the linear range, corresponding to 6.8×10^{-5} M, is 0.903.

3. There are at least two effective approaches to solving this problem.

APPROACH 1

Calculate the molar absorptivity and then use Beer's law to find the concentration at $A = 0.502$.

For the known solution:

$$A = \epsilon c l$$

$$A \div (cl) = \epsilon$$

$$0.339 \div (4.6 \times 10^{-5}\ \text{M})(1.0\ \text{cm}) = \epsilon$$

$$7370\ \text{M}^{-1}\ \text{cm}^{-1} = \epsilon$$

For the unknown solution:

$$A \div (\epsilon l) = c$$

$$0.502 \div (7370\ \text{M}^{-1}\ \text{cm}^{-1})(1.0\ \text{cm}) = c$$

$$6.8 \times 10^{-5}\ \text{M}$$

APPROACH 2

Set up a proportion equation and then solve for the unknown quantity:

$$\frac{A_1}{A_2} = \frac{c_1}{c_2}$$

We know three of the four values in this case:

$$\frac{0.339}{0.502} = \frac{4.6 \times 10^{-5}\ \text{M}}{c_2}$$

$$c_2 = \frac{(4.6 \times 10^{-5}\ \text{M})(0.502)}{0.339}$$

$$c_2 = 6.8 \times 10^{-5}\ \text{M}$$

4. Use problem 3 as a model. The concentration is 2.5×10^{-7} M.

5. (a) False. Transmittance is not linear with concentration.

(b) False. Transmittance is not linear with concentration.

(c) True.

$$A = -\log T$$

$$A = -\log(0.52)$$

$$A = 0.284$$

(d) True.

$$A = \epsilon cl$$

$$A = (855\ \text{M}^{-1}\ \text{cm}^{-1})(1.0\ \text{cm})(0.00036\ \text{M})$$

$$A = 0.308$$

(e) True.

$$A \div (\epsilon l) = c$$

$$0.188 \div (29{,}000\ \text{M}^{-1}\ \text{cm}^{-1})(1.0\ \text{cm}) = c$$

$$6.48 \times 10^{-6}\ \text{M} = c$$

(f) True.

$$A \div (cl) = \epsilon$$

$$0.388 \div (9.2 \times 10^{-5}\ \text{M})\ (0.5\ \text{cm}) = \epsilon$$

$$8435\ \text{M}^{-1}\ \text{cm}^{-1} = \epsilon$$

(g) True.

$$A = -\log T$$

$$A = -\log(0.39)$$

$$A = 0.409$$

(h) True. Transmittance and absorbance move in opposite directions.

(i) False. Absorbance is directly proportional to path length.

6. (a)

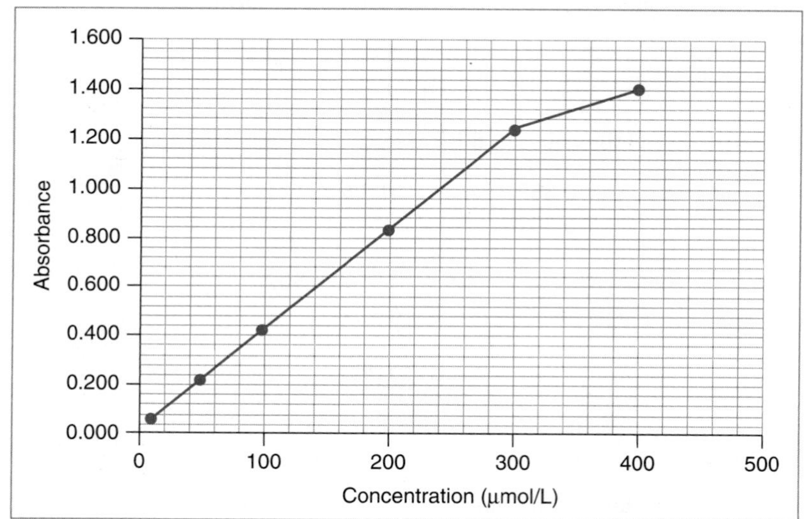

(b) The molar absorptivity is the slope of the line, which is described by Beer's law. Note that the path length has gone into the *x* value.

$$A = \epsilon \times \underbrace{c \times l}$$

$$y = m\,x \quad + b$$

$$m = \frac{1.230 - 0.041}{300 \times 10^{-6}\ \text{mol} \cdot \text{cm/L} - 10 \times 10^{-6}\ \text{mol} \cdot \text{cm/L}}$$

$$= 4100\ \text{L} \cdot \text{mol}^{-1} \cdot \text{cm}^{-1}$$

(c) There are three approaches to this question.

APPROACH 1

Visual interpolation. An absorbance of 1.080 corresponds to a concentration of 260 μmol/L.

APPROACH 2

Equation of ratios, as in problem 3.

$$\frac{A_1}{A_2} = \frac{c_1}{c_2}$$

$$\frac{0.821}{1.080} = \frac{200\ \mu\text{mol/L}}{c_2}$$

$$c_2 = 263\ \mu\text{mol/L}$$

APPROACH 3

Beer's law.

$$A = \epsilon\, c\, l$$

$$c = \frac{A}{\epsilon \times l} = \frac{1.080}{(4100\ \text{L} \cdot \text{mol}^{-1} \cdot \text{cm}^{-1})(1\ \text{cm})}$$

$$c = 0.000263\ \text{mol/L} = 263\ \mu\text{mol/L}$$

(d) No. Beer's law is valid only in the linear range of the graph. For this particular substance, the graph ceases to be linear above a concentration of 300 μmol/L, where *A* is 1.230.

(e) An absorbance value of 1.647 is off the standard curve. Diluting the solution by a factor of 2 or 3 would bring the absorbance value into the linear range. The corresponding concentration from the standard curve would then be corrected for the dilution.

(f) The final solution represents a 1:3 dilution. An absorbance of 0.757 corresponds to a concentration of 1.85×10^{-4} mol/L. Thus, we must multiply this concentration by 3 to give the original concentration, which is 5.54×10^{-4} mol/L.

7.

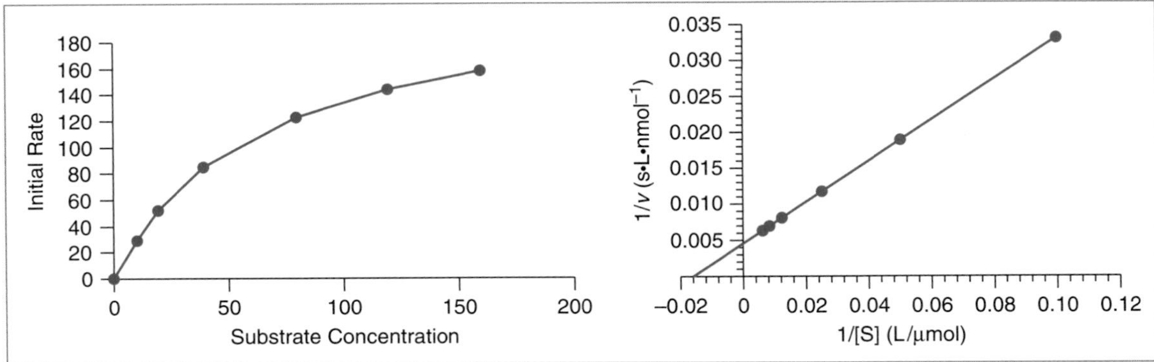

$$y\text{-intercept} = \frac{1}{V_{max}} = 0.0045 \text{ s}\cdot\text{L}\cdot\text{nmol}^{-1} \qquad x\text{-intercept} = \frac{-1}{K_M} = -0.016 \text{ L}/\mu\text{mol}$$

$$V_{max} = 222 \text{ nmol/L/s} \qquad K_M = 63\ \mu\text{mol/L}$$

8. The procedures are the same as those for problem 7 above. The constants are

$$y\text{-intercept} = \frac{1}{V_{max}} = 1.72 \text{ s}\cdot\text{L}\cdot\text{nmol}^{-1} \qquad x\text{-intercept} = \frac{-1}{K_M} = -0.059 \text{ L}/\mu\text{mol}$$

$$V_{max} = 0.58 \text{ nmol/L/s} \qquad K_M = 17\ \mu\text{mol/L}$$

9. (a) Enzyme #2 is more suitable. The K_M should be higher than the concentration of the substrate so that differences in concentration between specimens cause measurable differences in reaction rate. If you used enzyme #1, the substrate would be present at 5 to 25 times the K_M, which is in the plateau region of the curve where reaction rate changes little with substrate concentration.

(b) The concentration of substrate should be saturating, far above the K_M of 9 mM, so that the reaction rate depends only on the concentration of enzyme in the serum specimen.

10. The answer is 528 IU/L. The first step is to ascertain whether the reaction rate is constant. After the first 20 seconds, the difference from one time point to the next represents a rate of 0.081 per 20 s, or 0.243 per min.

Incubation time (s)	A_{405}	ΔA_{405}/20 s
20	0.033	
40	0.114	0.081
60	0.195	0.081
80	0.276	0.081
100	0.357	0.081
120	0.438	0.081

Every minute, the absorbance increases by 0.243. Thus, the second step is to convert this absorbance to a concentration. Beer's law accomplishes this:

$$A = \epsilon c l$$

$$c = \frac{A}{\epsilon l}$$

$$c = \frac{0.243/\text{min}}{(18{,}450\ \text{L}\cdot\text{mol}^{-1}\cdot\text{cm}^{-1})(1\ \text{cm})}$$

$$= 1.32 \times 10^{-5}\ \text{mol/L/min}$$

The concentration increases by 1.32×10^{-5} mol/L every minute, or 13.2 μmol/L/min:

$$\frac{1.32 \times 10^{-5}\ \text{mol/L}}{\text{min}} \times \frac{10^{6}\ \mu\text{mol}}{\text{mol}} = 13.2\ \mu\text{mol/L/min}$$

This enzyme activity came from a specimen that had been diluted 40 times (0.025 mL → 1.0 mL). Therefore,

$$13.2\ \mu\text{mol/L/min} \times 40 = 528\ \mu\text{mol/L/min} = 528\ \text{IU/L}$$

11. (a)

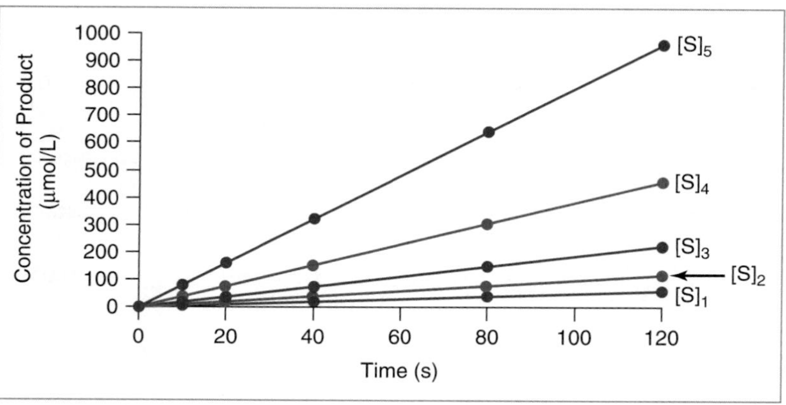

(b) The initial rate is the slope of the line at each starting substrate concentration in the above graph (before it enters a plateau). For example, the slope of the line at $[S]_3$ is

$$m = \frac{216\ \mu\text{mol/L} - 18\ \mu\text{mol/L}}{120\ \text{s} - 10\ \text{s}} = 1.8\ \mu\text{mol/L/s}$$

The slopes of the other lines are 0.50 at $[S]_1$, 0.98 at $[S]_2$, 3.8 at $[S]_4$, and 8.0 at $[S]_5$.

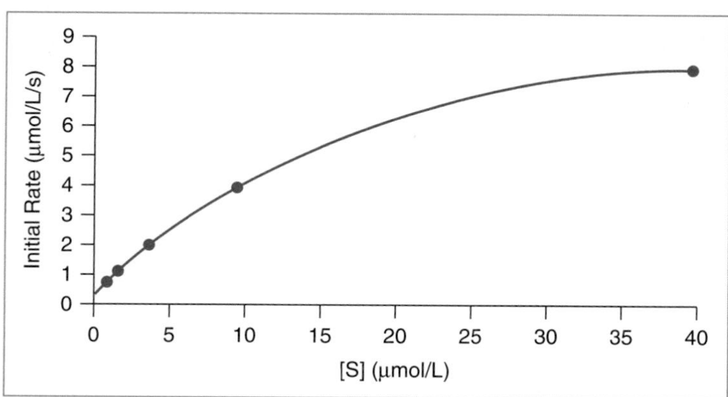

(c) The reciprocals of [S] and *v* are

1/[S] (L/μmol)	1/*v* ($s \cdot L \cdot \mu mol^{-1}$)
1	2
0.5	1.02
0.25	0.56
0.1	0.26
0.025	0.125

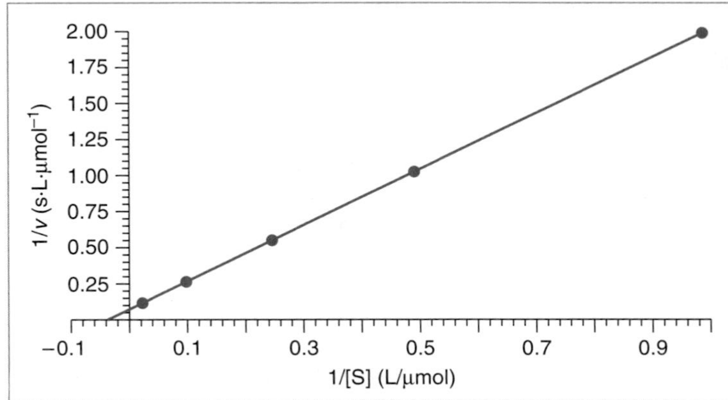

(d) By inspection of the curve in part *b*, it is nearly impossible to accurately evaluate V_{max} and, therefore, K_M. If we estimate V_{max} to be between 8 and 9 μmol/L/s, our value proves to be only about 60% of that from a Lineweaver-Burk plot (see below). A reliable curve-fitting computer program would return a better result, especially if we had gathered more data points.

On the Lineweaver-Burk plot, we directly read the values of V_{max} and K_M. Nevertheless, wisdom reminds us that these values are probably less accurate than those we would have obtained from a curve-fitting program on the original data.

$$y\text{-intercept} = \frac{1}{V_{max}} = 0.075\ s \cdot L \cdot \mu mol^{-1} \qquad x\text{-intercept} = \frac{-1}{K_M} = -0.039\ L/\mu mol$$

$$V_{max} = 13.3\ \mu mol/L/s \qquad\qquad K_M = 26\ \mu mol/L$$

12. The strongest acid has the highest K_a (lowest pK_a), and the weakest acid has the lowest K_a (highest pK_a).

Acid	pK_a
salicylic (*strongest*)	2.98
lactic	3.08
formic	3.75
valproic	4.60
acetic (*weakest*)	4.76

13. Use the Henderson-Hasselbalch equation to find the ratio of the concentration of conjugate base, $[HPO_4^-]$, to the concentration of acid, $[H_2PO_4^{2-}]$:

$$pH = pK_a + \log\frac{[A^-]}{[HA]}$$

$$10^{pH - pK_a} = \frac{[A^-]}{[HA]}$$

$$10^{7.0-7.2} = \frac{[HPO_4^{2-}]}{[H_2PO_4^-]}$$

$$0.631 = \frac{[HPO_4^{2-}]}{[H_2PO_4^-]}$$

$$0.631[H_2PO_4^{2-}] = [HPO_4^-]$$

The total concentration of the buffer is 0.10 M:

$$[H_2PO_4^{2-}] + [HPO_4^-] = 0.10 \text{ M}$$

Therefore,

$$[H_2PO_4^{2-}] + 0.631[H_2PO_4^{2-}] = 0.10 \text{ M}$$

$$1.631[H_2PO_4^{2-}] = 0.10 \text{ M}$$

$$[H_2PO_4^{2-}] = 0.0613 \text{ M}$$

and

$$[HPO_4^-] = 0.10 \text{ M} - 0.0613 \text{ M}$$

$$[HPO_4^-] = 0.0387 \text{ M}$$

Now, convert the concentrations into masses. The required mass of KH_2PO_4 is **8.34** grams:

$$1.0 \text{ L}\left(\frac{0.0613 \text{ mol}}{\text{L}}\right)\left(\frac{136.09 \text{ g}}{\text{mol}}\right) = 8.34 \text{ g}$$

The required mass of K_2HPO_4 is **6.74** grams:

$$1.0 \text{ L}\left(\frac{0.0387 \text{ mol}}{\text{L}}\right)\left(\frac{174.18 \text{ g}}{\text{mol}}\right) = 6.74 \text{ g}$$

14. Use problem 13 as a model for solving this one.

Required masses:

$$KH_2PO_4 = 1.31 \text{ g}$$
$$K_2HPO_4 = 2.67 \text{ g}$$

15. Use problem 13 as a model for solving this one.

Required masses:

$$KH_2PO_4 = 1.02 \text{ g}$$
$$K_2HPO_4 = 1.31 \text{ g}$$

16. First, use the Henderson-Hasselbalch equation to calculate the concentrations of the acid and its conjugate base (as in problem 13):

acetic acid = 0.129 M

sodium acetate = 0.0709 M

Next, calculate (a) the volume of acetic acid and (b) the mass of sodium acetate required for a final buffer volume of 1.0 L:

volume of acetic acid $$1.0 \text{ L}\left(\frac{0.129 \text{ mol}}{\text{L}}\right)\left(\frac{60.05 \text{ g}}{\text{mol}}\right)\left(\frac{\text{mL}}{1.049 \text{ g}}\right) = 7.38 \text{ mL}$$

mass of sodium acetate $$1.0 \text{ L}\left(\frac{0.0709 \text{ mol}}{\text{L}}\right)\left(\frac{82.03 \text{ g}}{\text{mol}}\right) = 5.82 \text{ g}$$

17. For the blood-buffering system, the Henderson-Hasselbalch equation is

$$pH = pK_a + \log\frac{[HCO_3^-]}{\alpha \times PCO_2}$$

which can be rearranged to

$$(10^{pH-pK_a})(\alpha \times PCO_2) = [HCO_3^-]$$

For specimen #1, the equation is

$$(10^{7.40-6.10})(0.0301 \text{ mmol/L/mm Hg} \times 40 \text{ mm Hg}) = [HCO_3^-]$$

$$24.0 \text{ mmol/L} = [HCO_3^-]$$

Specimen	$[HCO_3^-]$ (mmol/L)
1	24.0
2	23.5
3	23.7
4	20.8

18. pH = 7.38

19. pH = 3.57

20. **Patient 1.**

The patient is *alkalotic*. The cause cannot be respiratory because a high PCO_2 causes acidosis. Therefore, the cause is the high bicarbonate, making the condition *metabolic*. *Compensation is present* in the high PCO_2.

Patient 2.

The patient is *acidotic*. The high PCO_2 implies a *respiratory* cause. *Compensation is absent* in that the bicarbonate concentration is normal.

Patient 3.

The patient is *acidotic*. The low PCO_2 and bicarbonate concentration are consistent with a *metabolic* cause. *Compensation is present* in the low PCO_2.

21.

Patient	Anion Gap (with K^+)	Anion Gap (without K^+)
1	17	12
2	11	6
3	33	28

22. (a) 0.2 Osm/L

(b) 0.03 Osm/L (10 mM $CaCl_2$ = 0.01 M $CaCl_2$ = 0.03 moles of particles per L)

(c) 0.10 Osm/L

(d) 0.25 Osm/L

23. (a) Use Equations 6 and 7

Specimen	Osmolarity	Osmolality
1	294	295
2	285	286
3	315	317

(b) Subtract the calculated osmolality from the measured osmolality:

Specimen	Osmolality Gap
1	304 − 295 = 9
2	13
3	−7

24.

Specimen	[LDL] (mg/dL)
1	112
2	90
3	213

25. Convert to "centimeters" and "kilograms." Then use Equations 11 and 12.

Patient	H (cm)	W (kg)	A (m^2)	24-Hour Urine Volume (mL)	V_{urine}	$P_{creatinine}$ (mg/dL)	$U_{creatinine}$ (mg/dL)	Corrected Clearance Rate (mL/min)
1	149.9	69.75	1.65	1600	1.11	1.2	140	136
2	188.0	94.5	2.21	1830	1.27	1.9	128	67
3	177.8	82.35	2.00	1360	0.94	1.5	162	88
4	167.6	58.95	1.67	1780	1.24	1.4	155	142

CHAPTER 10

Practice and Contextual Problems

1. There would be 993 WBCs. The space in question has a volume of 0.15 mm^3. Therefore,

$$\frac{1\ \text{mm}^3}{0.15\ \text{mm}^3} = \frac{6620\ \text{WBCs}}{x}$$

$$x = 993\ \text{WBCs}$$

2. Using Equation 1 gives

$$\text{RBC count} = \frac{200\ \text{RBCs}}{0.02\ \text{mm}^3} \times 200 = 2{,}000{,}000\ \text{RBCs/mm}^3$$

Because the procedure was standard (all 5 "R" squares, 1:200 dilution), one can use the single factor (Table 10-1):

$$\text{RBC count} = 200 \times 10{,}000 = 2{,}000{,}000\ \text{RBCs/mm}^3$$

3. Using Equation 1 gives

$$\text{WBC count} = \frac{57\ \text{WBCs}}{0.4\ \text{mm}^3} \times 20 = 2850\ \text{WBCs/mm}^3$$

Because the procedure was standard (all four corner squares, 1:20 dilution), one can use the single factor (Table 10-1):

$$\text{WBC count} = 57 \times 50 = 2850\ \text{WBCs/mm}^3$$

4. A 40-fold dilution. The volume of a W-labeled square is 0.1 mm^3. Therefore, the cells would be present in the square at 50 per 0.1 mm^3, or 500 per mm^3. This concentration of cells is 40 times less than that of the whole blood (20,000 per mm^3).

5. Using Equation 1 gives

$$\text{RBC count} = \frac{166\text{ RBCs}}{0.02\text{ mm}^3} \times 100 = 830{,}000\text{ RBCs/mm}^3$$

Because the dilution was not standard (1:200), one cannot use the single factor.

6. Using Equation 1 gives

$$\text{WBC count} = \frac{36\text{ WBCs}}{0.4\text{ mm}^3} \times 10 = 900\text{ WBCs/mm}^3$$

Because the dilution was not standard (1:50), one cannot use the single factor.

7. Using Equation 2 gives

$$\text{MCV} = \frac{38}{4.7} \times 10 = 81\text{ fL}$$

8. Using Equation 2 gives

$$\text{MCV} = \frac{44}{5.1} \times 10 = 86\text{ fL}$$

9. The RBC count of 6.0×10^{12}/L is equivalent to $6.0 \times 10^6/\text{mm}^3$. Using Equation 2, therefore, gives

$$\text{MCV} = \frac{47}{6.0} \times 10 = 78\text{ fL}$$

10. Using Equation 3 gives

$$\text{MCH} = \frac{15.2}{5.4} \times 10 = 28\text{ pg}$$

11. Using Equation 4 gives

$$\text{MCHC} = \frac{13.9}{41} \times 100 = 34\text{ g/dL}$$

12. A factor of 1000 replaces the factor of 10. Thus, Equation 2 becomes

$$\text{MCV (fL)} = \frac{\text{Hct (L/L)}}{\text{RBC count } (\times 10^6/\mu\text{L})} \times 1000$$

For example, an Hct of 45% becomes 0.45 L/L, which is the same as 0.45 μL/μL. Substituting 0.45 μL/μL for an Hct of 45 divides the numerator by 100. To compensate for this, the factor of 10 in Equation 2 must be multiplied by 100, giving 1000.

13. Use Equation 10 to calculate the INR:

PT_{norm}	$PT_{patient}$	ISI	INR
12	21	1.22	2.0
12	16	1.91	1.7
12	21	2.0	3.1
12	24	1.5	2.8
11	19	1.35	2.1
11	30	1.1	3.0
11	23	2.2	5.1
11	10	1.0	0.9

14. Using Equation 1 gives

$$\text{platelet count} = \frac{91 \text{ platelets}}{0.1 \text{ mm}^3} \times 100 = 91{,}000 \text{ platelets/mm}^3$$

Because the procedure was standard (all 25 squares in center, 1:100 dilution), we can use the single factor (Table 10-1):

$$\text{platelet count} = 91 \times 1000 = 91{,}000 \text{ platelets/mm}^3$$

15. Using Equation 1 gives

$$\text{platelet count} = \frac{137 \text{ platelets}}{0.1 \text{ mm}^3} \times 100$$

$$= 137{,}000 \text{ platelets/mm}^3$$

Because the procedure was standard (all 25 squares in center, 1:100 dilution), we can use the single factor (Table 10-1):

$$\text{platelet count} = 137 \times 1000 = 137{,}000 \text{ platelets/mm}^3$$

16. Using Equation 1 gives

$$\text{platelet count} = \frac{208 \text{ platelets}}{0.1 \text{ mm}^3} \times 100$$

$$= 208{,}000 \text{ platelets/mm}^3$$

Because the procedure was standard (all 25 squares in center, 1:100 dilution), we can use the single factor (Table 10-1):

$$\text{platelet count} = 208 \times 1000 = 208{,}000 \text{ platelets/mm}^3$$

17. Use Equation 8 to calculate the percentage.

Reticulocytes per 1000 RBCs	Reticulocyte Percentage
37	3.7
106	10.6
9	0.9
233	23.3
13	1.3

18. Use Equation 9 to calculate the percentage.

Reticulocytes in Both Squares	RBCs in Smaller Square	Reticulocyte Percentage
40	260	1.7
18	194	1.0
105	168	6.9
17	233	0.8
129	173	8.3

19. Use Equation 5 to calculate the corrected count.

Reticulocyte Count (%)	Hematocrit (%)	Reticulocyte Index (%)
3.3	31	2.3
10.0	28	6.2
2.6	19	1.1
8.3	21	3.9
1.1	35	0.9

20. Use Equation 7 and Table 10-2 to calculate the RPI:

Reticulocyte Index (%)	Hematocrit (%)	Reticulocyte Production Index (%)
1.7	32	1.1
9.0	27	6.0
2.0	25	2.0
0.9	30	0.6
7.8	14	3.1

21. Use the two equations for the Rule of Three:

$$3 \times [\text{Hb}] = \text{Hct} \pm 3$$

$$3 \times \text{RBC count} = [\text{Hb}]$$

All except data set **c** satisfy the rule. The Hct for **c** should fall between 31.2 and 37.2.

22. The patient specimen is consistent with the presence of spherocytes. The normal specimen begins lysing at 0.50% and has lysed completely by 0.30%, whereas the patient specimen begins at 0.60%. The patient's curve is right-shifted relative to the normal curve.

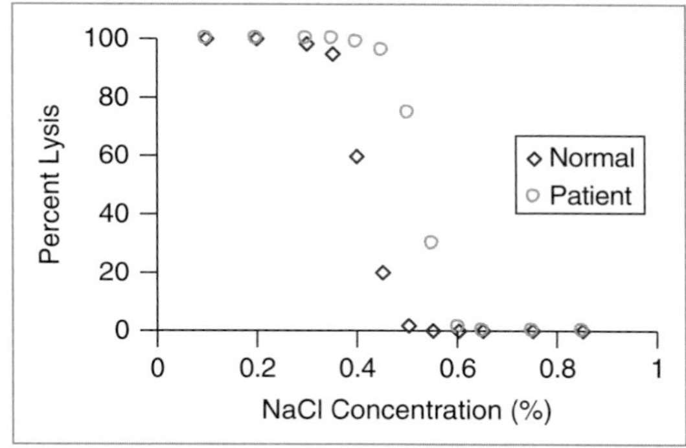

23. Use Equation 11 to correct the WBC count.

	Uncorrected WBC Count (cells/μL)	nRBCs per 100 WBCs	Corrected WBC Count (cells/μL)
(a)	18,500	14	16,200
(b)	5600	28	4400
(c)	2200	47	1500

24. Use Equation 1 to calculate the final counts. Alternatively, use the single factors (Table 10-1) because the procedure was standard.

	Raw Count			Final Count		
	RBCs (total in 5 squares on one side)	WBCs (total in 4 corner squares on one side)	Platelets (total in all 25 squares on one side)	RBCs (cells/mm^3)	WBCs (cells/mm^3)	Platelets (cells/mm^3)
(a)	193	72	136	1,930,000	3600	136,000
(b)	467	112	200	4,670,000	5600	200,000
(c)	250	400	61	2,500,000	20,000	61,000
(d)	590	231	277	5,900,000	11,600	277,000

25. Use Equation 1 to calculate the final counts. Consider the dilutions to have been nonstandard.

	Raw Count			Final Count		
	RBCs (total in 5 squares on one side)	WBCs (total in 4 corner squares on one side)	Platelets (total in all 25 squares on one side)	RBCs (cells/mm^3)	WBCs (cells/mm^3)	Platelets (cells/mm^3)
(a)	550 (dil. = 1:300)	200 (dil. = 1:30)	80 (dil. = 1:50)	8,250,000	15,000	40,000
(b)	360 (dil. = 1:100)	310 (dil. = 1:40)	95 (dil. = 1:50)	1,800,000	31,000	47,500
(c)	242 (dil. = 1:50)	95 (dil. = 1:10)	427 (dil. = 1:200)	605,000	2400	854,000
(d)	498 (dil. = 1:400)	400 (dil. = 1:30)	341 (dil. = 1:200)	9,960,000	30,000	682,000

CHAPTER 11

Practice and Contextual Problems

1. Day 5: R_{4s} (random error) Day 12: 2_{2s} (systematic error)
   Day 20: 4_{1s} (systematic error)
2. Day 12: $10_{\bar{x}}$ (systematic error) Day 20: 1_{3s} (random error)
3. Control 1: mean = 180 SD = 5.1
   Control 2: mean = 256 SD = 9.8

   Westgard Violations

   Day 4: 4_{1s} Day 7: 1_{2s} Days 13 & 14: 2_{2s} (control 2)
   Day 14: 2_{2s} (controls 1 & 2) Day 20: $10_{\bar{x}}$

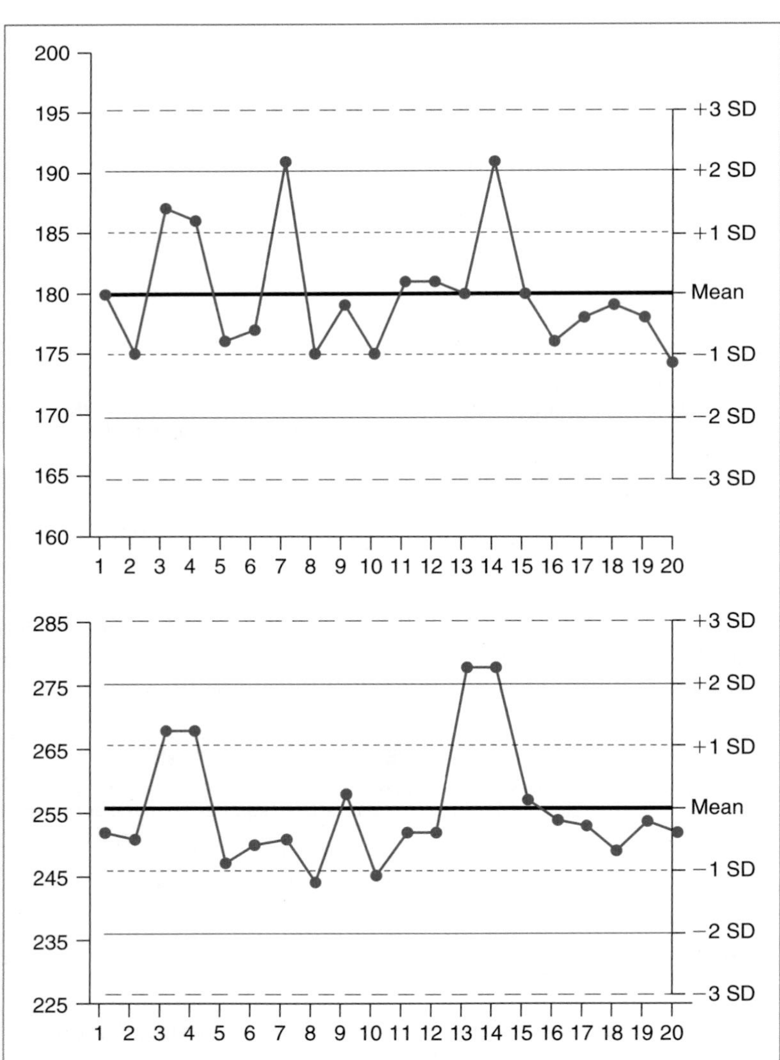

4.

	Na (mM)	K (mM)	Glucose (mg/dL)
Mean	149	6.6	100
SD	1.5	0.17	2.8
Question #1	Yes	no (4_{1s})	yes
Question #2	Yes	yes	no (1_{3s})

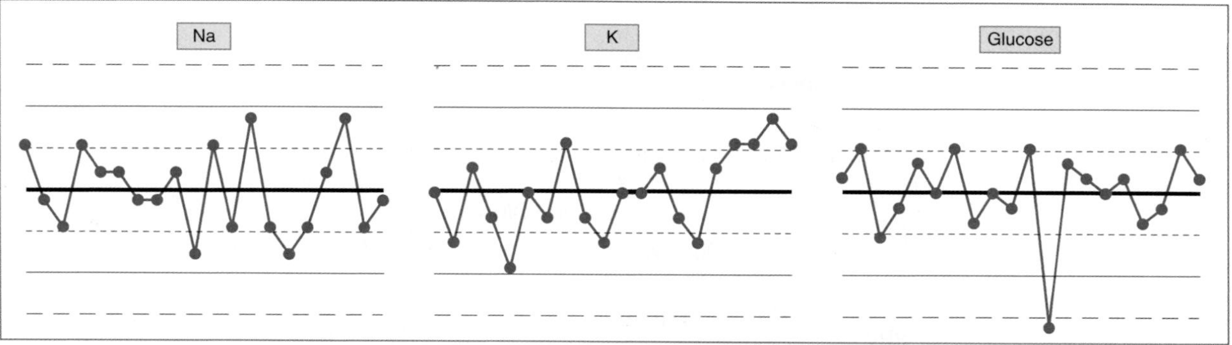

5. (a) The value of 45 is an outlier because it falls outside the range of $\pm 2s$, which runs from 35.8 up to 44.2. It is only a warning from the 1_{2s} rule—not a violation leading to rejection.

(b) There is an upward trend starting with the fourth new result (48). The final value of 57 is greater than 3*s* above the mean (56 mEq/L). Therefore, the run is rejected.

(c) There is a downward shift starting with the second new result (4.9). The final value of 4.3 is less than 4.4%, which is 2*s* below the mean. Therefore, the run is rejected.

6. (a) A violation of rule 2_{2s} means that both the current and preceding results exceed 2, but not 3, standard deviations above the mean. Therefore, the preceding result can be no less than 136 μg/mL and no greater than 139 μg/mL.

(b) A violation of rule 4_{1s} means that the current result of 134 is the last in a series of four results that are more than 1 SD above the mean. Therefore, each of the three preceding results can be no less than 133 μg/mL.

(c) A violation of rule $10_{\bar{x}}$ means that the current result of 128 is the last in a series of 10 results that lie on the same side of the mean. The 19th result in the entire sequence is the last one before the series of 10. Therefore, it can be no less than the mean, which is 130 μg/mL.

7. The run must be rejected for violating rule 2_{2s} across the two controls.

8. The run must be rejected because control 1 violates rule 4_{1s} and control 2 violates rule 1_{3s}.

9. The run may be accepted because there are no Westgard violations.

CHAPTER 12

Practice and Contextual Problems

1. (a) The prevalence is the number of persons with a condition expressed as a percentage of the total population tested. In this case, 10 of the 25 patients had bacteremia. Thus, the prevalence is 10 ÷ 25, or 40%.

(b) If the cutoff is 10×10^3 cells/mm^3, then all the patients with bacteremia would test positive for bacteremia by the leukocyte count. Thus, the sensitivity is 100%:

$$\text{sensitivity} = \frac{TP}{TP + FN} \times 100\% = \frac{10}{10 + 0} \times 100\% = 100\%$$

The specificity, however, is only 73% because 4 of the 15 patients without bacteremia would test falsely positive:

$$\text{specificity} = \frac{TN}{TN + FP} \times 100\% = \frac{11}{11 + 4} \times 100\% = 73\%$$

(c) Raising the cutoff to 15 would lower the sensitivity but increase the specificity:

$$\text{sensitivity} = \frac{TP}{TP + FN} \times 100\% = \frac{6}{6 + 4} \times 100\% = 60\%$$

$$\text{specificity} = \frac{TN}{TN + FP} \times 100\% = \frac{15}{15 + 0} \times 100\% = 100\%$$

(d) Equation 5 gives a positive predictive value of 71%:

$$\text{PPV} = \frac{(\text{sensitivity})(\text{prevalence})}{(\text{sensitivity})(\text{prevalence}) + (1 - \text{specificity})(1 - \text{prevalence})} \times 100\%$$

$$\text{PPV} = \frac{(1)(0.40)}{(1)(0.40) + (1 - 0.73)(1 - 0.40)} \times 100\% = 71\%$$

2. The answer to this question is the positive predictive value, which represents the likelihood that a positive test result is correct. There are at least two efficient ways to approach this problem.

APPROACH 1

Use Equation 7. The prevalence is 1 out of 85,000, which equals 0.000012, or 0.0012%:

$$\text{PPV} = \frac{(0.99)(0.000012)}{(0.99)(0.000012) + (1 - 0.99)(1 - 0.000012)} \times 100\% = 0.12\%$$

Thus, the probability that the man's positive test result is correct is only 0.12%, or 12 out of 10,000.

APPROACH 2

Reason through the problem step by step without using Equation 7. Out of every 85,000 people in the population, HIV is present in 1 and absent from the other 84,999. This means that HIV is present in 10 out of 850,000 and 100 out of 8,500,000. Because the sensitivity of the test is 99%, then, in a population of 8.5 million, 99 of the people with HIV will test positive, and 1 will test negative. Moreover, because the specificity is 99%, then the 8,499,900 people who do not have HIV will give 8,414,901 negative results and 84,999 positive. Using Equation 5 gives the positive predictive value:

$$\text{PPV} = \frac{TP}{TP + FP} \times 100\% = \frac{99}{99 + 84{,}999} \times 100\% = 0.12\%$$

3. (a) There are 514 subjects in the study (the sum of all the positives and negatives). By the new test, therefore, the prevalence is

$$\text{prevalence} = \frac{TP + FN}{TP + FP + TN + FN} \times 100\% = \frac{208 + 16}{514} = 44\%$$

(b) The sensitivity of the new test is

$$\text{sensitivity} = \frac{TP}{TP + FN} \times 100\% = \frac{208}{208 + 16} \times 100\% = 93\%$$

The specificity is

$$\text{specificity} = \frac{TN}{TN + FP} \times 100\% = \frac{280}{280 + 10} \times 100\% = 97\%$$

(c) The positive predictive value of the new test is

$$\text{PPV} = \frac{TP}{TP + FP} \times 100\% = \frac{208}{208 + 10} \times 100\% = 95\%$$

The negative predictive value is

$$\text{NPV} = \frac{TN}{TN + FN} \times 100\% = \frac{280}{280 + 16} \times 100\% = 95\%$$

4. (a) Using Equation 7, the PPV for the population of blood donors is 75%:

$$\text{PPV} = \frac{(\text{sensitivity})(\text{prevalence})}{(\text{sensitivity})(\text{prevalence}) + (1 - \text{specificity})(1 - \text{prevalence})} \times 100\%$$

$$= \frac{(0.999)(0.003)}{(0.999)(0.003) + (1 - 0.999)(1 - 0.003)} \times 100\% = 75\%$$

Using Equation 7, the PPV for the population in the substance-abuse clinic is 99%:

$$\text{PPV} = \frac{(0.999)(0.16)}{(0.999)(0.16) + (1 - 0.999)(1 - 0.16)} \times 100\% = 99\%$$

(b) Because the prevalence of HIV among the substance-abuse patients is 16% and there are 200 people in that population, 32 individuals are expected to have HIV:

$$0.16 \times 200 = 32$$

(c) The PPV from part *a* is 75%. Therefore, the number of correct positive results is

$$0.75 \times 1132 = 849$$

and the number of false positives is

$$1132 - 849 = 283$$

5. (a) The sensitivity and specificity of test *X* are

$$\text{sensitivity} = \frac{TP}{TP + FN} \times 100\% = \frac{51}{51 + 0} \times 100\% = 100\%$$

$$\text{specificity} = \frac{TN}{TN + FP} \times 100\% = \frac{317}{317 + 66} \times 100\% = 83\%$$

The sensitivity and specificity, respectively, of test *Y* are 72% and 99%.

(b) Test *Y* is more specific than test *X*. Therefore, when the result is positive, test *Y* is superior for ruling in salmonellosis.

6. (a) If specificity is the probability of a negative result in the absence of the condition, then its value in this case is 83% simply because a number of 2 or greater will come up 83 times out of every 100 with a healthy person standing nearby. (Of course, it will also come up 83 times out of every 100 with a sick person standing nearby.)

(b) A high value does not guarantee clinically meaningful information.

7. (a) 1 = TN   2 = FN   3 = FP   4 = TP

(b) The sensitivity decreases because the fraction of true positives goes down and the fraction of false negatives goes up.

(c) Moving the cutoff to three standard deviations above the pink mean amounts to an upward shift. The specificity increases because the fraction of true negatives goes up and the fraction of false positives goes down.

(d) Moving the cutoff to three standard deviations below the blue mean amounts to a downward shift. The sensitivity increases because the fraction of true positives goes up and the fraction of false negatives goes down.

8. (a) There are no false positives. Thus, this test is suitable for a condition in which false positives are unacceptable, such as a serious untreatable disease.

(b) In a serious treatable disease, the number of false negatives must be minimal. Thus, the cutoff should be moved toward the low end of the blue curve.

9. (a) The negative predictive value is the probability that a patient with a negative test result does not have cancer:

$$\text{negative predictive value (NPV)} = \frac{TN}{TN + FN} \times 100\% = \frac{399}{399 + 59} = 87\%$$

(b) The positive predictive value is the probability that a patient with a positive test result does have cancer:

$$\text{positive predictive value (PPV)} = \frac{TP}{TP + FP} \times 100\% = \frac{187}{187 + 514} = 27\%$$

(c) The efficiency is the probability that a given test result matches the diagnosis:

$$\text{efficiency} = \frac{TP + TN}{TP + FP + TN + FN} \times 100\% = \frac{187 + 399}{187 + 514 + 399 + 59} = 51\%$$

10. (LO 4) Solve Practice Problem 10 (a, b) in Chapter 8.

11. (LO 7) Solve Practice Problem 21 in Chapter 8.

12. (LO 7) Solve Contextual Problem 7 in Chapter 8.

13. 10.

Specimen	Conc. of Chloride (mEq/L)		Conc. Recovered (Eq. 9)	% Recovery (Eq. 10)
	Spiked Aliquot	Baseline Aliquot		
1	107	101	6	100
2	106	99	7	117
3	110	105	5	83
4	106	100	6	100
5	102	96	6	100
6	110	104	6	100
7	106	101	5	83
8	114	108	6	100
9	105	100	5	83
10	109	104	5	83
11	103	101	2	33
12	105	98	7	117
13	113	106	7	117
14	117	110	7	117
15	105	99	6	100
16	110	103	7	117
17	106	100	6	100
18	115	111	4	67
19	115	108	7	117
20	107	102	5	83

The average percent recovery is 96, which falls within the range of acceptability.

14.

$A1_C$ Conc. (%)			$A1_C$ Conc. (%) *(continued)*		
Method A	**Method B**	**A–B**	**Method A**	**Method B**	**A–B** *(continued)*
6.2	6.1	0.1	9.0	8.6	0.4
3.9	4.5	−0.6	4.6	5.0	−0.4
9.8	8.9	0.9	6.0	6.2	−0.2
5.0	5.1	−0.1	5.4	5.2	0.2
4.7	5.2	−0.5	4.7	5.0	−0.3
4.8	4.7	0.1	5.2	5.2	0
5.9	6.1	−0.2	6.6	6.9	−0.3
4.0	4.4	−0.4	7.9	7.8	0.1
13.2	13.8	−0.6	4.9	4.2	0.7
7.1	6.9	0.2	4.2	4.3	−0.1
4.5	4.2	0.3	12.2	13.0	−0.8
5.2	5.0	0.2	6.0	5.9	0.1
6.1	6.5	−0.4	5.1	5.1	0
4.9	5.0	−0.1	7.6	7.4	0.2
4.8	5.0	−0.2	4.6	4.4	0.2
10.7	10.3	0.4	4.8	5.0	−0.2
8.3	8.8	−0.5	5.0	5.0	0
			MEAN ($\overline{D}$) =		−0.0529
			VARIANCE (s^2) =		0.138
			n =		34
			t value =		−0.830
			(Equation 14 in Chapter 8, paired samples) $t = \dfrac{\overline{D}}{\sqrt{\dfrac{s^2}{n}}}$		

The calculated t value is −0.830, and there are 33 degrees of freedom. For $p = 0.05$, the critical value lies between −2.06 (25 d.f.) and −2.01 (50 d.f.). Therefore, we cannot conclude that the two methods differ significantly.

15.

The result occupying the 2.5% position is

$$2.5\% \times 162 = 4$$

which corresponds to a value of "0.26." The result occupying the 97.5% position is

$$97.5\% \times 162 = 158$$

which corresponds to a value of "1.39." Therefore, the reportable range is "0.26–1.39."

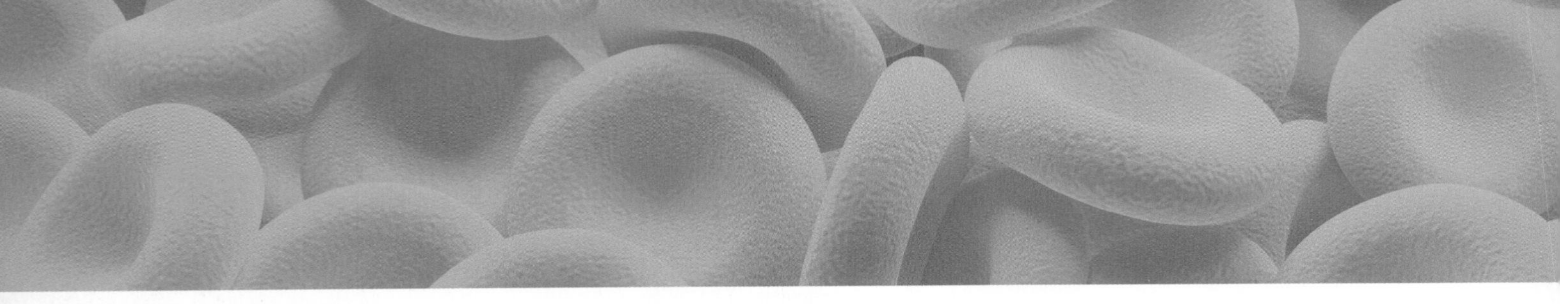

Glossary

Abscissa—the x coordinate of a point on a Cartesian graph.

Absolute uncertainty—the raw amount of uncertainty in a measurement.

Absorbance—the negative logarithm of transmittance. It is a measure of how much light a chemical substance absorbs (under defined conditions).

Accuracy—the degree to which a measurement or calculated result corresponds to its true value.

Acid dissociation constant (K_a)—a constant whose value captures the extent of dissociation of an acid under defined conditions.

Acidosis—the condition in which too much acid is present.

Alkalosis—the condition in which too much base (too little acid) is present.

Anion gap—the difference between the concentrations of the unquantified anions and the unquantified cations in the plasma. It represents the approximate concentration of unquantified anions that are not balanced by unquantified cations.

Antibody titer—the amount of antibody present in serum against a certain antigen, defined as the reciprocal of the highest sample dilution ratio at which antibody is detectable.

Antilogarithm—the inverse function of the logarithm; $\text{antilog}_b (\log_b a) = a$.

Aqueous—of or pertaining to water; being based on, or dissolved in, water.

Arithmetic mean—the sum of all the data values divided by the number of those values. It is the balance point of the data set, and the unique value that can replace every observed value in the data set without altering the total of those values.

Arithmetic scale—a scale on a graph on which each unit increase represents a linear increase in the number.

Associative property—in the context of addition and multiplication, the law that says that changing the grouping of numbers in an operation does not change the result: $(a + b) + c = a + (b + c)$ and $(a \times b) \times c = a \times (b \times c)$.

Avogadro's number—the number of elementary particles in one mole of a substance: 6.022×10^{23}) (some resources: 6.023×10^{23}).

Base—in an exponential expression, the number being multiplied by itself the number of times specified by the exponent.

Beer-Lambert law—the linear relationship among absorbance (A), molar absorptivity (ϵ), concentration (c), and path length (l): $A = \epsilon c l$.

Bias—constant error in a series of observations or calculations. In a method comparison, it is the difference between the average result from the new method and the average result from the reference method.

Buffered—resistant to changes in pH when acid or base enters the system in small amounts.

Calibrator—a solution of an analyte whose concentration has been determined to high accuracy, and is intended for use in the calibration of an analytical method.

Canceling—a way of reducing fractions by either dividing or multiplying both the numerator and denominator by the same number.

Cartesian coordinate system—a system for representing numbers as points on a graph and equations as geometric shapes. The name honors René Descartes (1596–1650), its developer.

Categorical variable—a variable that is not numerical.

Celsius scale—the temperature scale on which the freezing point of water is 0° and the boiling point is 100°.

Central tendency—the center of a data set; a typical value.

Characteristic—the part of a logarithm to the left of the decimal point.

Chromophore—a chemical substance that absorbs light.

Coefficient of determination (r^2 or R^2)—in regression, a number between 0 and 1, inclusive, that represents the proportion of the total variation in y that is explained by the variation in x.

Coefficient of variation—the standard deviation expressed as a percentage of the mean.

Common logarithm—logarithm with a base of 10.

Commutative property—in the context of addition or multiplication, the law that says that changing the order of numbers in an operation does not change the result: $a + b + c = c + a + b$ and $a \times b \times c = c \times a \times b$.

Complex fraction—a fraction in which the numerator and/or the denominator is itself a fraction.

Concentration—an expression of the relative amounts of solute and solvent present in a solution.

Confidence interval—a range that contains the true value of some parameter a large proportion of the time.

Conjugate acid—the corresponding acid formed when a base accepts a hydrogen ion.

Conjugate base—the corresponding base formed when an acid loses a hydrogen ion.

Constant systematic error—systematic error that is the same regardless of the analyte's concentration.

Contingency table—a table, in matrix format, that shows the frequency distribution of categorical variables.

Control—material used to generate quality control data. It chemically and physically simulates patient specimens that are typically run in the test under consideration.

Correlation—a mutual relationship, or association, between two variables.

Correlation coefficient (*r*)—in statistics, a number between -1 and $+1$, inclusive, that gauges the strength of the linear association between two measured variables. When $r = +1$, the correlation is perfect, the two variables move in the same direction, and all points lie on the line. When $r = -1$, the correlation is again perfect and all points lie on the line, but the two variables move in opposite directions.

Creatinine clearance—the process whereby the kidneys remove creatinine from the blood by glomerular filtration. The rate of this process is used to estimate the glomerular filtration rate.

Critical value—a predetermined value that serves as a threshold between failing to reject, and rejecting, the null hypothesis. Rejection occurs only if the calculated statistical value is more extreme than the critical value.

Cutoff—*see* Referent value.

Degrees of freedom—the number of independent values in a data set.

Denominator—the bottom number in a fraction; the number of equal parts into which the whole is being divided.

Dependent variable—the variable whose value is determined by the value of the other variable.

Diluent—a liquid (solvent or solution) used to dilute a solution.

Dilution factor—the value by which the concentration of a dilution is multiplied to give the concentration of the original solution. It equals the reciprocal of the dilution ratio.

Dilution ratio—the ratio of the initial volume to the final volume; the ratio of the final concentration to the initial concentration.

Dimensional analysis—a unit-conversion technique based on the fact that any quantity can be multiplied by "1" without its value being changed.

Directly proportional—changing in proportion to another variable.

Dissolve—to pass into solution.

Distributive property—the law that says that multiplication distributes itself over addition: $a(b + c) = (a \times b) + (a \times c)$.

Double-reciprocal plot—in the context of enzyme kinetics, a graph of reciprocal velocity ($1/v$) against reciprocal substrate concentration ($1/[S]$). It is usually called a "Lineweaver-Burk plot."

Efficiency—the probability that a binary test result, whether positive or negative, is correct.

Embedded zero—any zero that occurs between two nonzero significant figures.

End-point assay—an assay in which the signal (e.g., absorbance) is measured at a fixed time point and the rate is calculated from a standard curve, a single standard, or a proportionality constant (e.g., molar absorptivity).

Enzyme—biological macromolecules that catalyze chemical reactions in living systems.

Enzyme kinetics—the quantitative study of catalysis by enzymes.

Equivalent—one hydrogen ion in the formula of a chemical substance; one mole of positive or negative charges.

Equivalent weight—the amount of a substance that contains, theoretically combines with, or theoretically replaces 1 mole of hydrogen ions.

Exponent—in an exponential expression, the raised value specifying the number of times that the base is to be multiplied by itself.

Exponential notation—a system of writing numbers, particularly very large and very small numbers, in exponential form.

Exponential term—in the standard format of exponential notation, the factor containing the exponent.

Extrapolation—the act of predicting the value of one variable from the value of another outside the range of a standard curve.

Factor—in the context of multiplication, any number that is multiplying another number.

Fahrenheit scale—the temperature scale on which the freezing point of water is 32° and the boiling point is 212°.

False negative—a wrongly negative result for a patient who has the condition in question.

False positive—a wrongly positive result for a patient who does not have the condition in question.

Formula weight—the sum of all the atomic weights in the formula of a substance.

Friedewald equation—an equation for calculating the concentration of LDL cholesterol from total cholesterol, HDL cholesterol, and triglycerides. It is not reliable when the triglyceride concentration exceeds 400 mg/dL.

Glomerular filtration rate—the rate at which the kidneys are filtering blood through the glomeruli.

Graph—a visual summary of data depicting the relationship between variables.

Hemacytometer—a small device for manually counting blood cells under a microscope. It comprises two identical ruled glass platforms separated by an H-shaped moat.

Hematocrit—the volume of whole blood occupied by packed RBCs.

Henderson-Hasselbalch equation—an equation that relates pH, pK_a, and the concentrations of conjugate acid and base. It is useful for preparing solutions at selected pH values.

Hypertonic—having a higher solute concentration than that of a given solution.

Hypotonic—having a lower solute concentration than that of a given solution.

Immiscible—incapable of being mixed with something else.

Implied relative uncertainty—relative uncertainty that has been calculated from an absolute uncertainty assumed from the number of significant figures in a value.

Improper fraction—a fraction in which the numerator is greater than the denominator.

In range—falling within the defined limits of acceptability for a control result. The term itself is interchangeable with "in control."

Independent variable—the variable whose value is controlled or selected.

Initial rate—in an enzyme-catalyzed reaction, the rate of the linear phase, in which the rate of product appearance, or of reactant disappearance, is constant. It varies with the starting substrate concentration.

Insoluble—incapable of dissolving in a given solvent.

Interference experiment—a paired comparison in which one of two aliquots is spiked with a selected substance suspected of interfering with the assay; the other aliquot is not spiked.

International Normalized Ratio—prothrombin time that has been standardized so that the value does not depend on the instrument, controls, or reagent used.

International Sensitivity Index—a value that represents the sensitivity, or responsiveness, of a given thromboplastin preparation relative to the international thromboplastin reference.

International System of Units—adopted in 1960, a modern version of the original metric system, based on the number 10 and built on seven base units.

Interpolation—the act of predicting the value of one variable from that of another within the range of the standard curve.

Kelvin scale—the temperature scale on which the 0-degree point corresponds to the theoretical absence of all thermal energy. Each degree on the scale equals one Celsius degree, and a temperature on this scale is greater than the Celsius temperature by 273.15.

Kinetic assay—an assay in which the signal (absorbance, for example) is measured at each of several time points and the reaction rate is calculated from all of them. It is more accurate than either the endpoint or two-point assay.

Lag phase—the phase preceding linearity in an enzyme-catalyzed reaction. The rate is still increasing because of various processes that may be under way.

Leading zero—any zero that precedes the first nonzero digit in a number.

Least common denominator—the lowest number into which each of two denominators divides evenly.

Levy-Jennings chart—a graphical representation of control data over a certain period of time. It shows the relationship of each result to the mean and to multiples of the standard deviation.

Linear—of or pertaining to a straight line; having the properties of a straight line.

Linear regression—a technique that fits a straight line to a set of data points consisting of values for a dependent variable, *y*, and corresponding values for an independent variable, *x*.

Lineweaver-Burk plot—*see* Double-reciprocal plot.

Lipoprotein—an assembly of proteins and lipids that transport cholesterol and triglycerides (triacylglycerols) in the blood and other body fluids.

Logarithm—the exponent to which a specified base must be raised in order to produce a given number.

Logarithmic scale—a scale on a graph on which each unit increase represents an exponential increase in the underlying number.

Mantissa—the part of a logarithm to the right of the decimal point.

Maximal velocity (V_{max})—the highest reaction rate an enzyme can achieve under the specified conditions, substrate concentration included. It appears as the asymptote in the plateau on a plot of initial rate versus substrate concentration.

Mean—a measure of central tendency. The term itself usually refers to the arithmetic mean.

Mean cell hemoglobin (MCH)—the amount of hemoglobin per erythrocyte.

Mean cell hemoglobin concentration (MCHC)—the amount of hemoglobin relative to the erythrocyte's size.

Mean cell volume (MCV)—the average size of an erythrocyte.

Median—the midpoint of a data set.

Metabolic acidosis—acidosis with a metabolic cause, such as diabetes, diarrhea, or poisoning.

Metabolic alkalosis—alkalosis with a metabolic cause, such as diuresis or vomiting.

Metric system—a system of measurement established in 1791, based on the number 10. The term itself has become synonymous with "International System of Units."

Michaelis-Menten equation—the equation that relates the initial rate of an enzyme-catalyzed reaction to the starting concentration of substrate, describing a rectangular hyperbola, and following from the rapid-equilibrium model of enzyme catalysis proposed by Michaelis and Menten in 1913.

Miscible—capable of being mixed with something else.

Mixed number—a whole number with a proper fraction.

Mode—the most frequent value in a data set.

Molality—the amount of solute in solution per kilogram of solvent.

Molar absorptivity—the inherent ability of a chromophore to absorb light of a given wavelength. Its value is unique and constant under a specified set of conditions. It is also called the "molar extinction coefficient."

Molar absorptivity method—the use of the Beer-Lambert law to calculate the concentration of a chromophore. It is preferred when the analyte is too unstable for constructing a standard curve.

Molar extinction coefficient—*see* Molar absorptivity.

Molar mass—the mass of a substance numerically equal to its formula weight; the mass of one mole of the substance.

Molarity—the number of moles of a substance in 1 liter of solution.

Mole—the amount of a substance that consists of as many entities as there are atoms in exactly 12 grams of the element ^{12}C. That value is Avogadro's number.

Multirules—systems of rules governing the acceptability of control results by comparing those results to previous results. Their purpose is to keep the rate of error detection high and the rate of false rejection low. The Westgard system is the most common in clinical laboratories.

Natural logarithm—logarithm with a base of *e*.

Negative predictive value (NPV)—the probability that a negative test result is correct.

Nonlinear regression—a technique that fits a curve rather than a straight line to a set of data points consisting of values for a dependent variable, *y*, and corresponding values for an independent variable, *x*.

Normal distribution—a distribution that is symmetrical and bell-shaped, described by its mean and standard deviation. The probability of a value's occurring within one standard deviation of the mean is 68%; within two standard deviations, 95%; within three, 99.7%.

Normality—the number of equivalent weights of a substance in 1 liter of solution.

Null hypothesis—the hypothesis that there is no difference between two phenomena being compared (e.g., variances of two instruments, means of two data sets).

Numerator—the top number in a fraction; the number of equal parts under consideration.

Opposites—two numbers that lie at the same distance from 0 on the number line but in reverse directions.

Ordered pair—a pair of corresponding *x* and *y* values, specified in that order, that define a single data point on a Cartesian graph.

Ordinate—the *y* coordinate of a point on a Cartesian graph.

Osmolality—the number of osmoles of particles per kilogram of solvent.

Osmolality gap—the difference between the measured osmolality and the calculated osmolality.

Osmolarity—the number of osmoles of particles per liter of solution.

Osmole—a mole of osmotically active particles.

Osmosis—the phenomenon in which water passes through a semipermeable membrane from a hypotonic solution to a hypertonic solution.

Osmotic fragility—the susceptibility of erythrocytes to osmotic stress in a hypotonic medium. It is evaluated in a test for the presence of spherocytes.

Osmotic pressure—hydrostatic pressure caused by the difference between the concentrations of two solutions separated by a semipermeable membrane.

Out of range—falling outside the defined limits of acceptability for a control result. The term itself is interchangeable with "out of control."

Outlier—an extreme value in a data set.

***p* value**—the probability of observing, by coincidence alone, results more extreme than those that were actually observed (on the assumption that the null hypothesis is true).

Partial pressure—the pressure of an individual gas that is one of several gases in a mixture.

Percentage—the number of parts out of every 100 parts.

pH—the negative logarithm of the hydrogen ion concentration; a measure of the acidity/alkalinity of an aqueous solution.

Positive predictive value—the probability that a positive test result is correct.

Precision—agreement among repeated measurements or calculated results.

Prevalence—the frequency of a given condition in a population tested at a particular time.

Proper fraction—a fraction in which the denominator is greater than the numerator.

Proportional systematic error—systematic error that is proportional to the analyte's concentration.

Proportionality—the relationship between two variables in which one changes in proportion to the other.

Proportionality constant—the constant by which the value of one variable is multiplied to give the value of another variable.

Prothrombin time (PT)—the amount of time required for a plasma specimen to clot *in vitro* when mixed with a commercial reagent containing thromboplastin.

Quality control—a process for verifying the performance characteristics of a testing system, which includes reagents, electronics, and robotics. It consists of running special quality-control materials in the test being checked and then comparing the new results with previous ones.

Random error—error that arises from the normal vicissitudes of observation, which have no inherent pattern (e.g., imprecision in reading pipets, electronic noise in instruments, fluctuations in room temperature).

Ratio—a quotient of two numbers. It is the factor by which those two numbers differ from each other.

Ratio method—a unit-conversion technique involving an equation of ratios followed by cross-multiplication.

Reciprocals—two numbers whose product is 1.

Recovery experiment—a comparison for detecting systematic error in which each specimen is split into two aliquots, with one receiving the analyte in a known amount and the other receiving only diluent.

Red-cell distribution width (RDW)—a measure of the variation in RBC size in a given blood specimen.

Reducing—the process of simplifying a fraction such that the numerator and denominator are as small as possible, that is, until the only number divisible into both of them is "1."

Referent value—the value of a binary test result above which the patient is said to have the specified medical condition and below which the patient is said not to have it.

Regression analysis—the use of certain techniques to ascertain the mathematical relationship between a dependent variable and an independent variable.

Relative uncertainty—the fraction of a measurement's value represented by the absolute uncertainty.

Reportable range—the span of possible test results between the highest and lowest that are considered accurate.

Respiratory acidosis—acidosis caused by hypoventilation (airway obstruction, asthma, emphysema, etc.).

Respiratory alkalosis—alkalosis caused by hyperventilation (anxiety, certain drugs, high altitude, etc.).

Reticulocyte index (RI)—the reticulocyte count adjusted to the actual hematocrit.

Reticulocyte production index (RPI)—the reticulocyte index corrected for the premature release of reticulocytes in anemia.

Rounding digit—the digit that occupies the place to which a number is to be rounded.

Sample dilution—in a serial dilution, the dilution ratio of a given tube relative to the original sample.

Scientific notation—*see* Exponential notation.

Semilogarithmic plot—a plot in which one scale is arithmetic and the other is logarithmic.

Sensitivity—a measure of a test's ability to detect the medical condition in question in every patient who has the condition.

Serial dilution—a progressive series of dilutions in which each dilution is less concentrated than the preceding one, usually by a constant amount.

Shift—for control results, an abrupt move in which six or more consecutive data points all fall above or below the mean.

Significand—in the standard format of exponential notation, the factor containing the significant figures.

Significant figure—a digit that is known with certainty or that has been estimated.

Single-standard method—the use of only one standard to construct a standard curve. It is useful if the relationship is known to be linear.

Slope—for a straight line, the ratio of the change in the independent variable to the change in the dependent variable; the rate of change.

Slope-intercept form—an equation of a straight line in the form $y = mx + b$, where m is the slope and b is the y-intercept.

Soluble—capable of dissolving in a given solvent.

Solute—a solution component that is not the one present in the largest amount.

Solution—a homogeneous mixture of two or more substances that do not chemically react with each other.

Solvent—the component of a solution that is present in the largest amount.

Sparingly soluble—soluble in a given solvent, but only to a small degree.

Specific gravity—the ratio of the density of a solution to the density of water at 4°C.

Specificity—a measure of a test's ability to detect only the medical condition in question.

Specimen pairing—in a method comparison, the strategy of testing each specimen by each method. This creates a one-to-one correspondence between the methods for every specimen.

Standard—*see* Calibrator.

Standard curve—a graph showing the relationship between the known amount of an analyte (concentration, for example) and a measurable property of that analyte (absorbance, for example). By means of this relationship, one can determine an unknown amount of that analyte in a specimen from a single measurement of the property.

Standard deviation—for a data set, the square root of the average squared distance between the observations and the mean; the most common measure of dispersion in a normally distributed data set.

Statistically significant—unlikely to have occurred under the circumstances, possibly providing evidence for rejecting the null hypothesis.

Substrate—in an enzyme-catalyzed reaction, a reactant on which an enzyme acts directly.

Substrate-depletion phase—in an enzyme-catalyzed reaction, the later phase in which the rate is decreasing as the substrate supply is diminishing.

Systematic error—error that occurs repeatedly and cannot be minimized by averaging because all the data are inaccurate in the same direction.

***t* value**—the result of a *t*-test, comparing the difference that was actually observed between the means of two groups with the difference that would have been expected for randomly selected specimens.

Trailing zero—any zero that follows the last nonzero digit in a number.

Transmittance—the fraction of incident light that passes through a chemical substance (i.e., without being absorbed).

Trend—for control results, a gradual movement in one direction by a set of six or more consecutive data points.

True negative—a correctly negative test result for a patient who does not have the condition in question.

True positive—a correctly positive test result for a patient who has the condition in question.

Tube dilution—in a serial dilution, the constant dilution ratio from one tube to the next.

Two-point assay—an assay in which the signal (absorbance, for example) is measured at each of two time points and the reaction rate is calculated between them.

Unimodal—having only one mode.

United States Customary System of Units—a system of measurement in common use in the United States, rooted in the system of pre-1824 English units that had evolved from Anglo-Saxon and Roman units of measurement.

v/v—the number of milliliters of solute in 100 mL of solution, expressed as a percentage.

Variance—the average squared distance between observations. It is a measure of dispersion in a normally distributed data set, though used less commonly than the standard deviation.

w/v—the number of grams of solute in 100 mL of solution, expressed as a percentage.

w/w—the number of grams of solute in 100 grams of solution, expressed as a percentage.

y-intercept—on a graph, the point at which a line or curve intersects the *y*-axis.

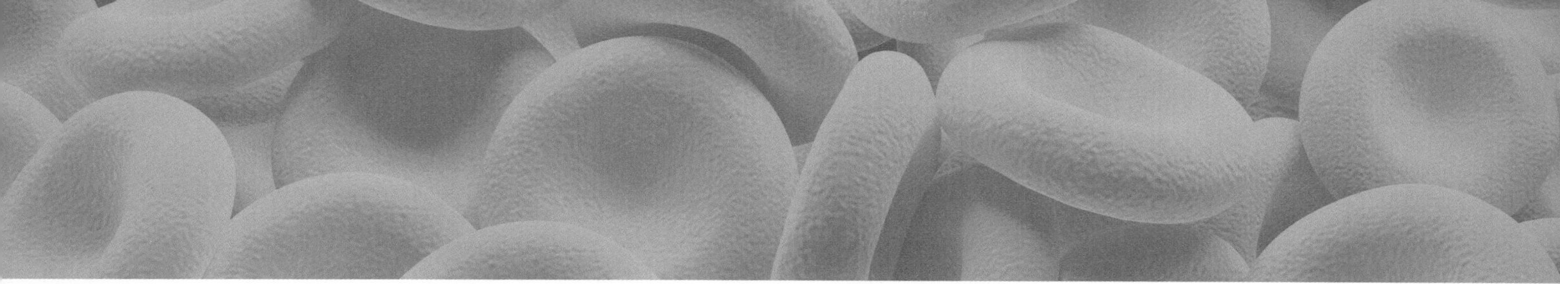

Index

M

N

O

P

Q

R